Veterans with a Vision

Studies in Canadian Military History

Series editor: Dean F. Oliver, Canadian War Museum

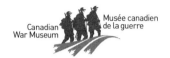

The Canadian War Museum, Canada's national museum of military history, has a threefold mandate: to remember, to preserve, and to educate. Studies in Canadian Military History, published by UBC Press in association with the Museum, extends this mandate by presenting the best of contemporary scholarship to provide new insights into all aspects of Canadian military history, from earliest times to recent events. The work of a new generation of scholars is especially encouraged and the books employ a variety of approaches – cultural, social, intellectual, economic, political, and comparative – to investigate gaps in the existing historiography. The books in the series feed immediately into future exhibitions, programs, and outreach efforts by the Canadian War Museum. A list of titles in the series appears at the end of the book.

The Sir Arthur Pearson Association of War Blinded

In 1918 some of the approximately two hundred Canadian blinded servicemen from the First World War helped create the Canadian National Institute for the Blind (CNIB). In 1922 they formed their own veterans' organization, the Sir Arthur Pearson Association of War Blinded (SAPA). These veterans were joined by war-blinded Canadians from the Second World War and the Korean War. Together they fought for improved pension and social legislation for the war blinded and for all disabled veterans and furthered the interest of Canadians with vision loss in general. Today, SAPA actively monitors and promotes veterans' rights and is a member of the National Council of Veteran Associations in Canada.

Veterans with a Vision

Canada's War Blinded in Peace and War

Serge Marc Durflinger

Published in Association with the Canadian War Museum
and the Sir Arthur Pearson Association of War Blinded

UBCPress · Vancouver · Toronto

20 19 18 17 16 15 14 13 12 11 10   5 4 3 2 1

Library and Archives Canada Cataloguing in Publication

Durflinger, Serge Marc, 1961-
   Veterans with a vision: Canada's war blinded in peace and war /
Serge M. Durflinger.

(Studies in Canadian military history, 1449-6251)
Includes bibliographical references and index.
ISBN 978-0-7748-1855-1 (bound); ISBN 978-0-7748-1856-8 (pbk.)

   1. Disabled veterans – Canada – History. 2. Blind – Canada – History. 3. Sir Arthur Pearson Association of War Blinded – History. 4. Canadian National Institute for the Blind – History. 5. Baker, Edwin Albert, 1893-1968. I. Canadian War Museum II. Sir Arthur Pearson Association of War Blinded III. Title. IV. Series: Studies in Canadian military history.

UB365.C2D87 2010   362.86'80971   C2010-900463-9

e-book ISBNs: 978-0-7748-1875-5 (pdf); 978-0-7748-5925-7 (epub)

Canadä

UBC Press gratefully acknowledges the financial support for our publishing program of the Government of Canada (through the Canada Book Fund), the Canada Council for the Arts, and the British Columbia Arts Council.

This book has been published with the help of a grant from the Canadian Federation for the Humanities and Social Sciences, through the Aid to Scholarly Publications Programme, using funds provided by the Social Sciences and Humanities Research Council of Canada.

Publication of this book has been financially supported by the Canadian War Museum and the Sir Arthur Pearson Association of War Blinded.

UBC Press
The University of British Columbia
2029 West Mall
Vancouver, BC V6T 1Z2
www.ubcpress.ca

En mémoire de

Marie-Lina Ste-Marie (*née* Gagné) (1896-1985),

my grandmother, who was blind

and for Bill Mayne

Contents

Illustrations

Following p. 200

Preface

She was aged and walked about the crowded six-room flat slowly and deliberately. Still, she got around surprisingly well and was able to do all she needed, never complaining. She cleaned, cooked, mended clothes, listened to television and radio programs, made numerous phone calls, and showed her children and grandchildren great love and affection. The widow of a wounded First World War veteran, she loved to laugh and had a terrific memory. She seemed to have a rather normal life for a woman in her late seventies. Except that she was completely blind. Her name was Marie-Lina Ste-Marie (*née* Gagné), but to me she was always simply "Mémé," my grandmother, a delightful, strong-willed woman who had a hand in raising me. I barely noticed that she could not see through her piercing blue eyes, and rarely gave a thought to the fact that she had never actually seen me. It was never an issue because her courage in overcoming her disability showed me at a young age that one did not need sight to have vision.

And so, when the opportunity presented itself to write this book, I leapt at the chance. It would not just be a fascinating and historiographically meaningful topic of enormous professional interest, casting new light on the experiences of Canada's war-disabled veterans; it would also be a subject that *mattered* to me. In some manner, I hoped that writing this book would pay homage to all of the country's blind, including my grandmother, and that researching the history of Canada's war-blinded veterans would take on an emotive personal dimension for me. This is precisely what has happened, which I hope is occasionally reflected in the pages that follow.

In May 2002, I gave a speech at the Royal Canadian Military Institute in Toronto. Despite the many people in attendance that evening, I could not help but notice the large number of Second World War veterans. One group of men, resplendent in their cardinal-red berets (which I did not recognize), especially stood out – because they were blind. These veterans were members of the Sir Arthur Pearson Association of War Blinded (SAPA) and some had come from the Sunnybrook Health Sciences Centre, home to hundreds of Canadian veterans requiring long-term care, to hear me speak. I was deeply moved by their presence. After I had delivered my address, I was introduced to a very distinguished gentleman. Bill Mayne, war blinded, was a long-serving member of SAPA's executive. We exchanged very sincere greetings and pleasantries, and then he was gone.

Some time later, Krysia Pazdzior, the Ottawa-based associate executive director of SAPA, telephoned me with a proposal. Thus began a series of conversations and meetings involving Krysia, Bill, Jim Sanders, at that time CEO of the Canadian National Institute for the Blind (CNIB), Richard Huyda, a dynamic CNIB volunteer and retired archivist, and others, that resulted in my writing this book on behalf of SAPA and the CNIB. The research began in 2005.

The documentary evidence allowing this history to be written has been staggering in volume and quality: a true cornucopia of material constituting both an historian's dream come true and the enormous and time-consuming challenge of deciding what to include and what to set aside. The archival material from SAPA's national office, superbly organized by Richard Huyda, consisted mainly of correspondence files, membership and statistical data, members' case files, financial statements, the highly detailed and enormously helpful minutes of the meetings of SAPA's executive and other committees maintained since 1922, numerous pamphlets, tracts, and minor publications published by SAPA in its eighty-five-year history, a complete run of the *SAPA Chronicle* (an especially informative newsletter begun in 1975), thick collections of newspaper clippings, numerous instructive photographs, and important audiovisual materials including oral history testimony.

The voluminous CNIB Papers, held at Library and Archives Canada (LAC), also have proven a treasure trove of rich and untapped historical material relating to Canada's war-blinded veterans. Like SAPA's archives, the CNIB Papers, covering the period from the institute's founding until the 1970s, consist of institutional and correspondence files, statistical data, financial statements, minutes of meetings, and numerous minor publications. A shocking amount of material deals directly with SAPA and the war blinded. The CNIB Archives in Toronto also yielded an immense quantity of pertinent material, while additional relevant sources were located in other manuscript and government record groups at LAC, especially the Edwin Albert Baker Papers.

Secondary sources supporting this research were a different story. Very little has been written on Canada's veterans, especially disabled veterans, and less still is available on Canadian veterans' organizations. Nevertheless, more than a hundred books and articles were consulted in the preparation of this book; most of these are listed in the select bibliography. In addition, although an extremely small number of Canada's more than 1.6 million twentieth-century veterans, the war blinded have written a surprising number of powerful and evocative memoirs. James Rawlinson's 1919 account of his military service and blinding during the First World War, *Through St. Dunstan's to Light*, is a minor classic. Of the four books written by veterans of the Second World War, David Dorward's little-known *The Gold Cross: One Man's Window on the World* (1978) is a beautifully written and deeply reflective memoir deserving of a much wider readership. John Windsor's *Blind Date* (1962) is also a moving and honest rendering of the shock of being blinded and the challenges that followed. Neil Hamilton, the lone blinded Royal Canadian Air Force veteran to have penned his reminiscences, wrote *Wings of Courage: A Lifetime of Triumph over Adversity* (2000), an unvarnished rendering of his tribulations in the postwar world and of the deep courage, and spousal love, required to persevere. Finally, the Honourable Barney Danson, a defence minister in the 1970s, wrote his memoirs late in life. *Not Bad for a Sergeant* (2002) reminds readers that near-total vision loss can occur even decades following the loss of a single eye in combat. The story of Canada's war-blinded veterans is an important one, and I feel privileged in having played a role in bringing their experiences before a broader public.

Acknowledgments

Many kind people have assisted me in preparing this history. The executive and staff of the Sir Arthur Pearson Association of War Blinded and of the Canadian National Institute for the Blind have been unfailingly co-operative and generous with their time. I would especially like to acknowledge long-time SAPA member Bill Mayne, whose passionate interest in the history of Canada's war-blinded veterans sparked this book project. Bill graciously took the time on more than one occasion to answer my many queries.

At my request, a CNIB-SAPA editorial committee was struck to review the manuscript, and I am grateful to Jim Sanders, Bill Mayne, Richard Huyda, Glenn Wright, and other occasional readers for their comments and encouragement. Jim Sanders, the CNIB's CEO, was always a source of support and good advice. Following his retirement in 2009, Jim, also serving as SAPA's executive director, very helpfully continued as the CNIB's contact with UBC Press and with me. Since the beginning of my involvement with the story of Canada's war blinded in 2004, Krysia Pazdzior, then SAPA's associate executive director, served as my contact. Having worked for SAPA for some twenty years, Krysia was always enthusiastic about this book project. Cheerful and generous, she helped me in many ways.

Richard Huyda, a retired photo archivist from Library and Archives Canada and a long-time CNIB volunteer, took on the demanding task of organizing SAPA's files and did so with great efficiency. He similarly helped organize the SAPA-related CNIB Archives in Toronto. His hard work made my research at SAPA's Ottawa headquarters and in Toronto much easier and more enjoyable. Equally important, Richard scanned nearly two hundred photographs and illustrations, including nearly all of those appearing in this book. I am indebted to him for this and for his encouragement and advice. Others of the CNIB-SAPA family to whom I owe thanks are Barbara Marjeram, Euclid Herie, Anne Michielin, JoAnne Mackie, Anne Sanders, John Andrew, and Laura Mayne. I would also like to acknowledge the assistance of Veterans Affairs Canada.

For the last fifteen years, I have benefitted from working along-side or consulting with Canada's finest military historians. The following have helped shape my understanding of Canada's military past, encouraged me, and, in most cases, provided me with research ideas for this book: Tim Cook, Terry Copp, Jack Granatstein, Jeffrey Keshen, Marc Milner, Desmond Morton, and Roger Sarty. Tim was also kind enough to give me a wonderful copy of *The Blinded Soldiers and Sailors Gift Book*, which I very much appreciated. I also acknowledge the help of University of Ottawa graduate students (as they were at that time) Nic Clarke and Sarah Cozzi, who offered useful research leads and good conversations. John Parry in Toronto gave freely of his precious time and sage advice throughout this project.

It was a pleasure to work once again with the skilled professionals at UBC Press. Given the needs of the visually impaired readership for this publication, the press agreed, with CNIB input and support, to produce a book different in font, font size, margin justification, and paper stock from its normal offerings. For their guidance through the publication cycle, I am grateful to Emily Andrew, Holly Keller, Melissa Pitts, and Peter Milroy. Sarah Wight did a superb job copyediting the manuscript, and Dianne Tiefensee was a meticulous proofreader and indexer.

I would like to gratefully acknowledge the assistance of Dean Oliver, Director, Historical Research and Exhibits Development,

Canadian War Museum, for agreeing to support this publication as part of UBC Press's prestigious Studies in Canadian Military History series.

To my wife, Janine Stingel, and my five-year-old son, Maxime, I express my love and gratitude for enduring with me through yet another book project.

Finally, I would like to offer my heartfelt appreciation to Canada's war-blinded veterans. Their story has profoundly inspired me.

Acronyms

AA	Amputations Association of the Great War
AVOC	Associated Veterans Organizations of Canada
BESL	British Empire Service League
BPC	Board of Pension Commissioners
BVA	Blinded Veterans Association (US)
CCA	Canadian Corps Association
CEF	Canadian Expeditionary Force
CFLB	Canadian Free Library for the Blind
CNIB	Canadian National Institute for the Blind
CPC	Canadian Pension Commission
DND	Department of National Defence
DPNH	Department of Pensions and National Health
DSCR	Department of Soldiers' Civil Re-establishment
DVA	Department of Veterans Affairs
EIA	exceptional incapacity allowance
HSB	Halifax School for the Blind
ICRC	International Committee of the Red Cross
MHC	Military Hospitals Commission
NCVA	National Council of Veteran Associations in Canada
NIB	National Institute for the Blind (UK)
PPCLI	Princess Patricia's Canadian Light Infantry
PRB	Pension Review Board

RCAF	Royal Canadian Air Force
SAPA	Sir Arthur Pearson Association of War Blinded (before 1942, Sir Arthur Pearson Club of War Blinded Soldiers and Sailors)
VAC	Veterans Affairs Canada
VAD	Voluntary Aid Detachment
WBTC	War-Blinded Training Committee
YMCA	Young Men's Christian Association

Veterans with a Vision

Introduction

Books written about the conflict record major political
decisions and their results; they speak of generals, and of
heroes. There is a paucity of literary tribute to those who
offered their youth to war; nor are there books which tell of
the disabled, the war blinded, the amputee, the burnt-out
veteran.

– David Dorward, blinded in Sicily, 1943

According to estimates provided by the Canadian National Institute
for the Blind (CNIB), citing information gathered by Statistics Canada,
in 2006 about 836,000 Canadians had suffered vision loss while
108,000 were registered as clients of the institute.[1] The standard
measure for visual acuity (the perception of detail) is the commonly
recognized Snellen chart. The different-sized letters printed thereon
are configured and shaped so that a person with normal vision can
read them all from a twenty-foot distance, hence the categorization
of 20/20 vision. In metric terms, this is expressed as 6/6, based on a
six-metre distance. However, an individual able to see only the top
line, consisting of the chart's largest letter, is rated at 20/200 or 6/60,
the second number representing the distance at which someone

with normal vision could read the same line. This is the boundary for determining legal blindness.[2]

But despite this large number of Canadian blind, only a handful can be classified as "war blinded," that is, those whose vision loss occurred while on military service in wartime, or whose post-service blindness was attributable to earlier wartime service. These men and women are to be distinguished from "blind veterans," that is, war veterans who, as a result of aging, disease, accidents, or other factors, lost their sight in a manner having nothing to do with their prior military service. This book is about Canadian war-blinded veterans, not blind veterans.

At the time of writing, Canada has been at war in Afghanistan since 2001. A new, albeit much smaller, generation of veterans is being created that will succeed those of the Second World War (1939-45) and the Korean War (1950-53). In addition to the 138 fatalities recorded through December 2009, Canada's approximately 600 wounded soldiers from the Afghanistan conflict include some severely disabled veterans. Among them are those with serious eye injuries. They join a small but influential group of blinded Canadian veterans from past conflicts whose courage and perseverance have helped reshape the way Canadians and Canadian government departments and agencies have perceived war disability in general and blindness in particular. The experiences of Canada's war blinded, from the South African War (1899-1902) to the present day, and the story of their work on behalf of all disabled Canadians as well as all Canadian veterans and their families, constitute an unexplored facet of Canada's social history.

Blindness is a poignant disability, and it is all the more so when those afflicted are a robust group of capable youth whose grievous injuries were sustained while on military service. In 1918 some of the approximately 170 Canadian blinded servicemen (and a handful of servicewomen) from the First World War (1914-18) were the driving force behind the creation of the Canadian National Institute for the

Blind. In 1922 the Canadian war blinded formed their own veterans' organization, an advocacy group closely linked to the CNIB, to see to their special needs as pensioned veterans and as newly blinded Canadians. The Sir Arthur Pearson Club of War Blinded Soldiers and Sailors (renamed in 1942 as the Sir Arthur Pearson Association of War Blinded, or SAPA) took its name from the wealthy British benefactor who, in 1915, established in London the St. Dunstan's Hostel for Blinded Soldiers and Sailors and assisted all the British Empire's war blinded to retrain for their new lives without sight. A generation later, these First World War veterans were joined by a comparable number of war-blinded Canadians from the Second World War.

Edwin Albert Baker, blinded at Ypres in 1915, was one of Canada's most remarkable veterans of the First World War. Known to royalty, world statesmen, and ordinary veterans, he acquired international fame as an eloquent advocate for the world's blind and especially for blinded veterans. Figuring prominently in this book, his story is intimately intertwined with the founding and growth of the CNIB and SAPA, and the successful social integration of Canada's war-blinded population. He served as the CNIB's managing director for four decades, was SAPA's secretary for nearly as long, and was among the first recipients of the Order of Canada, founded in 1967 as a Confederation centenary program; no one argued with the choice.

Baker and the other war-blinded veterans had been shocked upon their return to Canada to find that the lot of the blind was miserable and that their social status deprived them of their dignity. CNIB historian Euclid Herie has noted that until the twentieth century in Canada, "blind people were relegated to poverty, derision, pity, abuse, and social conditions that, with few exceptions, left them with a bleak promise for the future."[3] It seemed far-fetched that the blind could be educated and productive, and could form a part of mainstream society. Families took care of their blind, if possible. No institutions were fully capable of retraining newly blinded adults.

Young blind Canadians obtained a basic education and some vocational training at schools in Brantford, Halifax, and Montreal. Although
some became musicians or worked in trades, such as basket and
broom production, most remained in poverty.

According to American historian Frances Koestler, the traditional occupational sphere of the blind in the early twentieth century
could be a "life sentence" to a preordained menial occupation equated with blindness itself in much of the public's mind. Known as the
"blind trades," these occupied a scale from playing music and piano-
tuning to semi-skilled work including broom-making, chair caning,
and weaving, and down to more desperate ventures such as street
peddling or simply begging.[4] "They were feared, shunned, pitied,
ignored," Koestler begins her exhaustive 1976 study of blindness in
the United States. She goes on to state that "the belief that blindness
equals uselessness has prevailed so long and so firmly in western
culture that its traces have yet to be fully erased."[5]

Yet, given that the Canadian war blinded had sacrificed their
sight in the name of victory and higher ideals, a grateful public was
unwilling to accept that their heroes should suffer such humiliation.
Edwin Baker would not accept it for himself or for others. But would
employers be willing to take risks on blind employees? "Emancipation"
would occur with a change in attitude among the sighted, certainly,
but also among the blind themselves.[6] The blinded veterans, far more
organized and militant in their demands than the civilian blind, were
in the forefront of this change and acted as catalysts for their own
success. That they were significant actors and decision makers in
determining their futures and in advocating for access to sighted
society on the basis of ability, never pity, is a thematic thread running
throughout this work.

There have always been war-blinded and war-disabled veterans.
But having the state care for them, to an extent, and assume responsibility for their civil re-establishment is a decidedly twentieth-century
phenomenon. In 1254 French king Louis IX founded l'Hospice des

Quinze-Vingts in Paris, a refuge or almshouse for three hundred blind people. While the origins of this institution are open to some scholarly debate, it seems that King Louis was motivated to assist the blind by his devotion to some of his soldiers who had been blinded during the Crusades.[7] In 1813 Prussia offered some form of compensation for blinded veterans of the Napoleonic Wars, while Britain, in 1818, offered financial compensation and opened a special hospital for veterans suffering vision loss or "military ophthalmia." The first American legislation specifically pertaining to blinded veterans' compensation was passed in 1864, during that nation's Civil War, at which time a fully blinded veteran obtained the reasonably generous disability pension of twenty-five dollars a month.[8]

The First World War's massive casualties, including hundreds of thousands of maimed and severely disabled veterans, obliged governments to devise precedent-setting disability pensions and civil re-establishment schemes to assist them to find wage-earning work, which together could provide sufficient income for them to look after themselves. In the days before the development of the welfare state, such a plan – while significantly expanding the boundaries of state intervention in the lives of Canadians – lessened the likelihood that disabled veterans would become permanent public charges. Seen in this light, the pension and retraining programs were shrewd government investments both socially and fiscally. Promoting the veterans as productive and independent members of society also dovetailed nicely with contemporary social views of a man's role as his family's self-reliant breadwinner.[9]

Yet the First World War radically altered the country's social values and revolutionized the role of the state in people's lives. In part, these changes were driven by the need to care for the country's wounded and disabled veterans. Public views of the nation's blinded citizens also changed. If former soldiers could be retrained in occupations rarely opened to the blind in the past, why could not civilians be similarly trained? The occupational ghettoes of broom making and basket weaving could expand to more challenging, rewarding, and potentially lucrative skills. For most of the major combatant powers, including Canada, the First World War proved the watershed between the era when people feared and avoided contact with the disabled and the era when governments tried desperately to reintegrate disabled veterans into an employment stream leading to as normal a life as possible.[10] This trend continued even more strongly in Canada following the Second World War, with the re-establishment and life-course experiences of the war blinded standing out as successful examples of individual, institutional, and government co-operation in the areas of retraining, job placement, financial security, and social reintegration.

When Canada's war blinded came home to face their futures in the aftermath of the First World War, the prospects for the blind in Canada had changed dramatically since the outbreak of war in 1914. The federal government had assumed responsibility for its disabled soldiers, and the opening in 1918 of the CNIB's government-funded retraining facility, Pearson Hall, on Beverley Street in Toronto, gave the country's war blinded an opportunity to reintegrate into Canadian life, find stable employment, and regain a strong measure of independence. In fact, the CNIB's main role in its first few years of operation was to care for and retrain Canada's war blinded under contract to the Department of Soldiers' Civil Re-establishment, established in February 1918. Once most of Canada's war blinded had been retrained, by 1922, the CNIB maintained close bonds with them by providing perpetual aftercare services. At this point, the CNIB turned most of its attention to assisting Canada's far more numerous civilian blind. Public recognition of the blind as functioning members of society, sympathy for their plight, and, in the case of the returned soldiers, appreciation for their patriotic sacrifice, heralded a new beginning for the relationship between the sighted and the blind in Canada.

Increasingly, the assistance granted the Canadian veterans became an entrenched right, not a form of charity, and the government assumed greater responsibility for the returned men's perpetual care and welfare. The aid was universal, based in government obligation, and could not be denied through a means test or any other restrictive policy.

Pensions were always more generous to disabled veterans, including the war blinded, than was the slowly evolving government-funded financial compensation for the equivalent group of civilian disabled. In Canada, the war blinded also benefitted from some travel concessions and the free provision of specialized technical equipment. Noted American disability historian David Gerber believes that, in most Western countries, "disabled veterans consistently have been dealt with ... more generously than ... perhaps any other cohort in society." He further claims that despite advances in government aid to the civilian disabled, seemingly often driven by veterans' pensions legislation, "the gap has never closed between disabled veterans and disabled civilians."[11] This seems true of the Canadian experience as well. Like most historians of the blind, Gabriel Farrell similarly notes that in virtually all nations assuming responsibility for their war blinded, the latter serve as a model for the civilian blind seeking similar social benefits. Farrell refers to this as "veteran preferment," and notes that it has a "long history" in all categories of war-related disability.[12] In addition, he believes that the war blinded are given an exalted position among the disabled; this is certainly borne out by SAPA's experience.

"War blinded. Few phrases evoke a stronger response ... in which shock, pity, and guilt seek release through a passionate desire to make amends."[13] So writes Frances Koestler, further remarking on the "sad irony" that war, with its numerous blinded casualties, has tended to "arouse the conscience of the public to needs they comfortably ignore in peacetime." Support for the patriotically ennobled war-blinded veterans led to greater understanding and sympathy for all blind citizens. She refers to this as the "war-quickened aware-ness of blindness."[14] Euclid Herie makes clear that Canada exemplifies this phenomenon.[15] Canadian historian Susanne Commend also believes that Canadian government programs for the war blinded, and disabled veterans generally, noticeably advanced the profile and causes of the civilian disabled, with the latter eventually bene-fitting, for example, from advanced retraining methods and pros-thetic designs.[16]

But, as David Gerber notes, while positive ripple effects seem obvious, it remains difficult to ascertain the degree to which ad-vancements in the care and rehabilitation of disabled war veterans have stimulated government-sponsored benefits, over time, for simi-larly afflicted civilians.[17] The documentary evidence is fragmentary, and the causal link difficult to nail down. Accordingly, the present work, in concentrating on the war blinded, does not seek to argue conclusively that government-sponsored programs for disabled vet-erans *directly* led to the adoption of similar programs or legislation for the civilian sector. Nevertheless, in Canada at least, the CNIB-SAPA relationship was so close and intertwined that the veteran and civil-ian groups may have advanced the other's causes in roughly equal measure. Each group pressured the government for greater assist-ance, often collaboratively. In fact, for decades Baker and other war-blinded veterans, such as Harris Turner and Alexander Viets, SAPA stalwarts all, were also among the CNIB's leaders and decision makers. They simultaneously advocated for Canada's civilian and military blind, whose collaboration was probably closer than in any other na-tion. Certainly the war blinded themselves firmly believed that their pressure on government for improved social programs helped blind civilians. Canadian medical and disability historian Mary Tremblay has conclusively shown that, in the post-Second World War period, Canadian paraplegic veterans led the way for government-sponsored rehabilitation programs that quickly and directly benefitted civilian paraplegics.[18] Gerber considers this situation exceptional, and it is partly explained by the fact that the Canadian Paraplegics Association, a veterans' group, was willing to assist civilians and eventually opened its membership to them. This close Canadian civilian-veteran co-operation was not mirrored in the disability experience of the United States or other countries.[19]

Only broadly and tangentially does this book treat the correlation between the government's veteran and civilian programs and policies for the blind. For this, for social and policy developments affecting Canada's civilian blind, and for the shifts in public perception of the blind generally, the reader is referred to Euclid Herie's history of the CNIB and Marjorie Campbell's biography of Baker.[20] But the present work does show the influence of the war blinded on certain specific positive developments for the civilian blind, such as the founding of the CNIB and the war blinded's establishment of a scholarship foundation for blind youth.

If it was unusual for veterans' groups made up of single-disability members to align themselves with their civilian counterparts, it was equally odd for different and sometimes competing special-interest veterans' associations to closely co-operate in the pursuit of shared objectives. This makes the history of SAPA and the Canadian war blinded rarer still, because they not only reached out to the civilian blind but, under Baker's strong leadership, also forged a powerful alliance of disabled and pensioned veterans. While representing different needs, all shared the desire to obtain greater post-service benefits and entitlements. In 1943 SAPA played a leading role in creating, and became a charter member of, the National Council of Veteran Associations (NCVA), a remarkable grouping still in existence (with some fifty member organizations) and still displaying strong solidarity among its participating associations. The war blinded served as a hinge not just between the civilian and military blind but between disabled and non-disabled veterans, as this book seeks to document.

Over the last half of the twentieth century, the NCVA was frequently successful in pressing veterans' claims in briefs before parliamentary committees, royal commissions, the Canadian Pension Commission, the Department of Veterans Affairs, and other government agencies. SAPA formed part of a powerful lobby group. In general, the NCVA has been successful because of the joint petitions, mutually supportive goals, and close, fraternal co-operation of its members. Sometimes it co-operated closely with the much larger Canadian Legion, and sometimes its members stood alone in the struggle for greater veterans' benefits. Remarkably, given that Canada's war blinded were few in number, two SAPA members, Edwin Baker and William Mayne, the latter a Second World War veteran, have served as chairmen of the NCVA. "SAPA by itself could never have attained the high standard of pensions and benefits [the war blinded] now enjoy," wrote Mayne long after the war.[21]

In the 1920s, the war blinded felt the need to lobby the Dominion government for improved war disability pensions and other benefits to which they believed their war injuries entitled them and for which Ottawa had made little or no provision. It was in order to improve their negotiating position that they formed SAPA. Like the war blinded in most other countries, notably Germany,[22] the Canadians refused to be submerged in larger veterans groups such as the Great War Veterans' Association or, later, the Canadian Legion, preferring to remain a specific grouping, best able to articulate and promote their own interests. SAPA maintained its full independence as a member of the umbrella NCVA.

Because the war-blinded's injuries occurred in defence of the realm, their heightened visibility in general society might have prompted, in Gerber's phrase, "gratitude, generosity, and guilt"[23] among Canadians. But the war blinded were insistent on reminding Canadians and the government of their status as veterans, not allowing themselves to be seen merely as blind Canadians, the objects of well-intentioned pity. Instead, the war-blinded veterans helped *define* their social roles and the manner in which their fellow sighted citizens viewed and would remember them. As much as possible they seized their own destinies; most who came into contact with them did not offer pity, but rather admiration. The war-blinded veterans carved out their own place in society, being unwilling to be assigned a place by a potentially misunderstanding public and federal bureaucracy, no matter how genuinely sympathetic.[24]

As Gerber notes, "disabilities and disfigurements become a particularly significant marker for an individual's or group's social identity and self-understanding."[25] Canada's blinded veterans displayed a strong collective sense, having suffered similar fates at similar ages, often in similar wartime circumstances. They were young men leading vigorous lives at the time of their loss of vision. They still harboured their hopes and aspirations and they remained capable. They had not always been blind.[26] There was thus an instantaneous sense of community. Self-help comes easier under these circumstances, and Canada's war-blinded veterans maintained a very well-organized community, complete with regular social activities and large-scale national reunions. They also worked together to obtain generous government pensions and meaningful rehabilitation programs, while fiercely maintaining their individual and social independence. Successive federal ministers responsible for veterans, bureaucrats at all levels of the hierarchy, pension officials, and of course the CNIB validated the war blinded's finely developed sense of identity and facilitated their ability to mount unified, directed advocacy campaigns.[27]

Canada's veterans, especially disabled or wounded veterans, are generally ignored in the Canadian historical literature, while SAPA and the war blinded are virtually unknown outside of the few works pertaining to the CNIB.[28] Gerber, a leading international scholar of disabled veterans, has noted that the existing scholarly literature on veterans, disabled veterans, and government veterans' policy is shockingly sparse: "Disabled veterans are neglected figures in the histories of war and peace."[29] Although there are two published histories of the Royal Canadian Legion, works pertaining to Canadian veterans' organizations are also almost completely non-existent.[30] SAPA's story, and especially that of the Canadian war blinded as individuals, is a meaningful addition to the burgeoning field of socio-military history as well as to the rapidly developing professional and scholarly interest in disability history. While this book treats the experiences of Canada's war blinded in general, a major element of this study is devoted to the institutional history of SAPA and its eighty-seven-year involvement in ameliorating the lives of its members and improving the lot of all blind Canadians.

History is about people; so, too, is war. Wherever possible the narrative that follows seeks to highlight the human dimensions to the story of Canada's war-blinded veterans and to use the men's own voices, or at least their personal stories, to add immediacy, poignancy, and intensity to the text. I have sought to capture some of their spirit of perseverance because, in the end, the war blinded looked after themselves, and each other, very well. Typical is the example of Verne Russell Williams, who was severely wounded and blinded in 1944 while serving with the North Nova Scotia Highlanders in France. He raised a family but, due to his disabilities, was unable to work for most of his life. SAPA's fraternal assistance might have been essential to his overall well-being.[31] Many wounded men like him, living out their lives quietly, have been forgotten in our perhaps understandable desire to focus commemorative activities on those who did not return from Canada's wars. We know much about our war dead but next to nothing about our war wounded. But these hundreds of war-blinded veterans are the subject of *this* book, and I hope that this work will encourage further scholarship into the treatment and civil re-establishment of other groups among Canada's more than 200,000 war-wounded veterans of the twentieth century.

The first chapter introduces readers to Canada's first celebrated war-blinded casualty, the legendary Lorne Mulloy, who lost his sight during the South African War (1899-1902). It goes on to trace the re-establishment experiences of Canada's First World War blinded attending St. Dunstan's in Britain, with a focus on Edwin Baker, and explains the war blinded's fundamental role in creating the CNIB and their influence on government policy toward all Canadian war-disabled veterans.

Chapter 2 addresses SAPA's origins, goals, and activities in the 1920s and describes the challenges that confronted the organization and its war-blinded members. The focus is on employment retraining at Pearson Hall, the CNIB's Toronto facility, social reintegration and bonding, including the first of many large-scale reunions of war-blinded veterans, the provision of federally funded and CNIB-administered aftercare services, SAPA's emergence as a strong veterans' advocacy group under Baker's guidance, and the instilling in these mainly young men of a sense of personal independence and a will to carry on.

The economic crisis of the 1930s badly battered Canadians, including many veterans and especially the disabled. Chapter 3 de-scribes how the war blinded protected their hard-won pension gains and assisted each other through the fraternity of blindness, with the critical assistance of their families and some CNIB volunteers, mainly women. The blinded struggled to survive economically, strictly con-trolled eligibility requirements for SAPA membership, and participat-ed visibly in commemorative events, including the unveiling of the Vimy Memorial in 1936.

Chapter 4 deals with the years of the Second World War and shows how, with government assistance, the CNIB and SAPA planned for blinded veterans' civil re-establishment, reopened a rehabilitation and training centre (Pearson Hall), and established a residence (Baker Hall) in Toronto. This chapter also discusses the extraordinary part-nership between the CNIB, SAPA, and the Department of Pensions and National Health, replaced by the Department of Veterans Affairs in October 1944. The newly blinded veterans, some of whose stories are detailed in this chapter, were retrained to be functioning members of society and benefitted enormously from the experiences of the First World War veterans. The newcomers eventually took on leadership roles in the Canadian blinded and veterans' communities.

With hundreds of thousands of new veterans to deal with, the federal government was obliged to revisit its pension and rehabilitation policies, culminating in the extensive legislative package known as the Veterans Charter. Chapter 5 discusses this development and introduces some case studies of the post-1945 re-establishment process. It also explains SAPA's institutional growth to 1970 and its important role as a veterans' pressure group, detailing the large-scale, prominent war-blinded reunions that symbolized the tight bonds between those Canadians from two generations who had sacrificed their vision while on national service.

Chapter 6 introduces the evolving federal pension policies and programs as they affected the war blinded into the twenty-first century, details the complex relationship that developed between the CNIB, SAPA, and the Department of Veterans Affairs following the latter's assumption of responsibility for the delivery of war-blinded aftercare services, and describes the final SAPA reunions. This final chapter is also about the war blinded's legacy of hope for, and assistance to, the civilian blind, especially students. The perpetually funded F.J.L. Woodcock/SAPA Scholarship Foundation financially supports education and independence among Canada's blinded youth. This, perhaps more than any other single factor in their history, demonstrates that Canada's war-blinded were truly "veterans with a vision."

1 Canada's First War Blinded, 1899-1918

I was unlucky enough to get in the way of one of the shrapnel bullets. I felt a slight sting in my right temple as though pricked by a red-hot needle – and then the world became black. Dawn was now breaking, but night had sealed my eyes.

– James Rawlinson, blinded at Vimy, 1917

The modern political era for Canada began in 1867, when several colonies in British North America agreed to merge into a new Confederation. The resulting Dominion of Canada grew to vast geographic proportions in the following years, incorporating other colonies and, before the end of the century, attracting large numbers of immigrants, many from the British Isles, to settle its sparsely populated territory. Within a generation, the country's Atlantic and Pacific coasts were linked by a transcontinental railway. By 1900, most of Canada's 5.3 million inhabitants still lived in rural areas, although increasing industrialization led to greater urbanization and a denser concentration of road and rail networks. Montreal was Canada's largest city, with a population of 267,000 in 1901, rising to 406,000 in 1911; Toronto was a distant but growing second. Canada was a confident and comparatively affluent young country. In 1904, Prime

Minister Sir Wilfrid Laurier uttered his oft-repeated boast that "the Twentieth Century shall be the century of Canada." Most of his compatriots would have agreed.

Even though about 28 percent of Canadians were of French ancestry, Canada was very much a British country. It remained a British colony, a constituent part of the British Empire with no formal international status. The British monarch was Canada's sovereign, the national flag remained the Union Jack, and Canadian citizenship was unknown, all Canadians being British subjects. Until the 1950s, Canada's governor general was a British nobleman selected by London.

Since the 1870s, the British Empire had grown into an immense worldwide territorial and economic unit. Britain was the world's most powerful naval and commercial nation. Despite occasional violent opposition to British rule in some colonies, most Canadians of British ancestry considered the empire a progressive and stabilizing force in the world. Stirring popular accounts of imperial conquests filled books, journals, and newspaper articles, and promoted the idea that Britain's heroic armed forces fought for justice and higher ideals. Patriotism was a strong social principle. Duty to the empire and sovereign was primordial for many English Canadians and British immigrants residing in Canada. On the other hand, Canada's support for, and engagement in, British imperial rivalries and wars led to some domestic political and linguistic discord; imperialism was as divisive as it was unifying.

As a result of this ingrained sense of patriotic duty, all those serving or having served in the military stood highly in public esteem throughout the empire. Being a "Soldier of the Queen" was a noble pursuit and, given the often sacrificial nature of war service, received social acclaim not normally accorded to civilian vocations. It is within this context of late Victorian and Edwardian imperial and patriotic zeal that Canada embarked on its first overseas conflict and suffered its first publicized case of war blindness. The South African, or Boer, War (1899-1902) was fought over territorial and economic disputes between the British Empire and two small republics, the Orange Free State and the Transvaal, bordering Britain's colonies in southern Africa, whose European population consisted of Dutch colonists, known as Boers ("farmers" in Dutch). All told, Canada sent more than 7,300 troops to help Britain defeat the Boers.

Blinded in South Africa

In December 1899, at the age of twenty-four, Lorne Mulloy, an un-married school teacher from Winchester, Ontario, a fervent patriot, and a firm believer in the British Empire, volunteered for overseas service with the 1st Battalion, Canadian Mounted Rifles. He was shipped overseas to serve in South Africa. One year later, he was back in Canada a celebrated and decorated imperial and Canadian hero, the very model of courage, selflessness, service, and sacrifice. He had been presented to Queen Victoria, fêted by the Lord Mayor of Liver-pool, and hailed in the press throughout the empire.[1] Trooper Mulloy had achieved fame and earned these accolades through his cour-ageous actions in July 1900 during a desperate struggle with the Boers. But he had paid a price: he was permanently blinded by an enemy bullet that penetrated temple to temple. The poignancy of his condition led to an outpouring of national sympathy, while his determination to pursue his life's ambitions earned him admirers everywhere. Frequently known thereafter as "the Blind Trooper," Mulloy was Canada's first war-blinded casualty of the twentieth century.

Historian Carman Miller has referred to Mulloy, evidently the only fully blinded of 252 Canadians wounded in the South African War, as "a living monument to the cost of Canadian participation in the war."[2] Certainly Trooper Mulloy, winner of the coveted Distin-guished Conduct Medal, was easily the best known of Canada's dis-abled veterans from South Africa, among whom were also amputees and the seriously disfigured. Yet, despite his being a powerful symbol of war's devastating effects, the remainder of Mulloy's life was not all gloomy and, although no one knew it at the time, his impressive career set the standard for what Canada's war blinded could achieve given proper training facilities, government willingness to assist, and the support of an appreciative public. Mulloy proved that Canada's war blinded could be successful and productive citizens.

But Ottawa did not assume financial responsibility for South African War disability pensions, and Mulloy received a paltry British pension of eighteen dollars a month, not enough to make ends meet. While not exactly a charity case, as were most blind Canadians, proceeds from his many speaking engagements, like the seventy-three dollars he received in March 1901 following a lecture at a Methodist church near Cornwall, were no doubt helpful.[3] The heavy involvement of the state in regulating and paying reasonable military disability pensions would have to await the First World War.

In the meantime, the Canadian Patriotic Fund (CPF), a high-profile charity with royal patronage, was set up to assist those disabled or infirm as a result of service in South Africa, and to help their needy dependants. The CPF awarded Mulloy the comparatively enormous sum of more than four thousand dollars to pay his way through Queen's University in Kingston, Ontario, and Balliol College, Oxford. Although the CPF sought to dispense aid equally and had a two-thousand-dollar ceiling on gratuities to permanently disabled veterans, Mulloy's "ability, courage, and charm," not to mention the interest of Sir Sandford Fleming, chancellor of Queen's University, gained him special favour, according to historian Desmond Morton.[4] Mulloy's highly publicized wounding resonated emotively with Canadians, establishing the profile of the blinded Canadian soldier in the public's consciousness.

Newspaper accounts of his return to Canada suggest that society considered blindness a hopeless future. Even Mulloy felt that his "hopes, aims and aspirations [were] all cut down at a swoop, sudden and irreparable." He proved himself wrong. Perhaps ahead of his time, one letter-writer to a Kingston newspaper noted that the government should help the war blinded obtain meaningful employment, which, in Mulloy's case, "would make life under his great affliction more tolerable." Soon thereafter, the independent-minded Mulloy insisted that a determined blind man could enjoy a successful life. "Remember," he stated, "the three most important things are self-mastery, self-reliance and purposeful self-direction."[5]

Mulloy demonstrated, perhaps beyond all reasonable expectations in his era, the extent to which blindness could be overcome. His academic achievements, including a law degree in 1920, and life-long interest in public affairs showed that blinded soldiers could re-establish themselves in Canadian society. He married in 1911 and was employed at the Royal Military College of Canada as a professor of military history. During the First World War, with the honorary rank of colonel, he remained a prominent public figure, frequently appearing in support of recruiting drives and strongly endorsing compulsory military service. Not surprisingly, he was also a vocal advocate for the war disabled. Moreover, he sailed, golfed, and rode horses.[6] Lorne Mulloy was an early trailblazer for Canada's war blinded and the blind in general.

Canada's War Blinded of the First World War

In the period before the outbreak of the First World War, Canada's tradition of limited military pensions and care for returned soldiers or their survivors was based in parsimony; governments did not wish to assume extended or expensive responsibility for disabled veterans' pensions. For example, fully disabled "other rank" pensioners from the 1885 Northwest Campaign might obtain up to sixty cents a day at a time when a casual labourer needed at least one dollar a day for sustenance.[7] Although officers received greater government generosity, other disabled veterans were condemned to poverty unless family or friends could render assistance.

Canada's disabled pensioners were few in 1914, and there were no precedents for dealing with thousands of partially or fully disabled ex-servicemen.[8] In Britain, disabled soldiers begging on street corners reflected the appalling poverty of the unfortunate victims of war. Those who were blinded seemed especially sad cases. Few provisions existed for the care of the disabled who would soon be returning from distant battlefields. Moreover, no facilities offered specialized medical care or retraining for the maimed or sightless.[9]

In the United States, meanwhile, the outrageously generous and politically laden pensions awarded to Civil War veterans led to such financial excess that by the turn of the twentieth century the US government's very solvency was threatened. Canada would have to find a middle ground by adequately caring for its returned men, as the public would deem fit, without rewarding idlers anxious to benefit from a lax pension system. In fact, although many returned men would have to fight for their right to proper pensions, medical care, job training, and survivors' benefits, government involvement in, and responsibility for, their provision signalled revolutionary advancements in the role of the state in caring for Canadians. And, according to historians Desmond Morton and Glenn Wright, all Canadians ultimately benefited from the social programs that flowed from these precedents.[10]

In the summer of 1914, the First World War broke out following years of mounting political and military tension in Europe. On 4 August, after German forces invaded Belgium, whose security Britain had pledged to uphold, Britain declared war on Germany. Canada could not remain isolated from the conflict; constitutionally, and in the eyes of the world, it remained a British colony. When Britain was at war, so was Canada.

Canada's military response was outstanding. Through a Herculean effort, though not without political controversy, the nation mobilized for war. From a 1914 population of approximately

7.8 million, nearly 620,000 men and several thousand nurses were on active service during the war. Some 425,000 of these served overseas with the Canadian Expeditionary Force (CEF). Another 24,000 fought in the British air services, while 5,000 joined the Royal Canadian Navy. The cost to Canada in human lives was appalling: more than 60,000 soldiers lost their lives and another 138,000 were wounded in action. Thousands of others were injured in accidents or permanently weakened by the effects of disease.[11] Places such as Ypres, the Somme, Vimy, Passchendaele, and Amiens assumed enormous importance in the annals of the nation's military history and were etched in the collective memory of Canadians for generations.

Although the first contingent of Canadian troops was hurriedly shipped to Britain in October 1914, the first Canadian unit to see active service in the front lines was the Princess Patricia's Canadian Light Infantry (PPCLI), which saw action in the first week of January while serving in a British division. The 1st Canadian Division landed in France in February 1915 and entered the line at the end of that month at Neuve Chapelle. In April the Canadians were shifted to the Ypres sector, in Belgium.[12]

It was in the Ypres Salient, an Allied-held bulge extending into the German front line, that the Canadians conducted their first major operations. The more than 6,000 casualties suffered there by the 1st Canadian Division in April and May heralded the beginning of a steady stream of disabled veterans. Here, too, Canada suffered its first war-blinded casualty of the First World War: Lance-Corporal Alexander Griswold Viets, serving in the PPCLI, was blinded in May 1915. While he repaired a trench parapet, a German mortar bomb landed beside him, destroying his eyes and inflicting numerous wounds on his face, arms, and legs.[13]

Ottawa soon realized that taking an active role in recasting the lives of Canada's war disabled would be essential to their future success, and also precedent setting. The men's patriotic sacrifices and visible suffering could not be ignored. Prime Minister Sir Robert Borden agreed that the sheer number of returning wounded Canadians obliged the federal government to intervene with programs to care for them and assist with their rehabilitation. The Hospitals Commission (later the Military Hospitals Commission, or MHC) was established on 30 June 1915 to administer a system of medical and convalescent facilities in Canada for returned soldiers. Ernest Henry Scammell became its secretary.[14]

By September 1915, the military discharge depot at Quebec City was processing about a hundred wounded or ill soldiers every week. An increasingly effective Canadian Army Medical Corps and a well-organized casualty-evacuation system meant that a greater number of soldiers survived serious head wounds and other disabling injuries.[15] It was critical for the government to assist them to improve their physical condition and find employment, not only on compassionate grounds but also to show potential recruits that if injury befell them, they would be properly looked after with pensions, retraining, and proper medical care.[16] Besides, the best means of reintegrating wounded soldiers and preventing them from becoming a public charge was to assist them to become productive, wage-earning members of society.[17]

In 1915 a British parliamentary committee reported that "the care of the soldiers and sailors who have been disabled in the war is an obligation which should fall primarily upon the State: and the liability cannot be considered as having been extinguished by the award of a pension from public funds. We regard it as the duty of the State to see that the disabled man shall be, as far as possible, restored to health and that assistance shall be forthcoming to enable him to earn his living in the occupation best suited to his circumstances and physical condition."[18] Canada, too, accepted this principle and, with time, and not without growing pains, established programs, facilities, and a bureaucratic structure allowing disabled veterans to live and work in dignity. Few would benefit more from this change in attitude than Canada's returning war blinded.

By early 1917, of more than 13,000 patients administered by the Military Hospitals Commission in Canada, only 177 had suffered major amputations and only nine had been blinded – although many other Canadian blinded and amputees were being cared for in specialized British facilities. These returned disabled men gained immediate and widespread public support and sympathy.[19]

Sir Andrew Macphail of McGill University's Faculty of Medicine, the official historian of Canada's medical services during the war, noted that "wounds of the eye in war appear to be uncommon merely because they are so often fatal, being in association with more extensive lesions."[20] Nevertheless, by August 1917, the French were reporting some 2,400 totally blinded soldiers, and the British had suffered in excess of 1,300 before war's end. Soldiers of the British and Dominion forces suffering serious eye wounds were evacuated to an ophthalmology ward at No. 83 General Hospital at Boulogne, containing 150 beds.[21]

Many eye wounds causing partial or complete blindness resulted from contact with poison gas, especially mustard gas. Frequently, the full effects of gas exposure manifested themselves only years after the war, creating difficulty with pension claims based on wartime attributability. Immediately after exposure, gas casualties could contract subacute conjunctivitis, often successfully treated in the field by a combination of bandaging to shade against light, warm saline solution, and eye drops of liquid paraffin or atropine ointment.[22] But as eye casualties and incidences of blindness mounted among British and Dominion troops, so, too, grew the means of caring for these men and of retraining them to be independent. The organization created for this purpose, St. Dunstan's in London, England, epitomized innovation, resourcefulness, and courage.

St. Dunstan's Hostel for Blinded Soldiers and Sailors

At the outbreak of war in 1914, Britain's National Institute for the Blind (NIB) was headed by Arthur Pearson, a wealthy and energetic newspaper magnate. Pearson had for a decade been in failing eyesight, the result of glaucoma. By 1908, he no longer had sufficient sight to read or write properly. At the end of 1913 his eyesight failed completely, and he learned that he would be blind for life. Thereafter, his generous patronage of Britain's civilian blind was exceeded only by his devotion to the empire's war blinded.[23]

Immediately upon the declaration of war, the NIB offered its services to the British government. The institute's 1914 annual report, unquestionably from the pen of Arthur Pearson himself, notes that "all blinded soldiers and sailors will receive pensions from His Majesty's Government, but this must not form an inducement [for] them to live purposeless lives. Given a good training, blinded soldiers and sailors may become useful citizens." Here was Pearson's guiding wartime philosophy, which, with the help of the Red Cross Society and the Order of St. John, led to the creation of St. Dunstan's Hostel for Blinded Soldiers and Sailors – the world's leading readaptation centre for the blind.[24] The patriotic impulses unleashed by the war and the public's natural sympathy for its maimed and blinded veterans provided Pearson with the opportunity to help the blind on a scale hitherto unknown and to showcase their impressive capabilities and accomplishments. St. Dunstan's would serve as a model of rehabilitation and vocational training, affirming one of Pearson's mottos: "Lots of people see without perceiving; blind people learn to perceive without seeing."[25]

Among the first blinded Allied soldiers of the war was a Belgian whose eyes were destroyed by a bullet on the first day of the German siege of Liège in August 1914. He was sent to a London military hospital and, hearing of his case, Pearson visited him to offer encouragement. Not long after, two blinded British soldiers were treated at a military medical establishment in Chelsea, London. Pearson paid them a call as well. These visits sparked his idea to establish a dedicated facility to assist with the recovery and retraining of the empire's war blinded. A home was loaned to him for this purpose by a wealthy friend, but the volume of eye casualties soon outstripped the capacity of his Hostel for Blinded Soldiers and Sailors.

Pearson sought a spacious building with grounds on which to expand as the need arose. In March 1915, he secured St. Dunstan's, a spectacular and historic property of fifteen acres in Regent's Park owned by an American financier, Otto Kahn. Apparently, no estate in London was larger except Buckingham Palace, and the St. Dunstan's property was already well known throughout the United Kingdom. Ironically, even the German kaiser had been a prewar visitor. Returning to the United States, Kahn allowed Pearson unrestricted use of his estate, including the right to add buildings and alter existing structures. Pearson's new hostel and rehabilitation centre took the name of the original property: St. Dunstan's Hostel for Blinded Soldiers and Sailors – a name soon famous the world over.[26]

On 26 March 1915, 14 British war blinded were moved from the earlier cramped location to St. Dunstan's. A year later their number had grown to more than 150 in residence at St. Dunstan's and in annexes elsewhere in Britain. These included at least seven Canadians and some Australians and New Zealanders. "The Commonwealth family of St. Dunstan's had come into being," wrote St. Dunstan's historian David Castleton.[27] Pearson himself noted in 1919, with some exaggeration, that with "practically no exceptions all of the soldiers and sailors of the British Imperial Forces blinded in the war came under my care, in order that they might learn to be blind." He continued, "At the very moment when it would be most natural for them to be despondent I wanted them to be astonishingly interested. I wanted them to be led to look upon blindness not as an affliction but as a handicap, not merely as a calamity but as an opportunity."[28] Pearson's creed influenced two generations of Canadian war blinded and allowed them to participate fully in society and in life's pleasures. British officer Ian Fraser, blinded on the Somme in 1916 at the age of eighteen, recalled the psychological and emotional importance of St. Dunstan's: "My weakened link with the past snapped, but not before I was securely bound to the future. Fearfully and reluctantly at first, then more firmly, and finally with resolution, I crossed the bridge between the old world and the new. Pearson was waiting at the other end, his hand stretched out to help me."[29]

At Pearson's suggestion, the War Office sent all serious eye casualties to the 2nd London General Hospital at Chelsea on the Thames embankment (the former St. Mark's College for Women). Early in the war, most men were blinded from gunshot wounds, though subsequently splinters and blast effects from exploding artillery shells and grenades accounted for a higher proportion of eye casualties. Pearson met the new arrivals at the hospital and introduced them to the possibilities available at St. Dunstan's and to his philosophy that blindness need not be the end of a productive and happy life. The gift of a quickly mastered Braille watch proved that the road toward independence could begin immediately. The patients were regularly visited by cheery St. Dunstan's staff, a practice that Pearson insisted motivated the newly blinded into accepting vocational training and drawing strength from the company of others similarly disabled.[30] And there were many of them: at St. Dunstan's peak, following the terrible battles of 1916 on the western front, there were some eight hundred men in its care.[31] For his efforts, Pearson was knighted in 1916.

St. Dunstan's was a hostel, distinctly not an "institution" or a refuge. It was a functional place, where men could be retooled. It was financed through public subscription and received donations from all quarters, including many Canadians and the Canadian Red Cross. In 1918 Pearson wrote that "there are no expenses whatever in connection with a stay at St. Dunstan's; board, lodging and everything else is absolutely free."[32] Many of the instructors at St. Dunstan's were blind themselves, a morale boost for the men that contradicted the biblical view that "if the blind lead the blind, both shall fall into the ditch." The men were immediately trained in Braille and type-writing and offered various sorts of vocational training including boot repair, mat and basket weaving, poultry farming, telephone switchboard operation, and massage therapy (later known as physio-therapy). Training lasted from six to eight months for the less-complicated trades.[33] Those trained as joiners made small articles intended for sale, such as picture frames, tea trays, and ornamental tables. Those raising poultry were taught to distinguish different breeds of birds by touch alone and learned to operate incubators and manage the daily affairs of a poultry farm, including the simple carpentry needed to make coops and gates.[34]

Typewriting was of the greatest importance to the war blinded, as it gave the men the independent ability to communicate privately with others. The first letter was normally an "enormous thrill" for the writer and no less so for the recipient. "It is the first positive, active, useful thing that [a blinded soldier] ... can do for himself, and its morale effect is very great indeed," wrote Ian Fraser.[35] Once St. Dunstaners passed the typewriting course, they were rewarded with a typewriter as a gift.

The St. Dunstan's massage-therapy program lasted twelve to eighteen months and included basic but challenging courses in anatomy, physiology, and pathology, with all the body's bones made familiar to the students through touch. This was followed by more extensive training at the NIB and on-the-job experience at several hospitals in London. There then followed the examinations (the "most severe in the world," according to St. Dunstan's) held by the Incorporated Society of Trained Masseurs. To the spring of 1918, no St. Dunstaners had failed these examinations and one, Canadian Private D.J. McDougall of the PPCLI, had finished second in a field of 320. St. Dunstan's massage graduates were in high demand at mil-itary hospitals, where they assisted with wounded soldiers' physical rehabilitation.[36] More than 130 St. Dunstaners, including Canadians, became masseurs. Reflecting in 1961, following four decades of work at St. Dunstan's, Fraser, by then Lord Lonsdale, believed that "in no occupation have St. Dunstan's men been more successful than physiotherapy."[37]

St. Dunstan's also offered many recreational activities and morale- and team-building exercises, and many life-long friendships developed there. Female Voluntary Aid Detachment workers (VADs) provided "companionship" and, if required, "solace" to the men and also undertook many household tasks to help maintain the premises.[38] The VADs were nearly all unpaid volunteers who, Fraser remarked, "did not lend, but gave."[39] Moreover, the term "VAD" at St. Dunstan's included "the many kindly folk, who, while not belonging to any definite organisation, give a great deal of their time, their thought, and their sympathy to the blinded soldiers." The women accompanied the men on walks, read to them, organized entertainment, and "befriend[ed] them in countless other ways."[40] In fact, a number of romances blossomed between blinded soldiers and VADs, and several marriages resulted. By the spring of 1919, at least three blinded Canadians had married overseas.[41] These women's skills should not be underestimated. During the First World War, some Canadian St. John Ambulance VADs studied Braille in anticipation of assisting the war blinded. All obtained first aid and basic nursing certificates, although fully trained nurses were ineligible to be VADs. Near the end of the war, others completed courses at the University of Toronto's Hart House Military School of Orthopaedic Surgery and Physiotherapy, operated by the Department of Soldiers' Civil Re-establishment.[42]

As soon as a Dominion casualty was brought to St. Dunstan's, the normally tough-talking Sir Arthur Pearson wrote the man's wife or mother an encouraging and cheery letter, explaining the "manifold activities" available at the facility and that, as he himself was ample proof, blindness need not imply "mental or physical extinction."

Correspondence between Pearson and a man's family could continue for months or even the full length of the man's stay. This seemed to confirm others' impression that Pearson's "kindliness of heart was concealed under an autocratic manner."[43]

Many Canadian St. Dunstaners stayed in touch with their benefactor. Alexander Viets, the PPCLI soldier blinded at Ypres, was Canada's first graduate of St. Dunstan's, leaving in March 1916. Some months later he wrote a long letter to Pearson explaining his activities and business successes since returning to his hometown of Digby, Nova Scotia. He was soon busy selling magazine subscriptions, including some for the *Saturday Evening Post* and *Ladies Home Journal*. This allowed him to regain his confidence and return to selling insurance, his prewar occupation. "That was the work you advised me to take up again when I told you I had experience in it," wrote Viets. "I have the greatest reason to be thankful for having followed your advice." He moved to Toronto in October 1916 and became a successful agent for the Imperial Life Assurance Company of Canada. He wrote Pearson in 1919 that he was thriving: "Good health, a profitable occupation and a happy home are a combination that many a sighted man is not in possession of."[44]

Another Canadian St. Dunstaner, James Rawlinson, a private in Ontario's 58th Battalion, published his wartime experiences not long after his return to Canada. *Through St. Dunstan's to Light* (1919) is a straightforward account of what St. Dunstan's vocational training and sense of camaraderie could mean for a young man tragically and suddenly deprived of his sight. His might serve as a reasonably representative account of many blinded Canadians' experiences. Rawlinson was part of a working party behind the lines near Vimy Ridge in the early morning darkness of 7 June 1917. Caught in an enemy artillery barrage, he "was unlucky enough to get in the way of one of the shrapnel bullets. I felt a slight sting in my right temple as though pricked by a red-hot needle – and then the world became black. Dawn was now breaking, but night had sealed my eyes."[45]

In hospital in Boulogne, his left eye was removed, but he still clung to the hope that his right eye might yet be made good. Captain Sir Beachcroft Towse, VC, a blinded hero of the South African War, paid him a visit. Towse, who would head the NIB from 1922 to 1944, then "hit me harder than any Hun shell could hit a man. He snapped out in a voice penetrating, yet with a cheery ring to it: 'Well, you are blind, and for life. How do you like it?'" Wrote Rawlinson, "For about five seconds ... the night that sealed my eyes seemed to clutch my soul. I was for the moment 'down and out'; but I braced my spirits in the presence of this dominating man. I would show him how a Canadian soldier could bear misfortune ... I swore just a little to ease my nervous strain, and replied, 'That's a hell of a thing to tell a guy.'"[46] "Now the cruel fact had to be faced," he continued, "the only world I would see henceforth would be that conjured up by the imagination from memories of the past."[47]

During Rawlinson's treatment at the 2nd London General Hospital, some St. Dunstan's staff read the men newspapers and told them what St. Dunstan's could offer. But nothing could prepare Rawlinson for the occasion when Pearson, "one of the geniuses of the present age" and "a miracle worker," called on him at the hospital.[48] During that first meeting, "darkness seemed to vanish" and Rawlinson "knew full well that I should not be a burden upon anybody, sightless though I was." Before being discharged to St. Dunstan's, Rawlinson visited on a number of occasions to speak with the men already undergoing training. In the meantime, he learned some of the basics of Braille at the hospital. He was transferred to St. Dunstan's in August 1917 and stayed sixteen months, until December 1918. He qualified as a stenographer, taking Braille shorthand and typing it out on a regular typewriter at the rate of more than one hundred words per minute.[49]

Rawlinson recalled that at St. Dunstan's "nothing was compulsory except sobriety." But the care given the men there made them wish to "help others." The Canadian war blinded took on leadership roles in the blind community in general and were to become ambassadors for their disability. Alexander Viets wrote in the *St. Dunstan's Review* of 1917, "The care and education of the blind in Canada generally ... is in a very bad state ... [W]e think it will be through the returned blinded soldiers that considerable interest will be aroused, and when the war is over a lot of good can be done in ... educating and interesting the general public."[50] This proved correct.

Though probably never exceeding 10 percent of St. Dunstaners in residence, the Canadians maintained an esprit de corps and often stuck together, for example, in their own very successful rowing and tug-of-war teams. According to one British resident, while neither group formed cliques, as such, both the Australians and the Canadians "kept extra ties among themselves."[51] They also consoled and supported each other – as in the case of Rawlinson helping a twenty-year-old blinded Canadian who felt his life was over. The despondent young man responded well to encouragement and subsequently became an outstanding student.[52] One proud blinded Canadian, George Eades, led the contingent of five hundred St. Dunstaners who were reviewed by the king in Hyde Park on the day of the Armistice, 11 November 1918.[53]

"What I am, I owe to St. Dunstan's," wrote Rawlinson:

and while labouring here [in Toronto] my heart ever goes back to dear old England. I feel towards St. Dunstan's – and so do all the boys who have passed through her halls – as does the grown man for the place of his birth. She is home for me. I was born again and nurtured into a new manhood by her, led by her from Stygian darkness to mental and spiritual light, and my heart turns with longing towards her. At times separation from the genial atmosphere of this paradise of the sightless, from contact with the dominating, kindly presence of Sir Arthur Pearson and his noble assistants, weighs heavily upon my spirits. But there is work to be done here in Canada.[54]

The war blinded did, in fact, lead the way in organizing Canada's blinded population and in revolutionizing public perceptions of their disability.

Edwin Albert Baker

Edwin Albert Baker was a remarkable blinded veteran and advocate for the sightless everywhere. He was dogged, resourceful, energetic, charismatic, and utterly devoted to improving the lot of Canada's blind population, perhaps especially the veterans. His intimate association in the founding of the Canadian National Institute for the Blind (CNIB) and his lifetime leadership roles with the institute afforded it the national prestige and international acclaim that it might not otherwise have obtained.

Baker was born in 1893 in Ernesttown, Ontario, near Kingston, into a farming family. He graduated from Queen's University in 1914 with a degree in electrical engineering. Keenly interested in the military, he had served in the militia for five years prior to the outbreak of the war, at first in the 4th Hussars and later in the 5th Field Company, Royal Canadian Engineers. He was accepted for service in the CEF in February 1915, serving overseas as a lieutenant with the 6th Field Company, RCE, in the 2nd Canadian Division. Baker recalled that "as our ship pulled away from the harbour and put out to sea, a number of us leaning over the rail took what might [have been] for many of us a last look at the shores of Canada."[55] For Baker, this proved to be the case, though not in the manner that he had anticipated. He was in Britain by April and in Belgium by September 1915.

In October Baker commanded No. 3 Section of the 6th Field Company. He and his men spent the night of 9-10 October at Kemmel, about ten kilometres south of Ypres, perilously repairing severely damaged communications trenches linking rear areas with the front lines, and restoring a front-line trench destroyed by the detonation of a German mine. Baker was later awarded the Military

Cross, the French Croix de Guerre, and a Mentioned-in-Dispatches for his leadership and daring that night. The following evening, he led a party of five or six military engineers and up to sixty men pressed into fatigue duty to continue the work. He was arranging the rebuilding of part of the secondary line, perhaps thirty metres from the front line, when he entered a battered trench. It had been partially filled in with debris and fallen sandbags "so that it did not conceal anyone standing upright," recalled Baker. "I found myself with my head and shoulders above the top of the trench. A German star-shell lit up the desolate landscape ... I remember wondering if there was any possible chance of the enemy being able to see us. I think the last thing I saw was that bright, floating star shell for, as I watched, a bullet smashed through the bridge of my nose and left me to the mercy of the darkness and my friends." The bullet passed across his left eye and behind his right. "I've had it, boys!" was the first thing he uttered to those around him. He would never see again. He was twenty-two.[56]

Baker had known of blinded Trooper Lorne Mulloy before the war. But other than that one shining example, the blind people he had seen were either beggars or completely dependent, being awkwardly led around by family members. He felt condemned to such an existence. Like all cases of blindness, Baker was transferred to No. 2 London General Hospital, where he spent nearly ten weeks. Near the end of October 1915, Arthur Pearson visited and presented him with a Braille watch. Baker did not immediately realize that he had just encountered one of the great formative influences on his life and career. Not long after, Baker toured St. Dunstan's and engaged in a deep conversation with another war-blinded man. Thereafter, he was convinced there was life after blindness, and that it began at St. Dunstan's.[57]

By most accounts, Lieutenant Baker was the first Canadian officer to attend St. Dunstan's. Arriving on 2 January 1916 and staying until July, for a while he roomed with fellow Canadian Alexander

Viets and with New Zealander Clutha Mackenzie. But he soon moved to officers' quarters at 21 Portland Place, another home loaned to Pearson by a benefactor, where Pearson and his wife also stayed. Baker developed a very close, almost filial relationship with Pearson, who served as inspiration and mentor. While at St. Dunstan's Baker became an excellent typist, learned Braille, and easily passed the business course.[58]

Baker's distraught mother, learning of his plans and knowing little of St. Dunstan's, understandably wished for her son to come home immediately and, in December 1915, wrote Pearson to this effect. In a lengthy reply, Pearson reassured her that St. Dunstan's was the best possible place for Baker and that he was thriving. "There are numberless ways, some small, some great, in which he can be helped here in a manner which would be impossible in any home, however loving the care bestowed upon him." Pearson reported that Baker "already makes his way about with a freedom most unusual in one newly blinded." In January 1916, Pearson again wrote Mrs. Baker that her son was "showing the greatest aptitude of any Officer or man who has been blinded in the War ... His cheeriness and good humour are never failing, and he makes friends wherever he goes." Two months later, Pearson was even more pointed in his compliments: "He is quite the most confident, self-reliant man of all the 160 blinded soldiers with whom I have come into personal contact" since the opening of St. Dunstan's. Two years later, on hearing of Baker's appointment with the Department of Soldiers' Civil Re-establishment (DSCR) in Ottawa, Pearson wrote Mrs. Baker that "of all the twelve hundred soldiers who have now come under my care there is not one of them as well fitted for this work as is your capable and courageous son."[59] Nevertheless, when Edwin Baker was returned to his mother's arms at the Kingston train station in September 1916, she burst into tears, hugged him tightly, and exclaimed "Eddie! Eddie! My poor boy!"[60]

With a single man's pension of seventy-five dollars a month, Baker, determined and confident, set about finding work. He did not have to search long. By October 1916, he was working at the Ontario Hydro-Electric Power Commission in Toronto as a typist for a further seventy-five dollars a month. Soon thereafter he was promoted to preparing "trouble" reports from hydro substations.[61]

Edwin Baker was appalled to learn on his return that Canada had no training facilities even approaching those that Pearson had managed to set up at St. Dunstan's. There was no government employment placement program and no clear understanding of the needs of returned blinded soldiers; in fact, there was next to nothing at all in the way of support and aftercare.

Baker maintained an interest in the war and in patriotic activities. In October 1916 he spoke at Massey Hall, Toronto, at a fundraiser in aid of the Red Cross, and in the spring of 1917 he spoke at Victory Bond rallies. In April 1917 he was gazetted a captain.[62] He had become something of a celebrity, with the seriousness of his wound and his obvious capability earning him a public profile and widespread respect and admiration similar to that which Trooper Mulloy had encountered following his return from South Africa. Intentionally or not, Baker's growing fame helped him bring attention to the plight of Canada's returned war blinded. Dr. Charles Rae Dickson, honorary president of Toronto's Canadian Free Library for the Blind (CFLB), lauded Baker, "this brave lad," and noted at the time that the governor general, the Duke of Connaught, was impressed with Baker's "fine bearing and bright hopeful spirit."[63] In 1916 Dickson also met Alexander Viets and thought highly of him and the training he had received at St. Dunstan's.

Baker and Viets, close friends and collaborators, used the CFLB's Braille holdings and joined its management board in 1916. When they learned that the already pitifully small CFLB was to close and put its materials into storage for lack of funds, they decided to actively take up the cause of Canada's blind. Baker, Viets, Dickson, and Sherman C. Swift, the CFLB's secretary-general and librarian, obtained financial assistance from the Toronto Women's Musical Club and purchased a home at 142 College Street to serve as a new headquarters. They obtained donations of furniture and a piano, among other things, to make the new facility comfortable. This became Canada's first, informal, location where blinded soldiers returned from overseas could meet.[64] But far more was needed to properly organize Canada's blind population, and the returned soldiers would be in the forefront of change. Theirs was an achievement of profound importance to all Canadian blind: the establishment of the CNIB.

Initial Provisions for Canada's War Blinded

Despite their limited number, Canada's First World War blinded proved a challenge to Ottawa's system of re-establishing disabled veterans. For example, Ottawa dithered for more than two years over the formal procedures for the treatment, rehabilitation, and eventual repatriation of Canada's blinded soldiers. It simply was not clear what would happen to them upon their return.

As early as November 1915, Sir Frederick Fraser, a leading blind educator, had guardedly offered the use of the Halifax School for the Blind's facilities to the Military Hospitals Commission (MHC) as a potential alternative to sending Canadians to St. Dunstan's.[65] Fraser sought to make his school the premier retraining centre for the war blinded. But not all in Canada's blinded community agreed with the policy of shipping untrained and perhaps emotionally fragile blinded soldiers back to Canada – especially to a school designed for children. The CFLB, too, was interested in the plight of Canada's handful of returned blinded veterans. Rivalries between the two institutions were worsened by personality clashes and magnified as blinded casualties became more numerous and Ottawa hesitated over the best means of ensuring the men's rehabilitation.

In March 1916, the MHC promised to advise the CFLB of the arrival in Canada of all blinded soldiers but admitted that "at present the Commission has not a complete list of Blinded Soldiers who have returned."[66] On being pressed for the government's plans by Dickson, T.B. Kidner, the MHC's vocational secretary, implied that the problem of the war blinded was not significant given that perhaps fewer than a dozen Canadians were then in training at St. Dunstan's. Kidner confessed that "nothing has yet been considered" with respect to where the men officially would or should be retrained.[67]

Given the inadequacy of Canadian facilities, it was clear to these blinded civilians that the only realistic option was to send all Canadian blinded casualties to St. Dunstan's. In July 1916, Kidner wrote Swift that, henceforward, this would be the MHC's policy.[68] In fact, however, due to Canadian administrative confusion in Britain and contradictory signals from Ottawa, this would not actually prove the case until mid-1918. Some soldiers went to St. Dunstan's while others were shipped home by medical authorities lacking clear instructions. Some Canadian war blinded, erroneously assured of proper treatment at home, opted for a speedy return.

Sherman Swift and Charles Dickson made a formidable pairing in agitating for the best available treatment for Canada's war blinded. Dickson, a medical doctor, had worked for twenty-eight years in the field of electricity as it applied to medical practices. When he was accidentally blinded in 1908 in the course of X-ray and electrotherapy experimentation, he associated himself with the CFLB and with Swift, who had been a first-class scholar at McGill University.[69] Born in Kingston in 1858, Dickson had a long history of voluntary service and philanthropic work including helping form the Canadian St. John Ambulance Association and the Canadian branch of the British National Society for Aid of the Sick and Wounded in War, subsequently renamed the Canadian Red Cross Society.[70] A fervent patriot and imperialist, Dickson took on the cause of the war blinded as his own and, after meeting Viets, quickly accepted the merits of the St. Dunstan's philosophy. For the next twenty years he was to befriend virtually every blinded Canadian soldier.[71] Dickson firmly believed that the best teachers of the blind were other blinded people: "None but a blind man can appreciate the psychology of the blind," he wrote, explaining St. Dunstan's high rehabilitation success rate.[72]

Always on the lookout for any war-blinded veteran who had not been to St. Dunstan's and whom he could assist, Dickson stayed in close touch with the co-operative W.F. Moore, who worked with the MHC at the CEF Discharge Depot in Quebec City. Dickson also sought information on any returnees with eye conditions likely to lead to permanent blindness. In October 1916, for example, Moore sent Dickson the names of three soldiers invalided home suffering from retinitis pigmentosa. The CFLB had committed to trying to secure employment for as many returned blinded men as possible, filling a void where the government had yet to assume responsibility. For example, when Alexander Viets moved to Toronto, he was a house guest of Dickson's for several weeks while the CFLB helped him find work in the insurance world.[73] Although Dickson and Swift's responses were ad hoc and restrained by lack of funding, they offered more practical help than, as it soon transpired, was given returned soldiers at Fraser's Halifax school.

In 1916 and 1917, small groups of Canadian war blinded arrived at the Halifax School for the Blind (HSB) for vocational training at government expense. Most had arrived from Britain following combat- or disease-related blindness; some were suffering from blindness caused in training accidents or brought upon by service conditions. A few of these men had never left Canada. The Canadian Red Cross and the CFLB sent them Braille watches as encouragement. In the summer of 1917, these men formed a cross-section of those blinded while serving with the CEF. Private John Ross, born in Ireland and a resident of Missouri at the outbreak of war, was blinded at St. Éloi, south of Ypres, in April 1916 from a rifle-grenade blast that inflicted twenty-five wounds on his body. He was learning Braille, typewriting, and massage therapy. Private Peter Donaldson, born in Ayr, Scotland, and a resident of Fort William, Ontario, lost his sight from a gunshot wound in September 1916 while serving in the 28th Battalion at Courcellette on the Somme; he underwent similar training to Ross. Private Leonard B. Hopkins, born in Alberta, joined the 89th Battalion, but he was returned to Halifax in 1917 when it became apparent during training in Britain that his eyesight was failing drastically. Sergeant Alexander Graham, also born in Ayr and formerly of the Royal Artillery, transferred to the Canadian Garrison Artillery and lost his sight before the war, reportedly due to strain on his optic nerves. He entered the HSB in 1913 and graduated in 1917 as a piano tuner. However, he stayed on to render assistance to blinded soldiers in Braille and massage, and eventually trained as a masseur.[74] One soldier, Private Marion Smith, an American who enlisted in Alberta, was blinded while training at Valcartier, Quebec, and never sailed for France.[75]

Supported by Baker, Viets, and other war-blinded veterans, Swift remained as dogged as Dickson in pressing Ottawa for a firm commitment to send all Canadian war blinded to St. Dunstan's. In October 1917, Swift wrote Sir James Lougheed, president of the MHC, that he had heard "persistent rumours" that the Canadian war blinded were to be repatriated and not sent to St. Dunstan's, and that special facilities were to be built in Canada instead. He wrote that Baker and Viets were said to deplore such a move, noting that a Canadian version of St. Dunstan's could hardly be built overnight. According to Swift, about a dozen Australian war blinded had elected to be retrained at home in schools for blind children and the result had been "disastrous." "The blinded Australians finally rebelled and demanded to be sent ... to St. Dunstan's for scientific and enlightened training." Swift was adamant that any Canadian policy to deprive men of St. Dunstan's training would be simply "criminal." If the men returned to Canada without proper training, their desire to become independent would be stifled by a family naturally wishing to "pet, pamper and spoil" them. Moreover, since a number of British-born Canadian war-blinded had decided to stay in Britain following their St. Dunstan's rehabilitation and military discharge, bringing them home as a matter of policy seemed foolish.[76]

The main reason Swift wanted the MHC to send returned blinded Canadians to St. Dunstan's for proper training was that he believed Fraser's efforts at the HSB were not up to the task. Swift felt that Fraser was a self-aggrandizing attention seeker. He cautioned Lougheed about Fraser: "there is a movement now under way in Canada to induce our Government to bring blinded Canadian soldiers home." According to Swift, "already a spirit of discontent is appearing among the few blinded Canadians undergoing instruction" in Halifax. "They feel they are not getting all that is possible, nor all they deserve," a situation which would be remedied at St. Dunstan's. Officials at the MHC seemed unaware of any problems. Ernest Scammell wrote Dickson that the men in Canada were "progressing satisfactorily" and that he had no opinion on whether they should be returned to Britain to attend St. Dunstan's.[77] On this file, at least, the astute but overworked Scammell might not have done his homework.

Given that the government had pledged to assume the costs of retraining the war blinded, the CFLB did not solicit or accept money for their care. "People all over the country are sending in contributions, small and large," Swift wrote Scammell in November 1917. "Everybody nowadays persists in adding the word 'soldier' to the word 'blind,' many blind men are stopped in the streets and asked if they have been at the Front, a khaki color tinges the whole public view of the blind." This sensitization would serve Canada's blind population in the future. Swift sought MHC permission to accept such funds and, underscoring the CFLB's main interest in supporting

all blind Canadians, Swift reminded Scammell that "in a most important sense, the general cause of the Canadian blind is bound up with
the question of our blinded soldiers." In an effort to avoid embarrassment, the MHC opposed any public appeals but agreed that the
CFLB could use unsolicited donations to create a "trust fund" for the
war blinded.[78]

Canada's blinded were coalescing into an advocacy group,
stimulated by and seeking to derive advantage from the patriotic
impulses unleashed by the war. Also, the civilian blind strongly supported the war blinded. CFLB staff were of the opinion that the pension allotment for blinded soldiers was "utterly inadequate." Insisted
Dickson, "If the Government makes any mistake in the matter of
Pensions it should be on the side of cheerful liberality rather than
stinginess."[79] Swift argued that poverty led to stigmatization of the
blind as incapable and deficient – which in turn led to their poverty.
Accordingly, pension amounts had to be sufficient for the war blinded to live in dignity and be perceived by the public as contributing
members of society.[80]

The federal government ranked pensions according to the
severity of each soldier's disability, itself defined by the veteran's
capacity to earn a living. Pensions served as a form of "top-up" to
ensure an adequate (though often minimum) income. From Ottawa's
perspective, if pensions were too generous, veterans would have no
incentive to retrain or even work. And, as historians Morton and
Wright have noted, "the idea that the disabled could earn a genuine
living defied experience."[81] Moreover, if the pensions were indexed
to take into account a man's earnings, then what incentive would
there be for retraining? The CFLB lobbied the government on behalf
of individual soldiers. "The cry is for recruits and more recruits,"
Dickson wrote acidly to the Board of Pension Commissioners (BPC).
"Shall we say 'go' [and] if you fall you will get a soldier's grave, but, if
you are foolish enough to lose your sight, God help you, Canada
knows nothing about blind men!"[82]

Moreover, the BPC frequently ignored the lingering effects of injuries as the cause of veterans' deteriorating eyesight. For example, a Private Poirier had obtained a 40 percent disability pension for having lost an eye during the war. But as the sight in his other eye severely worsened in 1917, he lost his job with the Post Office. Poirier probably suffered from sympathetic ophthalmia, a condition associated with an existing eye injury or single-eye loss character- ized by a perforation or the presence of a foreign object. Frequently, over a period of months or years, the victim loses vision in the healthy eye as well. However, the pension board disagreed that Poirier's impending total blindness was attributable to war service and denied his claim for a pension increase.[83] Private William French, formerly of the Royal Canadian Regiment, lost an eye in a wartime accident at the Dominion Arsenal in Quebec City and received a pen- sion of a mere eleven dollars a month as a consequence. He subse- quently lost the sight of his remaining eye to sympathetic blindness but received no pension increase. Since French had been a soldier prior to the war and was enlisted as fit during the war, Dickson be- lieved that the board's notion that his blindness was caused by a pre- enlistment eye disease should be "disregarded." Similarly, Dickson wished to know why blinded Private W.D. McMillan, formerly of the 21st Battalion, residing in St. Catharines, Ontario, received a paltry twenty-two dollars monthly.[84] The system seemed devoid of gener- osity or compassion, was applied inconsistently, and exemplified the government's lack of experience in dealing with war-blinded veterans.

Continuing social class distinctions were also reflected in the pension system. Private Harris Turner, a prewar journalist from Sas- katchewan who was blinded at Sanctuary Wood in June 1916 while serving in the PPCLI, wrote in his magazine, *Turner's Weekly,* in Janu- ary 1919 that it was appalling that a man's rank would dictate the amount of disability pension he received. "That an officer with an arm off should get twice as much pension as a private with an arm off," he wrote, "is unfair, unjust, unsound, undemocratic, unreasonable, unBritish, unacceptable, outrageous and rotten."[85] He might have noted that the overwhelming number of Canada's growing war blinded were drawn from the non-officer class.

The situation for blinded soldiers at the Halifax School for the Blind, and the horrors of blindness itself, were thrown into high relief as a result of the tragic Halifax explosion in December 1917. Two vessels collided in Halifax harbour, and one of them, the *Mont Blanc*, was packed with high explosives. The resulting detonation devastated a good part of the city and killed nearly two thousand people. The HSB, located at Murdoch Square about three kilometres from the explosion, suffered massive superficial damage and all its windows were blown out. But there were no serious casualties among the staff or pupils. Wrote Sir Frederick Fraser, "The soldiers, many of whom have been on the battlefields of Flanders, declare that the most intense bombardments experienced by them were slight in comparison with the explosion." The school was pressed into service as an emergency hospital and a large number of Haligonians were treated there. Fraser, anxious to inform the CFLB that his work with blinded soldiers would continue, wrote Dickson that within five days of the explosion the special department charged with blinded soldiers' re-establishment was back in operation.[86]

Following on the heels of the explosion, Fraser launched a fundraising campaign for $500,000, to build a new facility in Halifax for the war blinded. He hoped to capitalize on the nation's sympathy for the stricken city, on the public's desire to assist the war blinded, and on the wide publicity allotted the large number of eye injuries that had resulted from the explosion. Fraser wrote Swift that more than two hundred Haligonians were blinded and that the HSB required the money to reorganize and see to their needs.[87] Overall, 5,923 eye injuries were reported, with 16 people losing both eyes and 249 one eye. Forty-one people were rendered completely blind in the explosion, at least three of them soldiers. Many eye injuries were sustained by women looking out their windows in the direction of the blast, which sent shards of glass into their faces.[88]

The turf war between the CFLB and the HSB had broader implications than the care of the war blinded. Talks had been ongoing for a year among the principal blind organizations to create a unified national group, the Canadian National Institute for the Blind. Fraser's reluctance to fold his operation into a larger one seemed to lead to his embellishing the success of soldiers' training in Halifax. One of Swift's contacts in the city, informally keeping an eye on the HSB, penned Swift a note in which he wrote that the soldiers were displeased and uncomfortable with their presence at the Halifax school. Some had taken up residence nearby rather than be quartered at the school and be subject to its many rules drawn up for children and young adults.[89] The men were told to obey all existing rules, including a 9:00 p.m. bedtime and no smoking or drinking. According to an earlier chronicler of SAPA's history, the men rebelled against these strictures and "reacted like good infantrymen and the resultant spree shook the school." The soldiers were speedily billeted at a hotel that was then destroyed in the Halifax Explosion.[90] In January and February 1918, Swift sent pipes and tobacco and games such as checkers and dominos for distribution to the eight blinded soldiers then under care at Halifax.[91]

Meanwhile, Ottawa took steps to establish a firm policy with respect to where Canada's war blinded would be retrained. Colonel Murray McLaren of the MHC visited St. Dunstan's to investigate whether Canadians should be sent there or redirected to Canada. He was impressed by what he saw and, in December 1917, reported very positively on St. Dunstan's. The MHC issued a press release about McLaren's visit, almost certainly in response to a letter published in the press by Baker, Viets, and Quartermaster Sergeant Bertram Mayell, PPCLI, all war blinded, against the establishment of facilities in Canada that would compete with St. Dunstan's. This was no time to be nationalistic. St. Dunstan's was obviously the place for the men to get the best care and civil re-establishment training. The MHC admitted that much stock would be placed in the three blinded veterans' opinions.[92]

In February 1918, two soldiers sent letters to Dickson complaining about conditions at the Halifax School for the Blind. Sergeant Alexander Graham, blinded in military service prior to the war and affiliated with the HSB for several years, wrote:

> The existing schools for the blind have not solved the problem of the adult blind, nor do they appear to have given the matter much attention. This statement is born [sic] out by the manner in which the re-education of blind Canadian soldiers has been carried out at this institution. The soldiers, while in England, were told that there were institutions in Canada equal in every respect to St. Dunstan's, and on the strength of this assurance they returned to the Dominion. They soon realized that they had made a great mistake in so doing. The ordinary school for the blind is about the last place to which blind soldiers should be sent ... I have heard nothing but praise of the work done by Sir A. Pearson in Great Britain. I have never heard a good word said about the work being done here.[93]

Graham went on to state that two of eight soldiers at the school were so disappointed that they planned to leave to enter American establishments. "Surely, Sir, we have a Pearson in Canada," he wrote, "and if he will step forth and take his proper place he will have the best wishes and practical support of all the soldiers here."[94]

British-born Corporal Abel Knight, thirty-three, married with a child, was wounded at Ypres in May 1915 while serving with the PPCLI. Dickson sent him a Braille watch and, in reply, Knight wrote the following:

In your letter ... you ask ... what professions we intend to follow. Well, after six months at this Institute, I can only reply that "I don't know." I came here last September enthusiastic and under the impression that I should meet men who have studied the blind adult question. My experience here has proved to me beyond all doubt that having got us here the officials at this Institute considered their labours ended.

Any complaint is met by the question, "What do you want to do?" I ask you, Sir, if Sir Frederick Fraser, after 45 years experience among the blind, does not know what a blind adult can do, how the devil can I, who was blinded by misadventure in the Ypres Salient, be expected to know?

... Until last month there were no Braille writers that would write in this place. I received my first lesson on a print typewriter two weeks ago, so am yet dependent on others to write my letters. True, a course of massage can be taken here, but I don't like that profession, nor am I prepared to become an itinerant vendor of scrubbing brushes.

The only thing achieved in my case here is the killing of all ambition ... my only desire now is to get home to my family, re-education or no re-education.[95]

With the creation of the CNIB only weeks away, it seemed an opportune moment to expose Fraser's work as unproductive and to encourage Ottawa to enter into a partnership with the new organization to ensure proper training at St. Dunstan's and to co-ordinate the retraining of the blind in Canada. Money was at stake, and Swift wrote a number of damning letters to potential HSB donors. Swift informed one of Fraser's American benefactors that "if after twelve months trial the net results of his attempt to readapt a dozen blinded soldiers to their new life are deep-seated resentment and openly expressed contempt of ... his methods, what assurance have we that his civilian protégés will not come to the same distressing conclusions?"[96]

For fear of breaking their confidence and inviting retribution against them, Dickson refused to send Graham and Knight's letters to Ernest Scammell at the MHC. Swift, however, was quick to notify Scammell of their existence, evidence of soldiers'"discouragement approaching despair." Swift reminded Scammell that the CFLB had, as early as 1916, insisted to the MHC that all blinded Canadians attend St. Dunstan's and pointed out that "the failure of our Government to see to it that our blind men were kept where they ought to have remained has resulted in such a scandalous state of things as now obtains in Halifax." "I am heartsick and discouraged over the whole business," wrote Swift.[97] The federal government had to act; its dithering was becoming public knowledge while the soldiers bore the brunt of the confusion and internecine rivalries among Canada's civilian blind.

The Canadian National Institute for the Blind and Retraining the War Blinded

After a year of planning, drafting a constitution, and consulting and negotiating with various organizations for the blind across Canada, the Canadian National Institute for the Blind was formally created in Toronto in March 1918. Dr. Charles Dickson was elected president (a post he relinquished in August to Lewis M. Wood) and became the general secretary. Edwin Baker served as vice-president, while Alexander Viets and Harris Turner joined the council, or executive committee. Later, blinded soldiers Lieutenant-Colonel T.E. Perrett of Regina and D.M. Ross of Toronto became members while Turner took a sabbatical. The fledgling organization's models were St. Dunstan's and Britain's National Institute for the Blind, and it incorporated the philosophy of independence promoted by the CFLB. Viets and Baker proposed Pearson as honorary president of the CNIB (he was already a patron), and Pearson accepted the honour.[98] The ties between the CNIB and St. Dunstan's were very close and would remain so. The war blinded had served as the impetus for the CNIB to form, they were heavily represented among its founders, and they served as the institute's first major clientele, with the retraining costs borne by the federal government. The war-blinded veterans' influence was thus felt immediately and was long lasting, especially in the case of Baker.

In a few years, the CNIB spread its services and the expertise it had acquired in assisting the war blinded to Canada's civilian blind. One blinded soldier remarked that "if as the result of our blindness the public will become interested in and have sympathy for the civilian blind, the affliction will have been well worth while." According to the CNIB's first published information sheet, "this admirable stand ... [had] the endorsement of all the war blinded." Moreover, "the great movement which has now been commenced for the Blind [i.e., the CNIB] may be regarded as a memorial to the gallantry and sacrifices of the Canadian soldiers who have lost their sight in the war."[99] But the organization was born of war and there was an official distinction between the war blinded and the civilian blind: the returned men received government support such as specialized training, pensions, some travel expenses, and some technical equipment.[100] It became the war blinded's and the CNIB's mission that these provisions be extended to cover all of Canada's blind.

On the other hand, in 1918, the CNIB's Sherman Swift wrote, "It is eminently true that our gallant blinded soldiers have recently focused public attention more directly upon the blind in general. It is not true that the needs of our soldiers gave birth to public interest in the blind." He saw the publicity given the war blinded as enhancing public understanding of the issues pertaining to all of society's blinded. Similar situations developed in France, where the Association Valentin Haüy looked after the war blinded, and in the United States. But Swift was proud of the work the civilian blind had undertaken before the war and noted that the existence of even a meagre civilian infrastructure for the blind had facilitated the readaptation of the recently war blinded. He estimated that the war blinded and their needs, and the availability of public funds to match these, had advanced the cause of the civilian blind by as much as twenty-five years. This "sudden injection into the veins of the blind body politic" had proven a "vitalizing stream." One advantage the war blinded brought to the broader blind community was that they had all recently had sight; the abilities they had acquired over their lives and their knowledge of the sighted world were extremely important in helping long-blinded Canadians.

Not all members of the CNIB were thrilled with the exalted status of returned blinded soldiers. Charles W. Holmes, hired in July 1918 as the first director of the institute, and clearly not on the friendliest terms with either Dickson or Swift, saw the war blinded as like any other blind people. He felt that blind persons' abilities and aptitudes should dictate their retraining schemes, not a hierarchical system valuing patriotic service in the first instance. In other words, a more apt civilian should have greater call on the demanding massage training course, for example, than a less promising soldier.[101] The difference, and some of the frustration, lay in the fact that Ottawa at the time recognized only its responsibility to pension the war blinded. Patriotic service favoured them, whereas the civilian blind had had little opportunity to serve their nation in time of war – or peace.

The institute's founders sought to establish a permanent, viable, and well-led organization catering to the needs of all Canada's blind. Such an organization could speak with greater authority and more realistically entice government subsidy and partnership in caring for the needs of the dozens of war blinded streaming home to Canada, some without benefit of St. Dunstan's training. It was these latter men's plight that most exercised Baker, and he and Viets sought to establish a smaller version of St. Dunstan's in Toronto to accommodate them. But the cash-poor institute required government assistance to set up a training program.

The matter of where to train Canadian blinded soldiers was still not settled. Pearson noted the case of a Canadian soldier whom he had visited at London's No. 2 General Hospital and who, in turn, visited St. Dunstan's and expressed a strong desire to attend. But he was earmarked for a speedy return to Canada. He went to see Pearson, explained the situation, and, through Pearson's personal intervention, was able to be taken on strength at St. Dunstan's. But, as Pearson put it, "If he had not had the sense to come and see me he would undoubtedly have been shipped back to Canada."[102] Dickson wrote Major-General G.L. Foster, the director of medical services overseas, noting that the CFLB (now part of the CNIB) was instructing three soldiers in Braille and typewriting and that "not one of these men was told about St. Dunstan's."[103] Even late in the war major communications problems existed overseas which resulted in needless delays in training.

In order to streamline the process of returning St. Dunstan's graduates to Canada, in May 1918 Pearson began informing local representatives of the Canadian Invalided Soldiers' Commission, part of the Department of Soldiers' Civil Re-establishment, of a soldier's upcoming graduation six weeks prior to the fact. This was to help ensure "suitable arrangements have been made for them when they arrive in Canada." Although the pieces were finally falling into place, an angry Pearson noted that there continued to be some "ridiculous efforts" at the repatriation centre in Folkestone to induce Canadians to return directly to Canada without benefit of St. Dunstan's. Already, according to Pearson, ten men were being detained there on a variety of "pretexts," rather than being sent to St. Dunstan's. One "frivolous" excuse offered was the need to supply glass eyes, which St. Dunstan's "could supply in five minutes."[104]

The creation of the CNIB and the authority with which it spoke on behalf of the war blinded helped enormously. Finally, on 31 May

1918, Walter E. Segsworth, the director of the vocational branch of the Department of Soldiers' Civil Re-establishment (DSCR), wrote Dickson at the CNIB that *all* Canadian war blinded willing to attend were to be sent to St. Dunstan's. None of Canada's war blinded were obliged to undergo retraining, but all who refused treatment at St. Dunstan's had to sign a waiver to this effect before two witnesses.[105] Segsworth was serving on the CNIB council as the representative of the Invalided Soldiers' Commission. Behind the scenes, Baker seems to have influenced the adoption of this long-desired policy. Baker was in the process of being hired by the DSCR to administer policies relating to Canada's war blinded. In February, the DSCR and the Invalided Soldiers' Commission had replaced the MHC in most functions: medical care, job retraining, and employment placement for its "graduates." Ernest Scammell had become the new ministry's assistant deputy minister.[106] Moreover, Segsworth agreed that any blinded soldiers in Canada wishing to go would be sent to St. Dunstan's with travelling expenses and vocational allowances paid by Ottawa. Major-General Foster, the Canadian Army director of medical services in Britain, was duly advised; there would be no more hasty returns to Canada.[107]

The CNIB immediately set to work to create programs for Canada's war blinded, registering as a war charity so that it could raise funds specifically for their welfare. It expanded the Braille and typewriting courses set up by the CFLB. Before the end of May 1918, five soldiers were in training. Moreover, as a clear example of its advocacy role, the CNIB communicated with all war blinded to inform them of their pension rights and began involving itself in securing employment for the returned men. By August, Dickson claimed that he was being "consulted daily ... by the staff of the Invalided Soldiers' Commission and by the Soldiers themselves."[108]

Sir James Lougheed, by this time the minister of soldiers' civil re-establishment, noted that the government's care for the blind was complicated by the development of blindness in some invalided soldiers and the absence of training standards in Canada. Accordingly, the DSCR's vocational department created a special branch for the war blinded and "secured the services of someone who was fully acquainted with all details in connection with the training and employment of blinded soldiers."[109] On 1 August 1918 the federal government appointed Captain Edwin Baker, vice-president of the CNIB, to the DSCR's vocational training staff as the secretary, Blinded Soldiers Department, "to take full charge of the Canadian Blinded Soldiers' problem," as one CNIB publication phrased it.[110] Essentially, the DSCR had created a blinded aftercare service that would be operated by the CNIB under contract with Ottawa. Baker was familiar with the care, rehabilitation, and employment prospects for the war blinded in both Britain and Canada.

The indefatigable Baker, only twenty-five, immediately set out to make St. Dunstan's positive philosophy into Ottawa's guiding policy. Baker moved to Ottawa and his influence was quickly felt. The DSCR contacted thirty-seven blinded veterans and offered them passage to St. Dunstan's. Twelve accepted, while twenty-five chose to wait for a suitable CNIB retraining facility to be established in Toronto.[111] Perhaps some of the latter did not wish to make the effort. St. Dunstan's imposed some self-discipline and drive on the men, something occasionally missing from their hitherto lax training regimen in Canada. Not everything went smoothly with early CNIB training. In October 1918, Charles Holmes, the CNIB director, wrote Baker that imposing a "serious ... business-like" vocational training routine on the men had led to difficulties: "two or three of these fellows are admittedly of very difficult disposition and out to make trouble ... The testimony is unanimous that the group which is already gone back to St. Dunstan's was away ahead of that which is still here in point of calibre, mentality, [and] social level." The tough-minded Holmes wondered how much "latitude" the CNIB should give the men in terms of "irregularity of attendance, indifference of application to work, and dictatorship in general as to what they will and will not do."[112] These were important questions, and Holmes and Baker worked to implement a process the DSCR, the CNIB, and the soldiers could live with.

A number of returned men with worsening vision problems were without St. Dunstan's or Canada-based training since they were not blind (defined as having less than 10 percent vision in each eye with corrective lenses) at the time of their discharge. But dozens of soldiers seriously aggravated or developed eye disorders while on service that progressively deteriorated following discharge. Baker saw his role with the DSCR as seeing to the "training and welfare of all blinded Canadian soldiers." He maintained files on all blind men and those on their way to becoming blind. Baker was anxious that the CNIB initiate some training of those returned soldiers with progressive blindness while they could still see. He felt that if these men were returned to their families, "little would be accomplished in the way of attaining independence," although "independence is a key to happiness" among the blind. Moreover, according to Segsworth, the best vocational training results were with men blinded immediately, and not gradually, since "there was not the mental strain of a long period of indecision and mental and physical re-adaptation."[113]

Baker conferred constantly with CNIB officials, met with as many of the blinded veterans across Canada as possible, offered them advice on pension claims, and kept their best interests in mind. He co-ordinated the furnishing of raw material if the men were producing items for sale and assisted with the marketing of their wares. In short, he "supervised the personal and business details in connection with every man who has graduated" or was enrolled in DSCR-approved training programs. It was Baker who decided whether the DSCR would pay to send a man to the CNIB for training, and what form this training would take. It was not always easy. For example, a Private Minnett "was rather hard to deal with," wrote Baker to Holmes, "as he had most impossible ideas regarding his future." Wishing to take a poultry-raising course at Guelph, Minnett could not conceive of a viable plan to undertake such an operation, and Baker "would not consent to his taking the course." Later, Minnett hoped to take up massage therapy but Baker felt he was unsuitable. Private Stevens was an "intelligent and practical man," but "if he had only a little more education," Baker would have recommended him for the demanding course in massage.[114] He tried to direct the men toward training programs best suited to their intellectual and physical capacities and their life experiences. It seemed a bit harsh at times, but the system had to be shown to work and, wherever possible, potential failure was identified and the men's retraining regimen redirected.

Corporal Charles Purkis, a war-blinded Canadian veteran of the 34th Battalion who had been trained at St. Dunstan's in 1918, instructed poultry farming to blinded veterans in residence at Guelph's Ontario Agricultural College. This was doubly convenient since Purkis hailed from Preston, close to Guelph. Specifically recommended by Pearson, Purkis, also a skilled carpenter, impressed Baker, who was no easy sell. By January 1919, Baker had sent five men to Purkis and his sighted assistant. Each man was provided with tools and "a small individual pen of fowl for which he will be responsible and thus secure actual practical experience." In November 1919, Purkis set up the poultry-farming course in Preston.[115] The Soldier Settlement Board facilitated the settling of the blind farmers and provided loans if needed. With the assistance of friends and relatives, the men selected locations for their poultry farms, normally on a plot of land varying from three to ten acres and near a suitable market.[116] This well-run program showed that Baker's initiatives were paying off; the war blinded *could* be retrained.

Canada's First World War blinded came from all walks of life and backgrounds, and the DSCR occasionally contracted with organizations other than the CNIB for blinded soldiers' training. In 1920 Segsworth, the DSCR's retiring director of vocational training, remarked that one of the blinded men, from the 2nd Construction Battalion, raised mainly in Nova Scotia, was "coloured," as were all the members of this segregated unit. He had successfully trained as a cobbler at the Halifax Technical School and lived in a section of Halifax "occupied by coloured people, and secures all their repair trade." Another man from Montreal's 60th Battalion had successfully completed a year-long course in broom making at the Montreal School for the Blind. Segsworth noted that he "suffers from shell shock, which has affected his mental capacity." The Montreal school employed him directly.[117]

Perhaps more typical was the case of Trueman Gamblin from King's County, New Brunswick. He had sold his woodcutting business and enlisted in 1915 at the age of twenty-nine. In July 1916, he proceeded overseas and by November had joined the 26th Battalion at the front. Gamblin later recalled, as recounted by his daughter, that during the storming of Vimy Ridge on 9 April 1917, "the last sunlight he remembers seeing was the brief break in the storm clouds in early afternoon of that day. A heavy shell exploding close by shattered the optic nerves in both eyes leaving him totally blind." Gamblin followed the usual medical route through Boulogne, St. Mark's Hospital in London, and then No. 2 General Hospital. Several operations to restore his vision were unsuccessful. He was trained in joinery at St. Dunstan's and returned to Canada in November 1918. He had married in Britain and he and his wife raised five children.[118]

By October 1918, 110 Canadian soldiers were known to have been blinded in the war, of whom about 45 or 50 were back in Canada. The breakdown of their place of training and their stage in the training stream provides a snapshot of the situation just prior to the cessation of hostilities:

19 graduates of St. Dunstan's
 3 graduates from Canada
38 in training at St. Dunstan's
15 in training in Canada
15 in hospital in Britain
 2 deceased in Canada

    15 unable or unwilling to retrain

    3 miscellaneous.

About 20 percent of these men had good guiding sight, another 20 percent had difficulty in getting about, 20 percent had light perception only, and 40 percent were "dark blind." The causes of blindness among them included gunshot and shrapnel wounds but also optic atrophy caused by exposure to poison gas, retinitis pigmentosa, detached retina, sympathetic blindness caused by the earlier loss of a single eye, facial wounds causing cataracts, spinal meningitis, existing vision problems aggravated by wartime service, and eye disorders contracted while on active service.[119]

By October 1918, 85 percent of the men trained or in training had been taught Braille and typewriting. Braille took on average five or six months to master sufficiently to pass a proficiency test. Upon successful completion of the typing course, students in Canada, as at St. Dunstan's, received the gift of a typewriter, which, according to Segsworth, would prove to be "one of his best friends during the rest of his days." Avocational training offered at St. Dunstan's, and in Canada, to build up manual dexterity (or "hand culture") and a sense of proportion and distance included basketry, netting, and mat-making. CNIB aftercare and follow-up visits were also begun with graduates.[120]

Blinded soldiers under the care of the CNIB mounted an impressive retraining and readaptation demonstration at the Canadian National Exhibition in Toronto in August and September 1918. They showcased their proficiency in reading Braille, typewriting, basket and tray making, scarf weaving, and rug making. Prime Minister Sir Robert Borden visited the men's exhibits, as did Ontario premier Sir William Hearst and Sir James Lougheed.[121] But despite the impressive showing, Canada's facilities for the blind were as yet unable to cope with the large number of war blinded. Only after the CNIB opened Pearson Hall, in December 1918, were the results even approaching satisfaction.[122]

Pearson Hall

Initially, the CNIB's DSCR-funded retraining programs were provided at CNIB headquarters at 142 College Street, Toronto, formerly the location of the CFLB. The institute's executive offices were at 36 King Street East. It became increasingly clear that a new facility was needed. The same site could serve as a "club" for the war-blinded men, where they could feel at home, meet other Canadians similarly disabled, and exchange counsel and information. At the 23 September 1918 CNIB executive committee meeting, Baker "suggested that suitable quarters be secured in the City of Toronto as a Club House for Blinded Soldiers in which those who desired might reside and those who resided outside might also come for social privileges." It was agreed that "steps in this direction should be taken," but an arrangement would have to be worked out with the federal government first.[123] Fortunately, Captain Baker worked at the DSCR and doubled as vice-president of the CNIB. The obvious conflict of interest in Baker's dual role seemed never to be raised. Clearly the DSCR found him a more useful employee *because* of his CNIB connection.

In October 1918, the CNIB leased an elegant Second Empire mansion at 186 Beverley Street, in a fashionable district of downtown Toronto, for $12,000, using funds made available by the federal government. The house was purchased outright for the CNIB for $38,000 the following year.[124] It had been built in 1876 for George Brown, a father of Confederation and founder of the *Globe* newspaper. It was located on a lot of 200 by 250 feet "within easy walking distance of several car-lines, but not immediately upon any of the noisy thoroughfares."[125] After remodelling, it served as the main retraining and rehabilitation centre for Canada's war blinded, adopting on a much smaller scale the philosophies and methods of St. Dunstan's. The CNIB took possession of the building in early November and welcomed its first resident a month later; fifteen men were expected almost immediately.

In January 1919, Sir Arthur Pearson was present for the official opening of the building named in his honour. It was a proud moment for all the Canadian war blinded, and perhaps especially for Edwin Baker, who was able to welcome his mentor to Canada's mini-St. Dunstan's, which Baker had been so instrumental in setting up. Pearson Hall was a testament to Pearson's work. On 6 January Pearson was the special guest at a banquet at Pearson Hall given by some twenty-seven war blinded from all over Canada, most of whom had been trained at St. Dunstan's. A reporter from a Toronto newspaper remarked that "the very air tingled with emotion." Alexander Viets rose and stated that "no mere words could voice our feelings tonight ... We welcome tonight not so much the man of title, friend of kings and queens and princes, but our old friend, the friend of the blind soldiers, the man with the big heart ... the man who came to us in our hour of gloom and pointed the way to the light." Other testimonials followed. When Pearson spoke, the same reporter noted that it "made an outsider feel an intruder on almost sacred ground." Pearson closed by reminding the veterans that they "must take particular care never to lose that feeling of seeing."[126] "I have never spent a more delightful evening in my life," Pearson later remarked, "than I spent listening to them telling of what they were doing and how they were doing it. ... [A] feeling of intense pride came into my heart." Several years later Baker recalled that Pearson "spoke that night of the men who owed so much to him, reminding them of the old St. Dunstan's days, of the great satisfaction it was to him of being privileged to assist them and of the hopefulness, optimism, and confidence he had as to their future and what he expected of them. He charged them to remember the St. Dunstan's axioms and to carry on in their respective spheres as normal men."[127]

Braving the January cold, Pearson formally declared Pearson Hall open on 7 January 1919. Baker's biographer hailed the event as a "milestone" in his life.[128] That evening a large public gala in Pearson's honour, and in honour of all war-blinded Canadians, was held at

Massey Hall under the auspices of the CNIB. The distinguished speakers were Sir James Lougheed, Sir William Hearst, Edwin Baker, and
Pearson himself. Baker referred to Pearson as the "greatest man the
world of the blind has ever known." He also emphasized that the
attention and assistance given blinded soldiers would benefit all
Canadian blind: "We blind soldiers also feel that the cause of the
civilian blind is our cause. We have been lucky enough to have had
a Sir Arthur Pearson, and we want to see every blind person given ...
as good a chance." Pearson later spoke to enthusiastic gatherings in
Hamilton, Montreal, Ottawa, and in the United States.[129]

Donations of every amount to help renovate the building
poured in from all sources, including Britain and the United States.
The Girls' Club of the T. Eaton Company in Toronto sent $1,000. In
May 1919, Toronto's Miss Alice Fisher sent $6.50 collected from her
bridge club, and in June the Montreal chapter of the Canadian Red
Cross Society donated $100. The same month Naomi Harris donated
$30, the proceeds from selling lilies of the valley on the highway in
Clarkson, just west of Toronto. In July Miss M. Thompson of Toronto
sent a cheque for $60.05, the proceeds from a bazaar given by a
group of children. "A deputation of these little children came to
[Pearson] Hall with the cheque," wrote Dickson to Holmes, "and were
greatly interested in meeting some of the men and in seeing the
Braille Writer." In 1921 the stewards and crew of the S.S. *Assiniboia*, a
Canadian Pacific steamer plying the Great Lakes, donated $30. "I may
say that a good percentage of our boys are returned soldiers and we
all deem it an honour to be able to assist your institute," wrote D.A.
Sutherland, the chief steward.[130]

Pearson Hall was financed in part from the CNIB's general
account and specific donations, but monies also accumulated in the
Blinded Soldiers' Fund, which consisted of unsolicited donations to
the CNIB to further its work on behalf of blinded soldiers. Helping
the war blinded was a popular charitable pursuit, and the fund grew
rapidly. In the first fourteen months of the CNIB's operation, to May

1919, the DSCR granted the institute $2,325 for vocational training, while the Blinded Soldiers' Fund received $4,852 in donations. Among the many contributions, ranging from $2 to more than $800, mainly from Ontario, were those from several chapters of the Imperial Order Daughters of the Empire, local Red Cross associations, corporations and businesses, such as the Dunlop Tire and Rubber Company ($50), regimental or military associations, and private citizens from all classes. The Canadian Women's Association for the Welfare of the Blind, which in April 1919 was renamed the CNIB's Women's Auxiliary, took on the responsibility of furnishing the building, mainly using publicly donated household goods.[131]

Social and entertainment committees were convened at Pearson Hall to organize Friday-night dances, parties, theatre nights, and other recreational activities. A player-piano was installed, as was a small gymnasium. Dedicated Red Cross VADs were assigned to help staff the centre and, according to a very early history of the CNIB, some bereaved women "found solace in caring for those who had lost sight during the Great War." Domestic arrangements were seen to by a house committee headed by Anne Clarke, the wife of Ontario's lieutenant governor. In its first annual report in 1919, the CNIB credited the members of this committee, the volunteer teachers and workers, and the "devoted" VADs with the successful functioning of Pearson Hall. Baker later recalled that the "loyal and active ... VADs rendered never-to-be-forgotten service throughout the whole training period."[132]

Men undergoing training at Pearson Hall received pay and allowances from the DSCR and were obliged to pay twenty-five dollars a month for their room and board. This money was then held in trust and returned to them in a lump sum on completion of their training. St. Dunstan's "graduates" could stay without charge from one to three months and thereafter pay twenty-five dollars a month.[133] Making Pearson Hall a hospitable drop-in centre for employed graduates of St. Dunstan's or CNIB training was excellent for the morale of the residents still undergoing training, some of whom were "fired with ambition to do as well" as those who had succeeded in life despite their disability.[134]

Dr. Charles Dickson became the first chairman of the CNIB's Blinded Soldiers Committee, overseeing the affairs of Pearson Hall, its residents, and trainees, and living there as well. Dickson's assistant at Pearson Hall was Roy Dies, brother of William C. Dies, a blinded Canadian soldier. William, serving with the 50th Battalion, had lost both eyes and his right arm during a 3:00 a.m. trench raid at Vimy on 13 February 1917. His last visual memory was of one of his comrades jumping into a trench and engaging German soldiers. Dies did the same and never saw again.[135] Roy had been working with the YMCA in England at the time of his brother's wounding and quit that position to help care for him and other wounded men at St. Dunstan's. "Sir Arthur Pearson says Roy Dies knows more about blinded soldiers and their needs than any other sighted man he has ever met," wrote Dickson in November 1918.[136] Bill Dies went on to become president of the Sir Arthur Pearson Club of War Blinded Soldiers and Sailors.

The CNIB reported that "without exception," every soldier trained at St. Dunstan's "possesses an independence and determination of character that is quite extraordinary."[137] Although the training at Pearson Hall was more modest and mainly intended for those not having attended St. Dunstan's, according to Sherman Swift, the new facility was "a very satisfactory replica in miniature" of St. Dunstan's and the name, Pearson, stood for "practically all that is good in the training and re-education of the military blind the world over." With the cessation of hostilities, and the flow of Canadians to St. Dunstan's down to a trickle, it was important that Canada take charge of its own retraining needs to meet the challenges of the postwar period.

By the spring of 1919, the CNIB estimated conservatively that about 125 Canadians had been blinded during the war, of whom perhaps 100 would be permanently resident in Canada, with most of the remainder in Britain. Later statistics showed that as of March

1919, some 1,347 Canadians had suffered some form of visual impairment as a result of their military service, though only 139, slightly more than 10 percent, required vocational retraining as a result of being judged 100 percent disabled due to blindness (though not necessarily 100 percent blind). Similarly, about 10 percent of Britain's 12,000 eye cases required training at St. Dunstan's. Of Canada's 139 blind cases, 46 had lost both their eyes.[138] Due to subsequent cases being discovered and the incidence of delayed blindness, by the early 1920s the tally of blinded men from the First World War approached 200, and this was far from the war's final tally. Of these, 92 received training at St. Dunstan's and most of the remainder trained at Pearson Hall.[139]

Pearson Hall was a great success. Nevertheless, occasionally it was difficult to deal with some of the men. James Rawlinson, for example, was possessed of a robust personality which rubbed many of his colleagues the wrong way. In January 1919 Baker, no fan of Rawlinson, who was then in residence at Pearson Hall, wrote Holmes that "the proposition of finding work for [Rawlinson] is rather a difficult one and rendered more so by his attitude in the matter. He takes the position that he should receive the preference in the appointment of a Braille teacher at Pearson Hall ... I do not think he possesses the necessary personality and disposition to make a success as an instructor. He is of a persistent and argumentative nature and rather inclined to be a grouch."[140] Fortunately, Rawlinson was hired by the DSCR office in Toronto, where he gave "entire satisfaction" according to Dickson.[141] Baker also recommended that Holmes organize outdoor exercises for the men to "eliminate the tendency towards moping" that some men exhibited. Despite the outpouring of public support and sympathy and Ottawa's willingness to pay for the men's retraining, life for these newly blinded young Canadians was far from easy.

To successfully meet their readaptation challenges and ensure adequate government support, Canada's war-blinded veterans were obliged to remain cohesive and vigilant, lest a grateful nation forget its heroes' postwar needs. Pension entitlements, medical care, and job retraining programs required constant improvements in the decades following the war's end. Frequently, special interest groups among the veteran population needed to have their voices heard above the rest. The war blinded were one of these groups. With spirited leadership, and the camaraderie of those with shared experiences, Canada's war blinded forged a new organization they could call their own. Throughout the 1920s and 1930s, and acting in close co-operation with the CNIB, the Sir Arthur Pearson Club of Blinded Soldiers and Sailors served its members' professional and personal needs and stood as a model of what a capable, willing, and dedicated group of veterans could accomplish.

2 The Sir Arthur Pearson Club of War Blinded Soldiers and Sailors, 1919-29

Does it matter? – losing your sight? ...
There's such splendid work for the blind
And people will always be kind,
As you sit on the terrace remembering
And turning your face to the light.

> – Siegfried Sassoon, *Does It Matter?*

At the conclusion of the First World War, Canada welcomed home the largest group of veterans the nation had ever known. Thousands returned physically maimed or psychologically scarred. Although most successfully reintegrated into civilian life, others never recovered and suffered enormous problems readapting. For some, the physical strains and painful memories proved too much, and death would arrive prematurely. As Desmond Morton and Glenn Wright have phrased it, the veterans still had to "win the second battle" – to overcome the trauma of their experiences and to obtain government disability pensions and other public or private assistance on the road to civil re-establishment. Unfortunately, Canada experienced a serious economic downturn from the end of 1918 until the early 1920s. This situation created increasing unemployment, rising poverty, government fiscal retrenchment, and a generally discouraging atmosphere for veterans, perhaps especially the disabled.

The Dominion government had attempted to prepare for the challenges of providing for returned soldiers. The Department of Soldiers' Civil Re-establishment (DSCR) was created in 1918 to deal with the veterans' return, reintegration, medical needs, employment training, and ongoing care. The Board of Pension Commissioners (BPC) administered Canada's complex pension system. Within this organizational context, Ottawa mandated the Canadian National Institute for the Blind (CNIB) to undertake on its behalf the difficult task of re-establishing Canada's nearly two hundred war-blinded veterans. The opening of Pearson Hall in 1918 and the creation of the Sir Arthur Pearson Club of War Blinded Soldiers and Sailors (SAPA) in 1922, closely affiliated with the CNIB, were natural corollaries to this process.

The 1920s witnessed the development of Pearson Hall as a re-adaptation and retraining centre and also as a residence for Canada's war blinded. It soon became the showpiece and headquarters of the CNIB, which the federal government subsidized to maintain veterans' aftercare programs. The war blinded generally performed well and frequently even excelled in their training and employment experiences, as in the case of massotherapist D.J. McDougall, discussed below. The war blinded's need to guarantee government pension regulations helped motivate them to form SAPA as an advocacy group and social club. The men kept in touch through frequent reunions and, as the decade came to a close, it was clear that Canada's war blinded had taken on leadership roles in promoting the cause of veterans in general, as well as the cause of all Canada's blind. Through his persistent advocacy and astounding capacity for work, Edwin Baker came to personify SAPA as much as he did the CNIB.

Aftercare and Re-establishment

Arthur Pearson described aftercare as a revolutionary concept in the care of the blind. He defined it as "the system of keeping permanently in touch with the men of St. Dunstan's."[1] In the autumn of 1917, young Captain Ian Fraser, a man in whom Pearson placed enormous faith, opened St. Dunstan's "After-Care Department," a phrase apparently first used at that time. Its role was to maintain contact with and serve the needs of St. Dunstaners following their "graduation." This practice was also adopted by the CNIB and Pearson Hall staff. In fact, once Baker joined the DSCR in 1918, Pearson felt nothing was "more appropriate and satisfactory" than that "on each side of the Atlantic" a St. Dunstaner was in charge of the aftercare of the war blinded.[2] "Ultimately, of course," wrote Fraser twenty-five years later, "the After-Care Department became practically the whole of St. Dunstan's."[3] Retraining the war blinded lasted for several years following the First World War; aftercare would last a lifetime.

In July 1919, Baker went to London to meet with the Canadian veterans whom the DSCR had sent to St. Dunstan's for training. There he joined the DSCR's director of vocational training, Walter Segsworth, and its assistant deputy minister, Ernest Scammell. Baker addressed the blinded men and outlined his role as the secretary of the Blinded Soldiers' Department at the ministry. He also met privately with each man to ascertain his condition, psychological as much as physical. Of course, he had been himself a resident of St. Dunstan's a mere three years previously. His own professional successes – and the fact that he had travelled to Britain alone – served as an inspiration. Baker also met with other blinded Canadian soldiers recuperating in a variety of medical facilities in Britain. One of the goals of the DSCR administrators' visit was to establish the best means of repatriating the war blinded to Canada upon their graduation from St. Dunstan's, by which time transportation arranged by the military would be scarce. Some of the war blinded had married, and arrangements were needed to allow spouses to accompany their husbands. As one DSCR official, Captain W.C. Nicholson, wrote Baker, "Your arrangements for the return of men from St. Dunstan's to Canada will fill a long-felt want, as the system of returning men and their wives by separate [ships] does not seem to be quite satisfactory." Eventually, some men returned aboard repatriation vessels under military authority while others travelled on civilian liners, as did the married couples.[4]

The return home could be difficult for some of the sightless veterans. In December 1918, F.G.J. McDonagh, returning aboard the hospital ship *Essiquibo*, recalled:

> I stood on the deck ... where along with other walking patients, I had gone to see Canada, to which we were returning after service in France and Belgium. As we looked, someone called out: "There she is" as Canada came into sight. The sudden emotional silence was shattered by the voice of one, who for a full moment, cursed and blasphemed everything which was dear to him, including his country and his Maker. We looked and said nothing. The voice came from a blinded soldier.

McDonagh, later a prominent veterans' advocate and friend of Baker's, claimed that his life-long interest in the welfare of blinded soldiers was the result of hearing that unidentified war-blinded veteran express his disillusionment and anger.[5]

In Canada, the DSCR's Blinded Soldiers' Department obtained information from military authorities respecting discharged blinded veterans, and Baker determined each man's retraining needs. He would then communicate with the CNIB and the superintendent of Pearson Hall to ascertain whether there was room for a new trainee in the specific area desired. Although Pearson Hall was a CNIB operation, and not a government entity, staff were obliged to report to Baker on the progress of the training program and on individual trainees. This must have seemed natural since Baker, the federal bureaucrat, was also a CNIB executive. Moreover, the CNIB remained responsible to Baker in its provision of soldiers' aftercare. To February 1920, according to Baker, "there has been no cause for complaint" from any quarter despite the fact that the institute's "aftercare and other arrangements were not wholly completed and are [in] the process of perfection."[6]

Beginning in June 1919, the DSCR initiated a series of five annual grants of $10,000 to the CNIB for the provision of services and aftercare to returned blinded soldiers. "Aftercare" was defined in that month's contract between the DSCR and the institute as "the provision of assistance in connection with all details which can be said to affect the comfort and earning capacity of the Canadian blinded soldier."[7] The CNIB used most of the DSCR money for settlement grants and loans to the returned men as well as for equipment and supplies provided to them. Smaller amounts went to maintain Pearson Hall. The CNIB was obliged to provide the DSCR with twice-yearly expense statements for the operation of the programs there and for the men's aftercare needs. Failure to do so could delay the payment of the grant, and the CNIB's early spotty record in sending in the required reports deeply concerned the department. For example, in June 1920 Baker wrote Captain McPhun, the CNIB business manager, that the department required a financial report and, until one was received, would not pay the next grant instalment.[8]

Dr. Charles Dickson had been named chairman of the CNIB's Blinded Soldiers Committee (i.e., put in charge of Pearson Hall) in December 1918, but he resigned this position effective June 1919, citing failing health. He was replaced by the sighted Captain Robert F. Thompson, MC, who was named head of the CNIB's renamed Blinded Soldiers' Department (later the Aftercare Office). According to an uncharitable character sketch of Dickson written in 1920 by Charles W. Holmes, the CNIB's first director, Dickson had suffered from "impracticality, lack of executive capacity, and temperamental idiosyncracies" during his tenure at Pearson Hall. Because of this, claimed the venomous Holmes, Dickson had earlier been replaced by Lewis Wood as head of the CNIB and had been obliged to yield Pearson Hall as well.[9] While administrative ability might have evaded Dickson, his and Sherman Swift's early efforts to assist the nation's war blinded helped lead to the creation of the CNIB and to an effective reintegration into civil life for the vast majority of Canada's war blinded, virtually all of whom came to admire and respect Dickson. Perhaps this, and not Holmes's assessment, should stand as the true measure of Dickson's importance to blinded veterans. In the meantime, the DSCR's Nicholson noted that he had been able to clear up "a great deal of business" with Thompson in short order.[10] In April 1920, Captain W.B. Powell, a sighted veteran of the 4th Battalion, replaced Thompson, who had fallen seriously ill. While Pearson Hall was generally functioning well, the CNIB annual report admitted that there had been some "difficulties to overcome"[11] in its first year and a half of existence, as the frequent changes at the helm suggest.

In January 1921, the CNIB *Bulletin* boasted with obvious exaggeration that 126 of 192 known war-blinded Canadian soldiers had been fully trained and were employed in their occupations "without one known case of failure."[12] Not all Canadian blinded veterans reintegrated seamlessly into civil society, especially those with multiple wounds. At the end of 1921, the DSCR ascertained that 2,888 Canadian veterans were in receipt of disability pensions for defective vision including blindness. The DSCR had deemed 197 of them eligible for retraining, of whom at least 135 were totally blind.[13] The majority lived in Ontario, particularly Toronto, about 20 resided in Quebec, 19 in British Columbia, 14 in Manitoba, 11 in Nova Scotia, 9 in Saskatchewan, 9 in Alberta, and 1 in New Brunswick, while up to 25 resided in Britain (usually their place of birth), several in the United States, and 1 in Belgium. The number living in Britain rose to 37 by 1923. Only a handful of the total had been officers, and 6 or 7 were French speakers. Almost all had served in the army although there were several former sailors.[14]

There existed some postwar confusion over the actual definition of "war blinded." Part of the problem was that the CNIB, and
later SAPA, adopted a stricter view than did the DSCR or the Board
of Pension Commissioners. The former felt that if a man was blinded
in action or lost his sight to an incapacitating degree (eventually
defined as worse than 90 percent blind in both eyes following cor-
rection) due to other service conditions, then he was war blinded.
The government view was based more on whether an eye casualty
needed the occupational and lifestyle retraining funded by the DSCR
and made available by the CNIB. Another problem in obtaining an
accurate number of war blinded was the occasional improvement in
and, more frequently, worsening eye conditions among veterans and
the difficulty of carefully monitoring these cases. This meant that
either of, or both, the CNIB and federal authorities might cease defin-
ing a veteran as blind or that, conversely, a man eventually losing his
eyesight due to a delayed reaction to wartime injury or disease
might never be considered war blinded. Accordingly, the overall
number of Canadian war blinded fluctuated as new cases developed
and as official or medical definitions changed.[15]

Even Edwin Baker, a hard-liner in the definition of war blindness, was confused. At the end of 1924, while serving as the CNIB's
general secretary (a position changed to managing director in 1931),
he wrote the DSCR, his former employer, about his frustrations at being unable to nail down a precise number of Canadian war blinded
from the First World War: "I must confess it is rather perplexing. It is
true [that the CNIB] trained a number of men who at the time had
been given the benefit of the doubt. In a number of cases we discovered that their vision did not warrant treatment on account of blindness. I am anxious to know whether they are still to be considered as
blinded soldiers on our lists or where and how we are to draw the
line." According to Baker, the DSCR seemed content to list men "who
were considered in one way or another at various times" to be sufficiently blind as to warrant aftercare training and treatment. The CNIB

and DSCR lists never matched. Yet, by the end of 1924, at least four veterans formerly classified as blinded had had their pensions revoked or severely curtailed as a result of a re-evaluation of their conditions. George Eades, on the other hand, who had trained at St. Dunstan's, was listed in CNIB records as having at least some "useful vision." He was not in receipt of a pension since his "night blindness" apparently had existed prior to his military service. Despite this, he received further CNIB training in Braille and poultry farming. In his case, the institute considered him war-blinded whereas the DSCR did not.[16]

By 1925, the DSCR paid 115 blinded veterans 100 percent disability pensions and attendance allowances – financial benefits awarded to those needing the services of an aide or attendant. Six more were rated as 100 percent disabled, though not necessarily 100 percent blind, but did not receive attendance allowances, and 34 others were considered 100 percent (or less) blind and were not in receipt of attendance allowance. Thirty-nine men were blinded to various degrees but either received no pension or received a pension attributable to other disabilities. A further ten men had died since the end of the war. This made a total of 204 war blinded as far as the DSCR was concerned.[17] In 1926 Baker visited the blinded soldiers in western Canada to ascertain their conditions. Several men could no longer formally be considered blinded, and, according to Baker's report to the DSCR, the CNIB's revised list stood at 156, not counting those deceased.[18] The disparity seems never to have been resolved.

In the summer and autumn of 1921, the CNIB's Captain Powell travelled the Dominion to visit as many blinded soldiers as possible – quite an undertaking given the vastness of the country and the relatively few war blinded. This was styled an "After-Care trip," and it became a common CNIB practice for decades to come. Powell visited more than 120 blinded men who had benefitted from retraining, checked on their circumstances, and judged the effectiveness of their training in obtaining them secure employment and in enabling them to "carry on." He reported on every case individually and also advised St. Dunstan's of the progress of its approximately eighty-five graduates residing in Canada. Powell noted that at least six showed "a lack of desire and ambition for any form of work" but also reported that there were no "cases of distress or any conditions even approaching hardship." Powell's optimistic report stated that "an exceedingly high percentage of the men are very successful [which] proves the wisdom of the training, care and settlement which was provided."[19] Baker noted that "all the men are working, and by far the greater proportion are forging ahead and making good." Still, a small minority of men remained unemployed or unemployable, and life could prove difficult for even those with jobs. Commenting on an aspect of the war-blinded veterans' activities which remained a hallmark of their community service into the twenty-first century, Powell reported to the CNIB that "a feature which may surprise and please you is the interest I found so frequently displayed by the Soldier toward the less fortunate amongst the Civil blind. In many cases this interest has taken the form of [tutoring] in Braille and typewriting and even home visiting and instruction in light handicrafts."[20]

By September 1924, and notwithstanding exceptions to the rule, SAPA admitted that the only two wage occupations to "provide a steady income to the majority of men engaged" were massotherapy and stenography.[21] On the other hand, by 1922 most of the businesses the CNIB had set up for the war blinded – tobacco and newspaper stands for the most part – proved to be successful ventures. Creating such jobs or placing men in wage-labour employment was one of the CNIB's most important aftercare provisions. Only a handful of men (less than 3 percent according to one 1924 report) were able to return to their prewar occupations. One man even owned a barbershop – but hired a sighted veteran as his barber! But there also had been a number of failures – which the CNIB attributed to the general economic downturn, a "lack of proper interest and co-operation on the part of immediate family," and a "tendency to extravagance" on the part of some blinded veterans. Still, most of the war blinded who had been trained in craft industries such as basketry or reed and rattan work (the most common occupation) seemed "contented," according to the DSCR's 1922 aftercare report. The CNIB supplied these men with their raw materials at cost price and helped sell their finished products; all profits reverted to the men and the CNIB absorbed any overhead costs. The CNIB purchased the products the men could not sell immediately. That same year, twenty-seven blinded veterans were unemployed for a variety of reasons ranging from physical incapacity to the tight labour market; however, few who had been trained seemed unwilling to work.[22]

There were some impressive personal accomplishments. British-born Captain J.D.C. Cochrane-Barnett of Winnipeg had been blinded by a bullet on the western front in 1916 while serving in the 28th Battalion. After training at St. Dunstan's he returned to Canada and successfully settled on a 1,400-acre Saskatchewan ranch, which he managed. He rode horses expertly and remained physically active on his property. He married in 1920 and, according to the *Manitoba Free Press*, he spoke "like a man full of joy of living and zest for doing things. The loss of his sight has not made him any the less a man of action."[23] Lieutenant-Colonel T.E. Perrett maintained his prewar employment as principal of the Saskatchewan Normal School and also as a provincial school inspector. (He resigned in 1926 and moved to Toronto.) Since his wartime blinding, Harris Turner had been a member of Saskatchewan's legislature and a publisher, and by 1921 he managed his own printing company. A.A. Archibald, who had suffered grievous facial wounds in addition to being blinded, worked as a stenographer with British Columbia's Department of Mines and Forests, while Charles Hornsby worked in the same capacity for Alberta's Department of Municipal Affairs.[24] These cases, some exceptional, provided the war blinded and the CNIB with some high-profile success stories.

In February 1920, the CNIB's Charles Holmes offered Baker, still at the DSCR, his explanations for the blinded soldiers' successes, especially in operating concession stands and other minor businesses.

"The average calibre of our returned men," wrote Holmes, "if they have not suffered any other disability than blindness, is considerably better than the average calibre of our blind civilians." Moreover, the war blinded's cause was greatly assisted by "the interest, support, and patronage of the public which is unquestionably given to any returned man with a disability in preference to a man without a disability or a man who has not suffered it overseas."[25] The war blinded were strongly supported institutionally, publicly, and privately but obviously earned any successes that came their way.

Aftercare came in many forms. One common example was the provision of essential supplies to war-blinded veterans. When they graduated from St. Dunstan's or Pearson Hall they took with them Braille watches and the typewriters that allowed them to communicate independently. Aftercare services supplied typewriter ribbons, paper, Braille paper, envelopes, and other stationery. For example, in October 1922, Whaley Austin, who had been badly mangled during the war, received one typewriter ribbon, 250 sheets of typewriter paper, 100 plain envelopes, and five pounds of Braille paper. Some men were clearly more active correspondents than others: D.J. McDougall received the most supplies throughout the 1920s, while men engaged in CNIB or SAPA business, such as James W. Doiron, J.W. Ogiltree, Alexander Viets, and Bill Dies, also obtained large quantities.[26] However, it was not until 1927 that the DSCR agreed to allow the repair costs for Braille watches, typewriters, and other equipment to be drawn from the aftercare budget. This had been standard in Britain since the war, but St. Dunstan's was financed through generous public subscriptions and could deploy its resources as it saw fit.[27] The CNIB also supplied the returned men with Braille literature and a monthly Braille magazine, *The Courier*. By the summer of 1920, B. Ross Swenerton, a war-blinded veteran employed by the CNIB, had taken on the duties of aftercare worker and salesroom manager for the institute.[28] Whatever their other CNIB duties, Baker and Swenerton would be looking after their own.

Edwin Baker had married Jesse Robinson on 16 December 1919 with CNIB president Lewis Wood serving as best man. The Bakers would raise three boys together. Wood, coveting Baker's expertise and work ethic, had been quietly lobbying him to leave the DSCR and return to the CNIB in an executive capacity. Baker was interested but reluctant to leave the department until he felt its blinded veterans' aftercare programs, which he was helping organize and oversee, were functioning more smoothly.[29] On the other hand, Baker's position with the department would be redundant once the war blinded had in large part been satisfactorily resettled. In fact, for a time in 1920, Baker did both jobs, serving the state as secretary and advisor to the Blinded Soldiers' Department, DSCR, and also, on a voluntary basis, acting as general secretary of the CNIB. In March 1920, the CNIB was thrilled to announce that Baker had been formally appointed its general secretary, a full-time, paid position, effective 1 October. His intimate knowledge of Ottawa's veterans' re-establishment policies and the enormous respect he enjoyed among the country's war blinded made him a near-perfect candidate. Minister of Soldiers' Civil Re-establishment Sir James Lougheed wrote Baker, "I desire to express to you my warmest appreciation for the splendid work which you have done in providing for the training of Canada's blinded soldiers under the auspices of this Department ... I would like to express my gratitude and trust that with your continued interest in this work in the future you will from time to time be available for advice." Similar feelings were expressed by E. Flexman, the DSCR's director of vocational training (having replaced Walter Segsworth): "I am extremely glad ... to know that you are ready and willing to be of any assistance possible to us, should we need your help." The deputy minister, N.F. Parkinson, echoed these desires.[30] The DSCR was pleased to note in its 1920 annual report that Baker remained "on strength of this Department in an advisory capacity." Baker would spend the next four decades assisting the war blinded and the civilian blind with the CNIB and SAPA.

Massage Therapy Education at Hart House and Pearson Hall

Blinded soldier massotherapists earned widespread praise during the postwar period and served as visible reminders that the war blinded could not only find employment, but could, in fact, become sought-after professionals. According to an early CNIB *Bulletin*, because of their acquired deft sense of touch, coupled with their imperviousness to visual distractions, blinded masseurs, more so than sighted ones, were seemingly able to harness their "powers of concentration" in the course of their duties. This challenging occupation was reserved only for exceptional candidates. The masseurs had to be in excellent physical condition, personable, and preferably younger than thirty-five. Edwin Baker felt it would help if they also displayed "tact, patience and unfailing courtesy."[31]

One particularly successful massotherapist exemplifies the potential of some of these disabled veterans. Private D.J. McDougall, from Orillia, Ontario, was wounded in the Ypres Salient in 1916 at the age of twenty-two while serving with the Princess Patricia's Canadian Light Infantry. He entered St. Dunstan's that November and graduated an acclaimed massotherapist, a man of whom Sir Arthur Pearson was particularly proud. Before returning to Canada, McDougall even worked briefly as a massage instructor at St. Dunstan's.[32] As early as March 1918, Pearson had acquainted the nascent CNIB with McDougall's talent and remarkable determination to overcome his disability. Lewis Wood wrote Pearson that the institute was "trying to figure out what sort of position can be obtained for him" in Toronto, and that the Military Hospitals Commission might employ him in one of their medical facilities. Failing that, Wood assured Pearson that the CNIB would "work him into the organization" somehow. McDougall was seen as a special case, a man whose success might help sensitize the Canadian public and government officials to the surprising career possibilities open to the war blinded.[33]

By August 1918, Edwin Baker, then taking up his new duties with the DSCR, arranged to have McDougall taken on by the School of Physical Therapy, Hart House, University of Toronto, at the excellent salary of $125 monthly, at first paid by the CNIB.[34] Hart House, which boasted superb facilities and specialized equipment, had been a recent gift from the Massey family and "became a showplace for rehabilitation," according to Morton and Wright. Only the best and brightest of the war blinded were able to train in massotherapy; the excellence of the graduates and the rigours of the program needed to be protected if they were to serve as models showcasing the war blinded's potential.[35]

It was intended that McDougall instruct only the war blinded and the civilian blind, with the institute supplying technical books in Braille. Yet the proficient McDougall was soon instructing classes of up to seventy sighted students in anatomy, pathology, and physiology. By then convinced of his exceptional abilities, the DSCR's Military School of Orthopaedic Surgery and Physiotherapy, also at Hart House, hired McDougall in December as a regular staff instructor, teaching massage to blind and sighted students.[36] The first two war-blinded Hart House massage graduates found work in military hospitals in Halifax and Calgary, though at the inadequate wage of $2.30 a day. Baker noted "considerable difficulty" in arranging a proper salary for the blinded masseurs hired by military hospitals in Canada. Matters quickly improved, however, due in no small part to Baker's exertions, and by January 1919, he was able to place massage graduates in the DSCR hospitals of their choice.[37]

Massotherapy was proving so effective in speedily rehabilitating patients in military hospitals and convalescent homes (many of the practitioners being blinded soldiers) that the profession anticipated a burgeoning demand in the civilian sector. But despite the blinded soldiers' evident proficiency, success in private practice was more difficult to attain. Lieutenant-Colonel Robert Wilson, a consultant with the DSCR facility at Hart House, was astonished that relatively few found employment outside of DSCR centres, since he felt that they were "amongst the most skillful" therapists he had encountered.[38] In an attempt to assist its high-profile graduates, the CNIB published articles and advertisements in medical journals to publicize the availability of the blind masseurs, though it is not known with what effect.[39] The irrepressible Dickson busied himself writing promotional literature for the blinded-soldier massage therapists. In the meantime, McDougall helped form a professional association of blind and sighted masseurs.[40] In late 1920, Corporal W. Williamson, trained by McDougall, sat for his examination under the auspices of the Canadian Association of Masseurs. Twenty-nine sighted masseurs and masseuses also took the exam. Williamson scored first place with a grade of 86 percent. The two sighted men who came in second and third had also been trained by McDougall.[41]

Effective 1 August 1919, the CNIB established a massage department at Pearson Hall and McDougall left his job at Hart House to supervise it, staying until July 1922. The talented McDougall then entered private practice, for a time operating out of Pearson Hall. At first his clients were mainly blinded soldiers, though eventually he also treated some civilian blind and sighted clients. Moreover, he enrolled in a BA program at the University of Toronto, where he stood first in his class.[42]

By April 1921, fourteen blinded-soldier masseurs were practising their profession. Hundreds of surgeons and doctors were familiar with their skills and prescribed massotherapy to their patients. By 1922, of the twenty-one blinded men trained as massotherapists, fifteen worked in DSCR hospitals, three were established in successful private practices, McDougall worked for the CNIB, one man had returned to England, and one had changed vocations and became a successful fruit farmer.[43] The CNIB received numerous letters from medical practitioners testifying to the men's excellence and the importance of massage in rehabilitating the injured and the maimed. "Blindness is but a slight handicap in the profession of massage," stated the CNIB *Bulletin*, reaffirming the claim that the touch sensitivity of the blind made them more skilled than sighted massotherapists.[44]

As wounded veterans' rehabilitation wound down and military hospitals became fewer in number in the 1920s, so, too, did firm job prospects for Canada's blinded massotherapists. By 1929, only seven remained employed in Canada. Not only was Baker thoroughly dismayed by this turnaround, but he was further outraged at some of the men's continuing low salaries, which were on a par with, according to Baker, "orderlies who scrub floors and provide bed utensils" in government-run veterans hospitals. A top-graded orderly made more (up to $1,680 a year) than a top-graded massotherapist ($1,500). These salaries ignored the men's professional status and seemed discriminatory. Ernest Scammell, then of the Department of Pensions and National Health (DPNH), which succeeded the DSCR in 1928, promised to look into the matter, though it is not clear what, if anything, was done.[45] The massage training program must be viewed as a success, however, not only for its tangible employment results but also for the confidence it instilled in the war blinded and the positive public attention it brought to their capabilities.

In 1925 McDougall abandoned his private practice and returned to Britain to study history at Oxford University at the graduate level on a "special" Rhodes Scholarship. An immensely proud SAPA sent him an official message of congratulations, and Baker noted that McDougall was the first totally blind student to obtain this honour. (Trooper Mulloy had been ineligible for such a scholarship a generation earlier.) SAPA viewed McDougall's success as all the more important "in view of the expressed purpose of the members of this Club to promote ambition to greater achievement, not only among blinded soldiers, but among [the] civil blind." McDougall graduated from Balliol College in 1927, obtaining the only First in Modern History awarded to a member of his college. He was the only scholar publicly congratulated by the examining board. Following two more years at Oxford, McDougall went on to an impressive career teaching early modern British history in the History Department at the University of Toronto.[46] Decades later, the historian Sam Hughes, a university colleague of McDougall's, recalled that McDougall was "by far the most eloquent lecturer of my experience in any university. He built up a substantial library in which he could direct his students to the position of a volume on his shelves and even to a page reference. Needless to say, the exercise of this feat of memory gave him the greatest pleasure."[47]

Pearson Hall Activities

In November 1919, the DSCR informed the CNIB that an Order-in-Council had been passed authorizing the institute to assume ownership of Pearson Hall and erect a vocational training building on the property. In fact, as the institute readily noted in that year's annual report, Pearson Hall had been "purchased and transferred to the Institute by the Dominion Government." This gift was worth $35,000.[48] To protect its investment, Ottawa retained the right to reacquire Pearson Hall at a fixed price of $50,000; this right was later relinquished under authority of Orders-in-Council PC 2094 (1928) and PC 293 (1929), at which time the building truly became the CNIB's, no strings attached. According to Baker, "The original idea ... was to ensure good faith on the part of the Institute in carrying out agreements on behalf of blinded soldiers."[49] Obviously the institute performed satisfactorily.

In the meantime, the CNIB showcased the building and its programs, attracting national attention to the cause of Canada's blind in general and the war blinded specifically. In February 1920, the Duke and Duchess of Devonshire, the vice-regal couple, visited Pearson Hall in company with the lieutenant governor, the Honourable Lionel H. Clarke, and his wife, Anne, head of the CNIB Women's Auxiliary. The duke took a personal interest since the vocational training annex then under construction behind Pearson Hall was mainly paid for with $50,000 in Red Cross funds at his disposal.[50]

Pearson Hall was a busy place, both professionally and socially. By May 1919, one hundred war blinded had returned to Canada. With its classrooms and library, Pearson Hall served as a training facility and residence for those still in the re-establishment cycle. In addition to Braille, typing, basketry, and various other crafts, the men at Pearson Hall also relearned some life skills made more challenging by being blinded, such as personal grooming, household mainten-ance, cooking, and shopping. They also obtained mobility and orien-tation training to offer them greater independence.[51]

As of 31 August 1919, nineteen blinded veterans were being trained at Pearson Hall, of whom seventeen were in residence. If Pearson Hall was full, or if a man desired to live in Toronto with his family and incur the expenses of food and lodgings, the CNIB made a monthly grant to "more or less place him on the same financial level as a man who lives [at Pearson Hall] at no expense to himself," ac-cording to Captain Powell, Pearson Hall's superintendent.[52] Because of congestion there, the CNIB rented a house at nearby 158 Beverley for classroom and vocational training, with Pearson Hall reserved for offices and housing.[53] On 10 November 1920, the new vocational training building, housing soldiers' workshops, was officially opened by the governor general, reportedly before no less than eight hundred invited guests.[54]

Additional staff was required, especially to teach Braille and typewriting, which were often taught individually. Private R. Adams, a fresh graduate from St. Dunstan's, offered a cobbling class, and English and French courses were available.[55] A snapshot of activities at Pearson Hall in May 1920 represents the varied instruction taking place there. Fifteen men were in training: three taking massotherapy, four boot repairing, two tobacco-store management, one stenog-raphy, one sales, and four poultry farming. Eight others were in the preliminary training stage while one had yet to begin. A typical day consisted of about five hours of instruction. More broadly, of the 185 veterans whom the DSCR had deemed eligible to that point, 54 were undergoing some form of training while that of 31 others was pending, either in Canada or at St. Dunstan's. A further 86 had graduated, while 14 were "unable or unwilling" to train. During the previous year, 46 men had undergone training by the CNIB at Pearson Hall and the poultry farm while two others had taken up residence without taking any formal instruction.[56] The training program was a major undertaking and an immense responsibility for an organization barely two years old.

Throughout the 1920s, social functions at Pearson Hall provided the opportunity for the war blinded, especially in the Toronto area, to gather in familiar surroundings. In September 1920, for example, 250 visitors, including quite a few Pearson Hall graduates, attended a sports day featuring competitions among the war blinded. Lieutenant Governor and Mrs. Clarke attended. The CNIB Women's Auxiliary organized a supper and tea, and a concert and dance in the Pearson Hall annex attracted 150 couples.[57]

The Pearson Hall House Committee, convened by Theresa Macdonald, and also consisting of Anne Clarke and Mrs. W.D. Riddell, was the source of wise advice and assistance both concrete and intangible, easing the men's sometimes difficult adjustment periods and ensuring maximum comfort for trainees and residents. Many individuals and organizations helped with the planning and execution of various entertainments, and Mrs. Macdonald referred to the Voluntary Aid Detachment workers (VADs) of the St. John Ambulance, in particular, as ever "faithful, valuable, and efficient" in this regard.[58] Some of them provided essential services: a number of men undergoing vocational training at Pearson Hall required daily eye treatments and, in the absence of a nurse, the VADs often applied various lotions and antiseptic solutions.[59] The women escorted the veterans on shopping excursions and outings, and some volunteers served as tutors. Mae Cameron, a teacher, successfully took charge of the French-speaking James W. Doiron, who at first experienced difficulty expressing himself in English. He became proficient enough to study massage under McDougall and pursued a successful career.[60]

The training program at Pearson Hall was winding down by the end of 1921, with only seven men in attendance as of 30 September. But training would continue, especially additional instruction for alumni and for new men who had not, for whatever reason, earlier availed themselves of the CNIB's services.[61] If new individual training was deemed necessary, the regular services and facilities of the CNIB, normally through its Home Teaching Department, would be sufficient for the task. Earlier that year, the DSCR had paid tribute to St. Dunstan's for the success of the Canadian program. N.F. Parkinson, the deputy minister, had written Sir Arthur Pearson that "anything that has been accomplished in Canada, the training and care of the blinded soldiers, has been due ... in a large measure to the example and initiative that was instilled into them while in your charge."[62] This might have been selling the CNIB and Pearson Hall a trifle short. In the spring of 1922, Pearson Hall became the headquarters and administrative centre for the CNIB's national headquarters and Ontario Division. By May, for the first time since its opening, no soldiers were on strength of Pearson Hall; W.B. Powell, with less to do, was promoted to CNIB business manager.[63]

The ongoing partnership between the CNIB and DSCR had been successful in that few of the war blinded seem to have had serious complaints about the treatment they had received. The CNIB certainly felt that its soldiers' training program had been a job well done, stating simply in the 1922 annual report, "The Blinded Soldiers problem, perhaps the most acute obligation arising from the War in connection with the Soldiers' Civil Re-establishment, was solved." The institute also offered high praise for the "unremitting attention" of DSCR officials in connection with programs for the war blinded.[64] In turn, in recognition of the time and effort the institute devoted to Canada's blinded soldiers, both Segsworth and Parkinson stayed on the CNIB council even after they had left the DSCR. Baker, especially, seemed to value Parkinson's counsel. Ernest Scammell joined them as the official DPNH representative in 1928, thereby ensuring as far as possible an alignment of institute and governmental policies.[65] The professional relationships and personal friendships remained close, a situation mirrored in the decades to come.

Throughout the 1920s, the DSCR, and its successor, the DPNH, continued to provide the CNIB with grants for blinded soldiers to cover expenses on a cost-recovery basis. Between 1925 and 1930, these amounted to an average of $5,371 annually, a not inconsiderable sum.[66] Some of this money was intended for loans to the war blinded – to help them get through an impasse or to assist if misfortune struck. For example, in 1919-20, six men received loans totalling $2,250. A. Hebbard was allotted $350 to cover the initial stock for his grocery business; J. Parker (whose earning potential was limited to basketry and netting) was loaned $100 to return to Edmonton; and L.S. Hitchcock received $19.83 to pay for "a small supply of hammock netting string and string bag twine to enable him to start remunerative spare-time employment." Such loans were normally paid back in regular installments.[67] Between 1924 and 1932, CNIB loans to the war blinded averaged $1,974 annually, with the high-water mark being 1924, when $5,048 in loans were made. In the corresponding period, the CNIB loaned on average $1,102 annually to the civilian blind, for whom the federal government was not financially responsible.[68] In 1924 loans to the war blinded were valued at six times those to the far more numerous civilian blind. Of course, some of these loans, frequently granted under emergency conditions, were never paid back. The same year the institute even carried a line item of $3,000 in its annual budget "in reserve for doubtful loans."[69] Not all of Canada's war-blinded veterans landed on their feet.

The Death of Sir Arthur Pearson

On 8 December 1921, Edwin Baker received a warm letter from Sir Arthur Pearson, in which he reviewed the St. Dunstan's philosophy:

> When I lost my sight it seemed to me that the one thing neces-
> sary to ameliorate the condition of blind people in every pos-
> sible way was to try and get a little spirit into them, and a little
> commonsense into those who wanted to help them, to throw
> away as much as possible everything to do with affliction,
> helplessness and dependence, and to use every possible
> means to infuse a spirit of real life and equality with the sight-
> ed world, both into those who could not see and into those
> interested in their welfare.[70]

What neither man could know was that Pearson had written his own testament. The next day, to the shock and grief of St. Dunstaners everywhere, he died suddenly at the age of fifty-five. According to Ian Fraser, Pearson's successor at St. Dunstan's, "The manner of his death was the cruellest irony. It was a blind man's accident ... He slipped while stepping into his bath, struck his head on the tap, fell forward unconscious, and drowned."[71]

No Canadian was more devastated than Edwin Baker. He immediately sent a telegram to Lady Pearson: "Words cannot express sorrow felt at news of Sir Arthur's death. Deepest sympathy for yourself and Neville [son] in great bereavement."[72] The December issue of the CNIB *Bulletin* published some moving tributes, including an unsigned one by Baker:

> Sir Arthur came to me in my darkest hour and brought with
> him an atmosphere of hope and optimism. He fathered me
> through my discouragements and despairs, and started me

back to my native Canada refitted to carry my share of work
and responsibilities ... The torch which he lighted and started
on its way has been seized by the eager hands of those who
knew and loved him so well ... I personally feel the loss of a
very dear friend and benefactor.[73]

According to Fraser, Pearson "was like a father to his great
family ... The attachment of St. Dunstaners to their late chief was
very strong and personal."[74] On hearing of Pearson's death, Prime
Minister Arthur Meighen cabled Lady Pearson, "The Government of
Canada convey to you deepest sympathy in the sad loss of your distinguished husband, and desires to express its profound appreciation of the work which he did for blinded Canadian soldiers at St.
Dunstan's during the Great War and for the further interest which he
took during his lifetime in the Canadian National Institute for the
Blind, this having been of incalculable service to Canadian Soldiers."[75]
Approximately 1,200 war-blinded veterans attended Pearson's funeral in London. Wrote Fraser, "I do not suppose that so large a number
of blind men have [ever] been gathered together before." Canadian
St. Dunstaners sent a wreath to his funeral consisting of a large
maple leaf made of yellow flowers.[76]
    A large memorial service "of Gratitude for the Life, Sorrow for
the Death, [and] Honour for the Memory" of Sir Arthur Pearson was
held in Massey Hall, Toronto, on the afternoon of Sunday, 18 December 1921. The service was held under the auspices of the CNIB, but
the impetus for it came from "the Soldiers of the C.E.F. who were
Blinded in Action and Trained at St. Dunstan's." Lieutenant-Colonel
Henry Cockshutt, the lieutenant governor of Ontario, chaired the
service while the band of Toronto's 48th Highlanders provided the
music. Baker delivered a ten-minute address on behalf of Canadian
St. Dunstaners, and Reverend Sydney Lambert, head of the Amputations Association of the Great War (AA) and a close friend of Baker's,
was among those offering prayers.[77]

On 1 October 1922, Lieutenant Governor Cockshutt unveiled a memorial tablet honouring Pearson that was prominently placed just inside the main entrance to Pearson Hall. About forty Canadian war blinded, attending a local reunion, were present for the ceremony. The tablet consisted of Pearson's head and shoulders in relief alongside the St. Dunstan's torch with the motto "Victory Over Blindness" wrapped around it. There followed the words, "Erected by the members of the Canadian Expeditionary Force blinded in the Great War." Canada's war blinded had raised $383 among themselves to fund the tablet – just enough. D.J. McDougall, who headed the fundraising campaign and arrangements for the tablet, provided a powerful address in which gratitude and devotion to Pearson shone through. "We feel," said McDougall, "a certain amount of pride in erecting a tablet upon which the world may gaze, and the world may know that we, the men Sir Arthur loved, do not forget."[78]

Pearson's philosophies and methods had been spread throughout the Commonwealth by returned St. Dunstaners who had established similar organizations either specifically for the war blinded or for the blind in general. Nowhere was this more the case than in Canada, with Edwin Baker and Alexander Viets being key players in the CNIB's founding in 1918 and in the founding of SAPA in 1922. Similarly, in New Zealand, Baker's friend from St. Dunstan's days, Clutha Mackenzie, blinded at Gallipoli, eventually played an important role in New Zealand's Jubilee Institute for the Blind. During the Second World War he also established a rehabilitation program for India's war blinded. The Australians at first set up organizations for the war blinded in each individual state, with the St. Dunstan's message of hope and achievement espoused especially by blinded veterans Charlie Hills and Elmer Glew. Eventually, they established a federal group, the Australian Blinded Soldiers' Association. In South Africa, St. Dunstaner Michael Bowen, blinded at Ypres in 1917, was elected to Parliament and helped establish the South African National Council for the Blind.[79] The Canadians' story was part of a wider

Commonwealth experience based on shared service and fates. All these men were steeped in the St. Dunstan's tradition and heeded Pearson's call to assist themselves – and then others.

The Sir Arthur Pearson Club of War Blinded Soldiers and Sailors

Shortly after Pearson's death, Canadian war-blinded veterans formally organized themselves into an association distinct from, but intimately affiliated with, the CNIB. Not surprisingly taking the name of their revered benefactor as their own, in April 1922 they formed the Sir Arthur Pearson Club of War Blinded Soldiers and Sailors (SAPA).[80] SAPA was at once a patriotic veterans advocacy group and a social club promoting camaraderie among those sharing the same disability.

Creating SAPA was also a means of distinguishing Canada's relatively small number of war blinded from the civilian blind who formed the bulk of the CNIB's clientele. This was especially the case in 1922, at which time veterans' training at Pearson Hall virtually ceased. Nevertheless, the war blinded made their presence and influence felt in the institute. For example, of the twenty-five members of the 1920 CNIB council, five were blinded soldiers: Edwin Baker, T.E. Perrett, D.M. Ross, Harris Turner, and Alexander Viets. Two years later the ratio had not diminished, and was further bolstered by the addition of D.J. McDougall to the CNIB staff as instructor in massage.[81] The close bonds between SAPA and the CNIB were not mirrored in Britain; in the same year SAPA was formed, St. Dunstan's formally split from Britain's National Institute for the Blind, a change perhaps accelerated by Pearson's death.[82] However, the Canadian civilian and military blind opted to work as part of the same team, a process facilitated by the formidable presence of Baker and other veterans in both groups.

It was not known how long Pearson's work and influence would survive him in Canada, thereby giving added reason to create a homegrown special-interest group as quickly as possible. J. Harvey Lynes, who had enlisted at the age of sixteen and had been blinded in action at Bourlon Wood, near Cambrai, in late September 1918 while serving in the 21st Battery, Canadian Field Artillery, recalled years later that he felt something should be done to perpetuate Pearson's memory. While Pearson Hall already served the purpose of memorializing its namesake, the formation of SAPA appears at least in part motivated by a desire to honour Pearson.[83] Lynes was an unlikely founder, if indeed the organization's founding should be attributed mainly to him. In fact, given Lynes's intermittent participation in the organization's early years, Baker's hand was almost certainly more in evidence in creating SAPA than the surviving documentary evidence suggests. Lynes had been a failure at St. Dunstan's, unable to pass his typing or Braille tests and drinking far too much for Pearson's liking. Following his return to Canada, Lynes had also run afoul of Pearson Hall administrators for his poor behaviour there, and in 1920 Captain Powell expelled him for three months. This was a very rare occurrence. However, Lynes shaped up and was successfully trained as a masseur by McDougall. In 1921 he was employed at a military hospital in Toronto at the good salary of $110 a month.[84]

Perhaps reflecting his changed attitude, in March 1922 Lynes invited four of the best known of Canada's war blinded, Edwin Baker, D.J. McDougall, Bill Dies, and Alexander Viets, all St. Dunstaners, to a meeting in Toronto to explore the possibility of forming a veterans' group with its own identity and goals but that would remain closely linked to the CNIB. All were in favour of proceeding, and Lynes was named chairman of a Constitution Committee to draft the embryonic group's objectives and membership rules.[85] Lynes's committee agreed that SAPA sought "the perpetuation of the memory of the late Sir Arthur Pearson ... and the furthering of the interests of the blind of

Canada in general and of blinded soldiers and sailors in particular,"
thereby succinctly enshrining the principles by which SAPA would
abide throughout its history. Additionally, the club would provide for
the recreational needs of its members and operate on strictly non-
partisan and non-sectarian principles. Membership was open to all
war-blinded Canadians whether they had seen Canadian or imperial
service, and to all blinded British veterans resident in Canada. The
club levied a one-time registration fee of fifty cents but charged no
annual dues. Its Executive Committee consisted of a president, vice-
president, secretary-treasurer, and four other members not holding
specific offices.[86]

SAPA's founding meeting was held on 7 April 1922 at Pearson
Hall with fifteen men present, among them Baker, McDougall, and
James W. Doiron. The organizers had contacted as many of the Canadian war blinded as possible, but the inaugural general meeting
consisted mainly of those residing in the Toronto area. The constitution was accepted and Lynes was named the group's first president;
Baker became vice-president and Doiron secretary-treasurer.[87]

The first item of business was to write to Lady Ethel Pearson
requesting permission to use her husband's name for the club and to
request her official patronage. Lady Pearson granted both requests.
Among SAPA's other inaugural patrons were the vice-regal couple,
Lord and Lady Byng of Vimy, Lieutenant Governor Cockshutt, Anne
Clarke, Dr. Dickson, and Lewis Wood. The organization's first honorary
members were a careful cross-section of military, social, and business
leaders, selected to represent Canada's different regions and both
sexes: Brigadier Victor Odlum, N.F. Parkinson of the DSCR, Colonel
Hamilton Gault, millionaire founder of the Princess Patricia's Canadian Light Infantry, Lady Eaton, and the heads of most of the
major service institutions active in Canada.[88] There were no French-
speaking Canadians among them, however. J.P. Lynes, brother of
J. Harvey Lynes, was appointed SAPA's honorary secretary and, with

rare periods of absence, served as the recording secretary at the group's meetings for the next half-century. He was often the only sighted person present.

There were additional reasons for the group's creation. Bill Mayne, a Second World War veteran who at the time of writing has been a member of SAPA for nearly sixty-five years, felt that the war blinded banded together to avoid being integrated and blurred into the broader community of Canada's civilian blind. Mayne wrote that they founded SAPA "fearing their interests and identity would be lost in the rapidly expanding CNIB services for the civilian blind and believing they ... could best negotiate for improvements in disability pensions and other benefits and, to benefit from strength in numbers."[89] Given the veterans' community's perceived need for solidarity during pension negotiations, and its occasional confrontations with federal government authorities, SAPA's origins must also be seen as having strong advocacy roots. Canada's war blinded were first and foremost veterans, entitled to special privileges as a result of their service and disablement. A special-interest group would help maintain the men's public profile.

Is it a coincidence that SAPA was founded less than a month after CNIB headquarters, formerly at 36 King Street East, moved to Pearson Hall in March 1922? Certainly the CNIB *Bulletin*, of which Baker was editor, felt that this move was a positive development that would help bond the disparate groups within the CNIB, namely the civilian blind clients of the institute and the blinded soldiers at Pearson Hall. The veterans had become a comparatively small CNIB constituency, though they had a guarantor in Baker. Despite the taking over of Pearson Hall by CNIB office staff, blinded soldiers continued to benefit from a ground-floor dining room and club room, essential since a small number of them remained in residence. Moreover, the travelling war blinded in need of a welcoming and familiar place to stay would always be accommodated.[90] SAPA, too, was headquartered there.

Factors outside the confines of Canada's blinded community also influenced the creation of SAPA. Very much *au courant* with developments among Canadian veterans and immensely knowledgeable about pension regulations and DSCR procedures, Baker undoubtedly noticed that several special-needs and disabled veterans' organizations were forming in Canada. These men felt inadequately represented in the councils of the larger veterans' groups, such as the Great War Veterans' Association, and perceived a pressing need to serve as their own advocates. In October 1921, the Amputations Association of the Great War (later the War Amputations of Canada) was founded, with Captain the Reverend Sydney Lambert elected president. Lambert had lost a leg while serving as a private in the 50th Battalion. The same month, the Invalided Tuberculous Soldiers' Welfare League met as a body for the first time.[91] Perhaps the Canadian war blinded felt that the time was at hand to further their own interests on a formal basis. Baker and Lambert had become close friends, with Baker joining the Amputations Association and Lambert accepting SAPA's invitation to become the organization's honorary president.[92]

SAPA's funding became an immediate issue. According to Harvey Lynes's recollections six decades after the fact, despite widespread views in the club that public fundraising would be successful, neither Lewis Wood of the CNIB nor Baker, who served in executive capacities with both groups, wanted SAPA to compete for funds that the institute might raise for the benefit of all of Canada's blind.[93] Similarly, half a century later, Bill Mayne, while an official of both the CNIB and SAPA, noted that

> immediately upon formation ... there appeared the possibility of conflict between the Club and the CNIB. The Club ... was in need of money to carry out its program of making [it] a viable, functioning body, maintaining contact with the war blinded of Canada, providing the social and business gatherings so

necessary to the well-being of blinded veterans, and carrying
on its negotiations ... with the Government of Canada with respect to ... veterans' benefits. The Club membership was small
in number and scattered from coast to coast ... it appeared the
logical source of income was from public appeal.

On the other hand, the CNIB was also "in dire need of funds and was
seeking public support."[94]

But, as Mayne pointed out, because SAPA was expected to "experience great difficulties in financing its operations and that simultaneous appeals to the general public for funds would be detrimental
to both appeals ... an understanding was reached ... that CNIB would
finance the Club's business and social operations through the Aftercare Funds, thereby leaving the field of public appeal and any other
fund raising activities to the Institute." This arrangement certainly was
known to, and seemingly met the approval of, the DSCR.[95] Accordingly, as the CNIB *Bulletin* noted, "The Club is made up entirely of
blinded soldiers, [and] the Institute is, from its Blinded Soldiers' Fund,
providing for expenses of its social activities."[96] The CNIB also agreed
to underwrite the new organization's anticipated modest operating
costs, still using funds provided by the DSCR. Even the greater expenses associated with the SAPA members' reunions were funded
indirectly by the DSCR through the CNIB – an extraordinary use of
departmental funds that tacitly recognized the critical importance
of peer socialization in the re-establishment process. As the SAPA
minutes clearly reveal, Baker was the key to SAPA receiving financial
assistance from the CNIB and DSCR. Looking back on a lifetime of
partnership between the two organizations, Lynes heaped praise on
the CNIB and noted that the institute was at all times "anxious to do
anything to help the members of our group."[97]

Patriotic or charitable groups and individual Canadians gave or
bequeathed money to the CNIB's Blinded Soldiers' Fund for the use
of SAPA members. All donations were welcomed given the high

costs of operating Pearson Hall and seeing to the men's needs. For example, in the year ending 31 May 1920, expenses were $21,425, not counting $7,945 spent on vocational instruction to blinded soldiers and $1,584 for training at the Preston poultry farm.[98] The annual $10,000 subsidy plus a further $6,916 vocational training allowance from the DSCR that year did not cover the institute's outlay. However, the fund recorded the whopping income of $30,795, including $10,000 from the Canadian Red Cross and an equal amount from the Canadian War Contingent Association. Other donors included numerous Red Cross chapters across Canada (and even $130 from one in Peru), church groups, sporting teams, Imperial Order Daughters of the Empire chapters, one of which purchased musical instruments for use at Pearson Hall, and some lesser-known entities such as the South Porcupine Patriotic Society ($150) and the Women's Auxiliary of the Boston Canadian Club ($130).

In 1921-22, with most monies left over from wartime and immediate-postwar patriotic funds expended, donations to the Blinded Soldiers' Fund dropped to $2,457. Again, the donors were scattered widely, though most were from Ontario. The largest grant was a bequest of $1,000 while the lowest was $2. Many of the 1921-22 donors were women's and girls' organizations: the Girls Sunshine Club of Provost, Alberta, gave $70, the Janey Canuck Club of Mount Albert, $9, and the Five Women's Club of Toronto, $6.75.[99] Fundraising and public donations remained important to the CNIB's operations and the soldiers' rehabilitation. In 1926-27 the fund received $410, mainly from church groups. A year later, $601 had been added, generally from individuals, whereas in 1928-29 donations amounted to an impressive $1,202, including a bequest of $1,000. There were regular donors throughout the interwar period: Miss Margaret Lazenby of Buffalo, New York, gave $27 annually while Miss Margaret Hoskin gave $12 every year. Miss Agnes Cotter of Montreal was also a regular subscriber to the fund.[100] In short, Canada's war-blinded veterans were not forgotten by either the government or grateful citizens.

Throughout the remainder of 1922 SAPA's executive met infrequently. Yet the association contacted as many of Canada's 100 percent disabled war-blinded veterans as possible to inform them of their automatic membership in the organization.[101] At a general meeting in September 1922, Baker outlined the CNIB-DSCR aftercare program and invited members to discuss their needs with him. Baker's genuine compassion for the blinded men is palpable in the SAPA minutes. There was also a clear desire to circulate information and seek publicity for the club's existence and activities, including sending material to the *St. Dunstan's Review*. Close co-operation with the CNIB was a foregone conclusion.

The early affairs of SAPA were not without friction. Bill Dies mentioned the "apparent lack of confidence between members and urged a better spirit."[102] This almost certainly referred to the antics of Harvey Lynes, whose difficult personality rankled some other members. D.J McDougall was elected SAPA president at the organization's first annual general meeting (AGM) in February 1923, and Baker wrote in April that "the boys [were] well satisfied" by this change in leadership. Six months later Baker again faulted Lynes, noting that he had a very poor attitude and that he was "at outs with practically all the men."[103]

In September 1923, Bill Dies was elected SAPA president with Baker continuing as vice-president and Doiron as secretary-treasurer. The other permanent members of the Executive Committee were selected as representatives from Canada's different regions. The executive agreed that regular SAPA business was to be handled by Toronto-area members of the executive with the opinions of the regional representatives to be solicited in the event of major issues arising.[104] Most executive members were returned by acclamation every year in amicable voting carried out by the twenty-five to

thirty-five SAPA members present at the AGMs – a number that
doubled if the AGMs coincided with reunions, as in 1926 when sixty-
one members were present. Without Lynes's active involvement, the
men seemed to get along better, and in 1926, Alexander Viets, SAPA
president at the time, expressed his pleasure that the club was operating in such a "harmonious atmosphere."[105] By 1924 SAPA's executive
meetings were more professional and businesslike, and dealt far less
with the affairs of individual members or Pearson Hall social activities
and more with critical matters such as pension reform and employment prospects for members. The organization was coming into its
own as a bona fide veterans' advocacy group.

Because aftercare and most recreational costs were borne by
the DSCR through the CNIB, SAPA had few significant expenses. The
CNIB took care of most of SAPA's operating needs and the latter's
financial statements recorded few receipts or expenditures. In September 1924, SAPA had $237 in the bank. A year later there was only
$57 available – a shoestring budget to say the least. Money would be
even harder to come by in the 1930s.[106]

Flowers and small gifts to mark special occasions accounted
for most of the group's spending, and SAPA members had a number
of people to thank every year. In 1925 "sincere and heartfelt expressions of appreciation" were sent to the indefatigable women of the
Pearson Hall House Committee and the VADs, "all of whom have
taken such a keen interest in the welfare and activities of the ... Club
and who have done so much to render successful and enjoyable the
various functions arranged." Among the annual activities they organized were an Armistice Day dance, a Thanksgiving dance, a Christmas
party, and various special events or visits.[107] Attendees at the annual
SAPA Christmas dinners at Pearson Hall normally included up to
twenty war blinded, including invariably the group's executive, and
invited guests from the DSCR or DPNH, the Amputations Association,

and other organizations. House Committee members Misses Sutherland, Graham, and Burns also devoted much care and time to organizing these events, with the men's wives, including Jesse Baker,
playing important supporting roles.[108] These events helped solidify
ties and inject a semblance of normalcy into the men's social
experiences.

At the 1926 AGM, members present voted "an expression of
sincere appreciation" to N.F. Parkinson, deputy minister of the DSCR,
through whose sincere care and attention a solid relationship had
developed between SAPA and the department.[109] The antagonisms
marking relations between some veterans' groups and the federal
government were absent in SAPA's dealings with the DSCR. But the
extensive funding and retraining extended to the war-blinded veterans, relatively few in number, made them a group apart.

Inexplicably, the late 1920s appear as something of a moribund
period in the organization's normally dynamic history. There was virtually no movement in the bank account or any significant official
activity by SAPA. The Executive Committee rarely met; no meetings
are recorded in the group's minute books between September 1925
and October 1926, for example, and none are shown to have taken
place for the next several years. There were still AGMs, however, and
in 1927 James W. Doiron was elected president. Along with J.B.A.
Renault of Montmagny, Quebec, Doiron was one of SAPA's few
French-Canadian members. Both men were also among SAPA's
very few naval veterans, Renault having served as a sub-lieutenant.
Alexander Graham became vice-president and Edwin Baker assumed
the position of secretary-treasurer – a post he held for some thirty
years.[110] While the association's presidency alternated between
members, Baker's permanence made him synonymous with SAPA,
perhaps its de facto leader, as had also become the case with his
work at the CNIB.

SAPA Reunions

Canada's war blinded met in large numbers during formally organized SAPA reunions. For many, these reunions created lasting memories, forged camaraderie, and served as uplifting occasions. To some extent, SAPA patterned its reunions on the St. Dunstan's model of holding local annual reunions in centres across Britain. The St. Dunstan's Aftercare Department organized the reunions as social occasions and opportunities to exchange information and bring to light situations requiring attention; the men could also gripe in convivial surroundings.[111] Or, as Baker phrased it several years later, without specifying the nature of any of the men's complaints, from SAPA's perspective the reunions "enabled the more reasonable to iron out the criticisms of the unreasonable."[112] The SAPA reunions served a double purpose: in lieu of organizing an expensive aftercare trip across Canada, regular meetings of SAPA members offered Baker and others at the CNIB an opportunity to gauge how the men were coping. In fact, the DSCR report of its activities and services pertaining to the war blinded referred to the reunions as "alternatives" to aftercare trips.[113]

Instead of the September sports day in 1921, the war blinded organized a three-day reunion for men living in Ontario – the first of the so-called local or Pearson Hall reunions. The Pearson Hall VADs organized a well-attended dance complete with orchestra and the House Committee put on a dinner. On the following day, sixty-four blinded men and escorts enjoyed a boat excursion to Port Dalhousie on Lake Ontario and then motored to St. Catharines for tea, returning late that evening. This excursion was courtesy of the Knights of Columbus, while the Rotary Club provided cars to enable the men and their escorts to enjoy day trips all over the Toronto area.[114] Even though the war had ended three years previously, the war blinded enjoyed something of a privileged status in the veterans' community, and in the thoughts of many Canadians, as this generosity attests.

This first reunion was a great success and encouraged SAPA to plan more ambitious reunions as a tonic for some of the men's occasional discouragements or loneliness, and for the pleasure of renewing friendships.

With the co-operation of the CNIB and its Women's Auxiliary, a national reunion was held at Pearson Hall from 29 September to 1 October 1922. Some forty-six SAPA members attended from Ontario, Manitoba, and Nova Scotia, twenty-four of them from the Toronto area alone. Quite a few brought their wives or other escorts, and all SAPA executives were present, especially given that the closing act of the reunion was the unveiling of the memorial tablet at Pearson Hall in honour of Sir Arthur Pearson. Dr. Charles Dickson gave the main address at the reunion, in which he urged extremely close co-operation between the blinded soldiers and the CNIB. The men attended the theatre and, as in the previous year, partook of organized motor trips around town. The ample grounds of Pearson Hall were used for an impressive sporting program, the highlight of which was a tug-of-war between the St. Dunstan's and Pearson Hall old boys, with Pearson Hall winning, although the Canadians had evidently been the St. Dunstan's champions. Taking advantage of the presence of so many members, SAPA, formed only six months previously, held a general meeting at which the men were advised and encouraged to contact Edwin Baker who, as the general secretary of the CNIB, was also in charge of soldiers' aftercare.[115]

The Canadian war blinded's interest in the 1922 reunion led to another the following year. The roll of the 7-9 September 1923 reunion in Toronto lists seventy attendees, among whom forty-five were from Ontario.[116] This was the largest gathering yet of Canadian war blinded. Travel and accommodation for forty-two of the men and their escorts were covered from the CNIB aftercare budget, with departmental approval, at a cost of about four thousand dollars – an important admission by the DSCR that the reunions and other social activities served a therapeutic aftercare purpose. There was a sports day and garden party at Pearson Hall, with the mayor of Toronto, G.A. Maguire, presenting prizes to the winners of the sporting events. One hundred men and escorts enjoyed a harbour cruise and on the evening of Saturday, 8 September, a party of seventy-two attended a show by the Dumbells, the famous First World War Canadian veterans' entertainment troupe, and a further forty went to the Canadian National Exhibition. More practically, many of the men found time to drop by the DSCR's Christie Street Hospital for eye examinations, to be fitted with new artificial eyes, and to obtain other medical services and information.[117]

Another important goal of the reunions from SAPA's, the DSCR's, and the CNIB's perspectives was to sensitize the men to the considerable efforts being made on behalf of Canada's war blinded. As a result of the reunions, stated the 1923 DSCR Report, "It is felt that the men now have a better understanding of the ... cooperation existing between the DSCR and the CNIB. They also realize to a far greater extent the important part played by the Institute in their affairs and the great good that can be accomplished if they accord their undivided sympathy toward efforts on behalf of the civilian blind." These words were probably penned by Baker.

The success of these reunions encouraged SAPA to embark on a triennial reunion schedule. The 9-12 September 1926 Reunion was again held in Toronto, with Pearson Hall as usual the main gathering point. It was the site of the official welcome, a tea on the lawn, the SAPA annual general meeting, an evening concert, and a dance. The men also went to a picnic lunch and supper at Eldorado Park, just outside the city, travelling in specially reserved streetcars. There, the blinded veterans engaged in sporting competitions such as the shot put, potato sack and three-legged races, the broad jump, and other similar competitions. Later they attended a show by the ever-popular Dumbells at the Royal Alexandra Theatre. On the last day of the reunion, a service was held at Pearson Hall in memory of Sir Arthur Pearson.[118] Most subsequent reunions consisted of similar activities.

This one was organized and sponsored by the DSCR, the CNIB, the Pearson Hall House Committee, and the VADs.

Planning reunions for war-blinded veterans was no easy task, and SAPA invested an enormous organizational effort in their execution. One government program assisted the task: in 1922 transportation subsidies for the war blinded were enacted by Order-in-Council PC 1929, thus enabling the soldiers' escorts to travel for free.[119] For the 12-18 September 1931 reunion, the SAPA executive and other members living in the Toronto area, the Pearson Hall House Committee and VADs, and some CNIB and DPNH resources were all mobilized to co-ordinate the arrival, stay, and departure of dozens of veterans and their escorts. In fact, a SAPA transportation officer was named to the task and Canadian National Railways assisted in arranging transit for the blinded veterans. Some forty-eight SAPA members from all over the country attended and, counting escorts, mostly wives, but also sisters, children, and friends, there were about a hundred people to accommodate, a typical number for most interwar reunions.[120]

Illustrating the strong ties between the two veterans' organizations, SAPA planned this reunion to coincide with the annual convention of the Amputations Association of the Great War, held at the Royal York Hotel. All SAPA members were welcome to register for the AA convention and were eligible for certain privileges and activities that the AA had organized for its own members. For example, free theatre attendance was arranged with the Famous Players Corporation, though the blinded veterans were obliged to wear their Amputations Association convention badge. This badge also ensured free admittance to concerts and activities at the Canadian National Exhibition grounds. SAPA co-ordinated some of its activities with the AA at the Royal York Hotel, including concert recitals, receptions, and a memorial service. The Lions and Kiwanis Clubs also held luncheons for the SAPA and AA men, fifteen spots being specifically allotted to the war blinded. Showing solidarity, the blinded and amputee soldiers marched from the South African War memorial on University Avenue to the cenotaph at Toronto City Hall, where they laid wreaths to honour fallen comrades.[121] It was a stirring and emotive sight and a testament to the will of Canada's disabled veterans to co-operate but also to get on with their lives.

The War Blinded outside Canada

It is interesting to note the experiences of the First World War blinded in other countries. In Britain, there were more than 2,000 war blinded in the postwar period. In the 1920s, with the emergence of hundreds more cases of veterans' blindness, St. Dunstan's remained extremely busy and enormously relevant and had earned an international reputation as a centre of excellence for the care and rehabilitation of the war blinded. It was not government funded but relied for the continuation of its operations on fundraising and the obtention of legacies. These were not easy tasks in the turbulent economic times of the interwar period, but under Ian Fraser's dynamic leadership and with some severe budget cuts, St. Dunstan's survived and was on firm financial footing by the later 1930s.[122]

Germany was without benefit of a St. Dunstan's equivalent, and most retraining was carried out in local civilian centres for the blind. Of Germany's 3,500 war blinded, only about 500 had taken St. Dunstan's-like courses. In March 1916, a group of 37 German war-blinded veterans in Berlin formed an organization not unlike SAPA, the *Bund der Kriegsblinden Deutschlands*. This group even published, in German, the uplifting history of St. Dunstan's, demonstrating the fraternity of the war blinded across national and even adversarial barriers. Germany's war blinded pioneered the use of dogs to assist with mobility. By 1930, 1,600 German war-blinded veterans used guide dogs. Germany also led in integrating the war blinded in industry, where they worked alongside sighted workers. In 1918, with the war still ongoing, about 40 were employed in the examining and packing departments of various munitions plants. After the war, large firms were obliged by law to employ disabled veterans at the rate of between 1 and 2 percent of their active workforces. In the 1920s, the firm of Siemens was a national leader in this respect, and, in one department alone, 80 war blinded worked alongside some 300 sighted workers.[123]

Approximately 3,000 French soldiers were blinded during the war. Eugène Brieux, the Frenchman appointed to organize the re-training of his country's war blinded, noted that "for some wounded our responsibility is over when their wounds [heal], but with the blind it only begins ... They need to be prepared for their new life."[124] On 24 August 1914, the Hospice des Quinze-Vingts, a Paris centre for the blind established in the thirteenth century, became a military hospital treating eye wounds, with the blind remaining on strength of the institution. On 29 March 1915, only three days following the founding of St. Dunstan's, the Société des Amis des soldats aveugles (Friends of Blinded Soldiers) was established to assist the first forty French war-blinded veterans who had taken up residence in a con-verted old home in Reuilly, near Paris, that served as an annex to the Quinze-Vingts. Here, the men convalesced, retrained as blinded men, and learned some shop work. Reuilly became France's St. Dunstan's. However, since most of France's growing numbers of blinded veter-ans were rural conscripts with a fierce desire to return home, military authorities decentralized their rehabilitation system by opening seventeen smaller training centres in the provinces. Accordingly, the majority of that country's war blinded trained in the centres closest to their homes.[125]

French disabled veterans' groups formed during the war and specific blinded soldiers' organizations emerged in the postwar period: the Union des Aveugles de guerre and the Mutilés des yeux, the latter attaining some ten thousand members though not all were blinded.[126] In addition to this, in 1914 the American philanthropist Winifred Holt established the Committee for Men Blinded in Battle and the next year founded the first in a series of "lighthouses," centres for rehabilitation and recovery for the French war blinded. Their motto was *Ex tenebris lux,* "From darkness light."[127]

The situation in the United States was far less satisfactory than in the Commonwealth, Germany, and France. The approximately 450 war-blinded American servicemen, a figure rising to 726 by 1941 as a result of the service-related ocular deterioration of other veterans, were without benefit of a voluntary, non-regimented training facility like St. Dunstan's or Pearson Hall. Morale and motivation lagged badly at Evergreen, the ninety-nine-acre facility outside Baltimore that had been intended to emulate St. Dunstan's. This was far from the case. One enduring problem was that the men remained on strength of the military and were subject to its discipline while receiving far less in service pay than would have been the case had they been discharged and in receipt of their disability pensions. Moreover, Evergreen's mainly civilian (and often sighted) teachers could not command the men's respect like the war-blinded teachers and administrators at St. Dunstan's and, often, Pearson Hall.

The US war blinded formed a SAPA-like organization, the United States Blind Veterans of the World War. But unlike its Canadian counterpart, the American group was rife with internal dissension and discord. For example, even though the US government had set aside funds for the establishment of a permanent national training centre for the adult blind, because of heated factionalism, the US Blind Veterans was unable to decide whether this would serve all American blind or merely the war blinded. Shockingly, the money was never spent.[128] This sorry situation was contrary to the CNIB's and SAPA's basic principles of advocating on behalf of *all* Canada's blinded. The American war blinded seemed less well trained, disappointingly disunited, and perhaps poorly led.

In short, if St. Dunstan's was a world leader in the readaptation of the war blind, Canada's system was not far behind, and its well-organized war-blinded community quickly emerged as national leaders in promoting disabled veterans' causes.

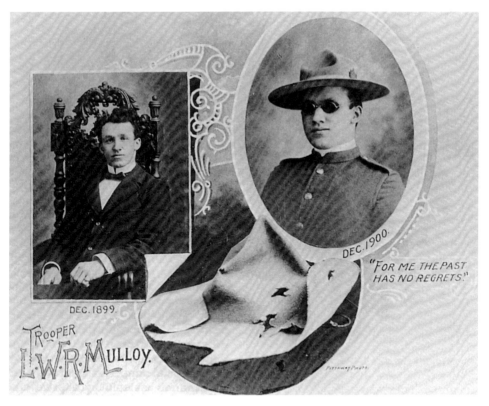

DEC. 1900.

"FOR ME THE PAST HAS NO REGRETS."

DEC. 1899.

TROOPER L.W.R. MULLOY.

1 Trooper Lorne Mulloy, serving with the Royal Canadian Dragoons, was blinded in July 1900 during the South African War. His astonishing subsequent career successes set the standard for what Canada's war blinded could achieve. *Library and Archives Canada (LAC), C-14081*

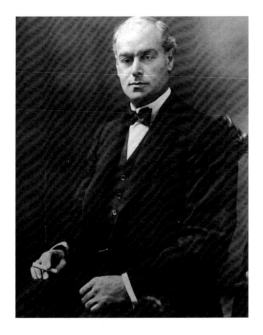

2 Sir Arthur Pearson (1866-1921), an energetic British newspaper magnate and philanthropist, was rendered completely blind in 1913 by glaucoma. His devotion to the empire's war blinded led him, in March 1915, to establish St. Dunstan's Hostel for Blinded Soldiers and Sailors. *St. Dunstan's Collections & Archives*

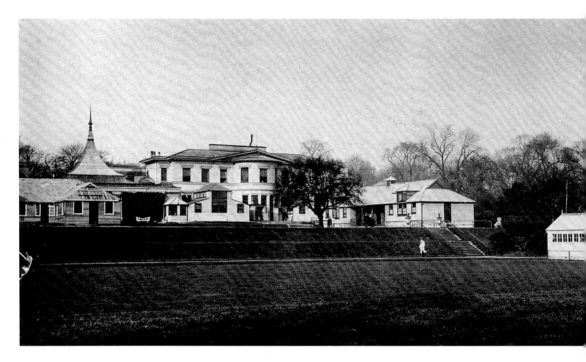

3 The sprawling facilities of St. Dunstan's Hostel for Blinded Soldiers and Sailors in Regent's Park, London, c. 1915. St. Dunstan's quickly established itself as the world's leading wartime readaptation centre for the blind.
St. Dunstan's Collections & Archives

4 Artist Craven Hill's sober First World War illustration (c. 1916) captures both the anguish of sudden blindness and the hope inspired by St. Dunstan's. *St. Dunstan's Collections & Archives*

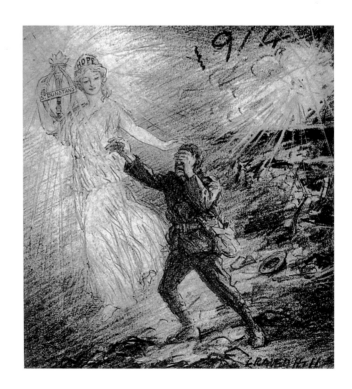

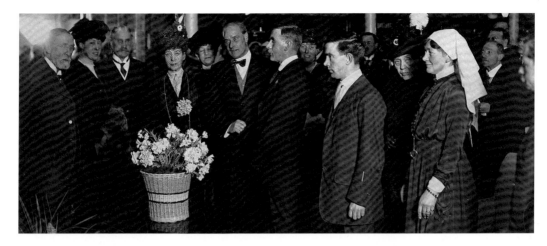

5 Queen Alexandra visits St. Dunstan's, c. 1919. The basket containing the carnations was made by one of the blinded soldiers in the centre of the photo and presented to her. Canadian Prime Minister Sir Robert Borden is third from left, Sir Arthur Pearson is fifth from left. At far left is Sir George Foster, Canada's minister of trade and commerce. *St. Dunstan's Collections & Archives*

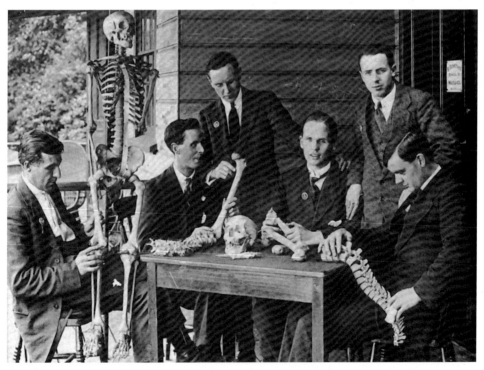

6 During and immediately following the First World War, more than 130 war-blinded soldiers, including Canadians, trained as massotherapists at St. Dunstan's School of Massage. Graduates were in high demand at military hospitals, where they assisted with wounded soldiers' physical rehabilitation. *St. Dunstan's Collections & Archives*

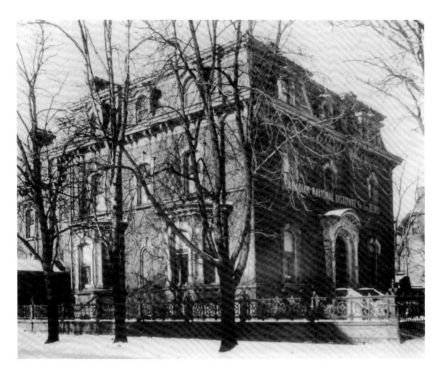

7 Pearson Hall, 186 Beverley Street, Toronto, was acquired by the CNIB in 1918 as its headquarters. It served as a training facility and residence for war-blinded veterans until 1922, after which the veterans enjoyed recreational activities there. *CNIB Archives*

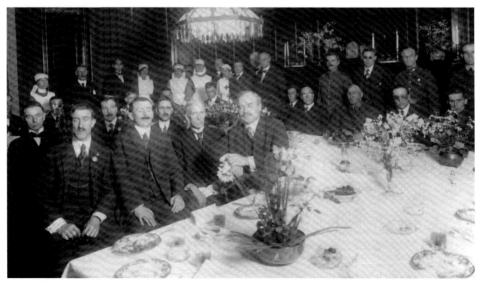

8 On 6 January 1919, Sir Arthur Pearson attended a banquet at Pearson Hall given in his honour by some twenty-seven war-blinded Canadians from across the country, most of whom had been trained at St. Dunstan's. He is standing at the centre-rear, wearing a bow-tie. *CNIB Archives*

Public Testimonial

IN HONOR OF

Canadian Soldiers Blinded in the War

AND

Sir Arthur Pearson, Bart., G.B.E.

Founder of St. Dunstan's

UNDER THE AUSPICES OF

THE CANADIAN NATIONAL INSTITUTE FOR THE BLIND

MASSEY HALL

TUESDAY, JANUARY 7TH, 1919, AT 8 P.M.

Chairman

HON. W. J. HANNA, K.C.

Speakers

SIR ARTHUR PEARSON, BART., G.B.E.
HON. SIR WILLIAM HEARST, K.C.M.G.
HON. SIR JAMES LOUGHEED, K.C.M.G.
CAPTAIN E. A. BAKER, M.C., Croix de Guerre

Musical Programme

Mr. Colin O'More, Tenor   48th Highlanders' Band

9   On 7 January 1919, a large public gala in Sir Arthur Pearson's honour was held at Massey Hall, Toronto. The list of distinguished speakers is a testament to the public profile attained by the CNIB and the war-blinded veterans. *CNIB Archives*

10   Voluntary Aid Detachment (VAD) members posing on the steps of Pearson Hall, c. 1919. Mainly affiliated with the Red Cross or the St. John Ambulance, and partially trained as nurses, these women provided invaluable assistance of every kind to the war blinded during the men's training at Pearson Hall. *CNIB Archives*

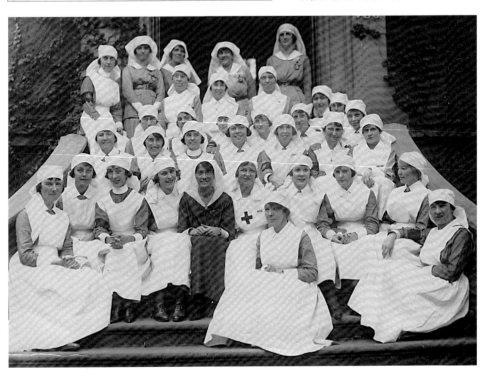

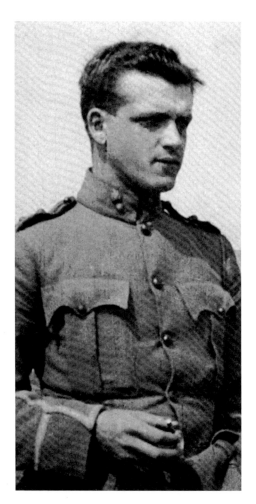

11 Lieutenant Edwin Albert Baker (1893-1968), 6th Field Company, Royal Canadian Engineers, at Valcartier, Quebec, 1915. Baker, blinded near Ypres in October 1915, was a driving force and inspiration behind the founding of the CNIB (1918) and the Sir Arthur Pearson Club of Blinded Soldiers and Sailors (SAPA, 1922). *CNIB Archives*

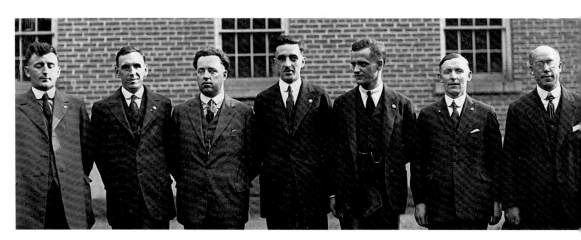

12 Some Canadian war-blinded veterans in the 1920s: from left, Alexander Graham, D.J. McDougall, J.W. Doiron, J. Harvey Lynes, E.A. Baker, W.L. Williamson, and A.G. Viets. *CNIB Archives*

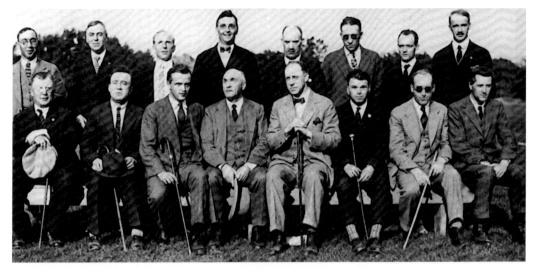

13   Some Canadian graduates of St. Dunstan's, including Edwin Baker, third from the left, front row. The photo was probably taken at SAPA's 1932 local reunion in Toronto. *CNIB Archives*

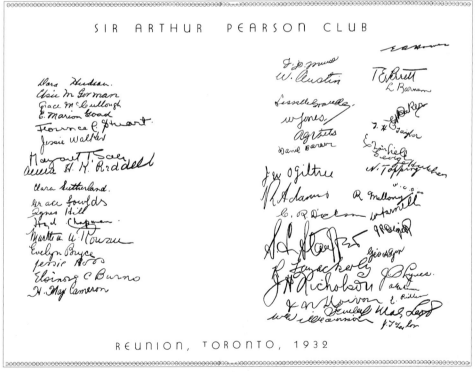

14   Evocative souvenir signatures by the thirty-one war-blinded attendees at the 1932 SAPA local reunion. On the left, the names of the members of the Pearson Hall House Committee, VADs, teachers, volunteers, and friends. At right, the men's signatures plus those of Dr. Charles R. Dickson and SAPA's sighted recording secretary, J.P. Lynes. *SAPA Archives*

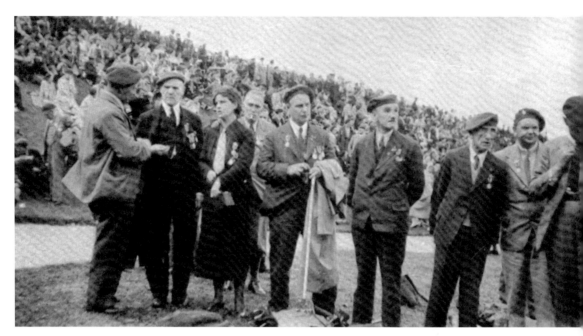

15 A group of Canadian war blinded await the arrival of King Edward VIII on the occasion of the unveiling of the Vimy Memorial, 26 July 1936. *Royal Canadian Legion*

16 Dr. Charles Rae Dickson (1858-1938), early advocate for the blind and war blinded, was briefly the first head of the CNIB in 1918 and in charge of Pearson Hall from December 1918 to June 1919. *CNIB Archives*

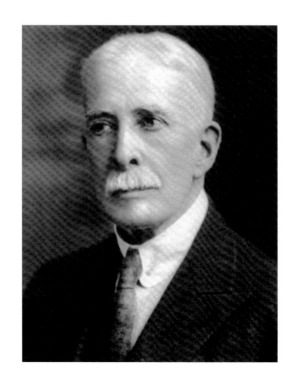

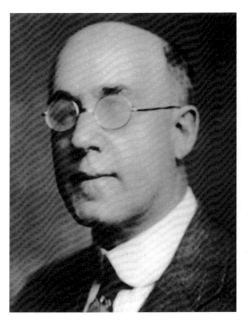

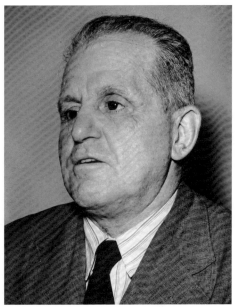

17   Alexander Griswold Viets (1878-1949), a founder of the CNIB and an executive of the institute and SAPA for three decades. Viets was possibly the first Canadian to be blinded during the First World War, while serving with the Princess Patricia's Canadian Light Infantry in February 1915. *CNIB Archives*

18   Bill Dies (1887-1968), a stalwart of the Canadian war-blinded community and an executive member of SAPA for nearly half a century. *CNIB Archives*

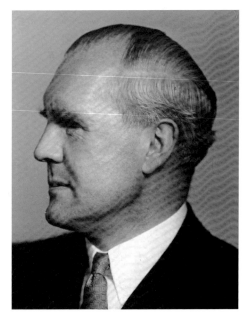

19   Sir Ian Fraser, Baron Fraser of Lonsdale (1897-1974), blinded on the Somme in 1916. His astounding administrative ability led to his appointment as head of St. Dunstan's following Pearson's death in December 1921, a position he held for more than fifty years. *St. Dunstan's Collections & Archives*

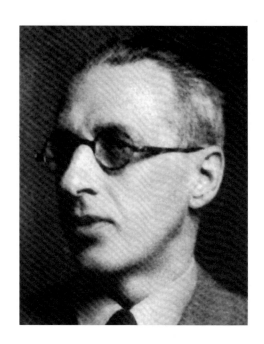

20 J. Harvey Lynes (1896-1985), blinded in France in 1918, was one of the founders of SAPA in 1922 and the organization's first president, a position he held again in the early 1940s. This photo was taken in 1943. *CNIB Archives*

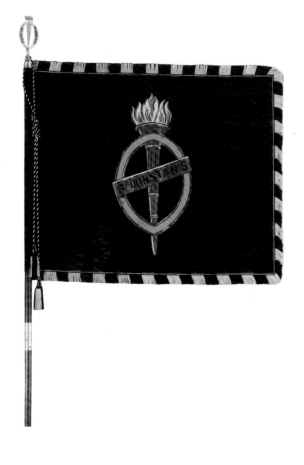

21 St. Dunstan's presented this standard to SAPA in December 1934, on the anniversary of Sir Arthur Pearson's death. It quickly became perhaps the organization's most cherished item. *SAPA Archives*

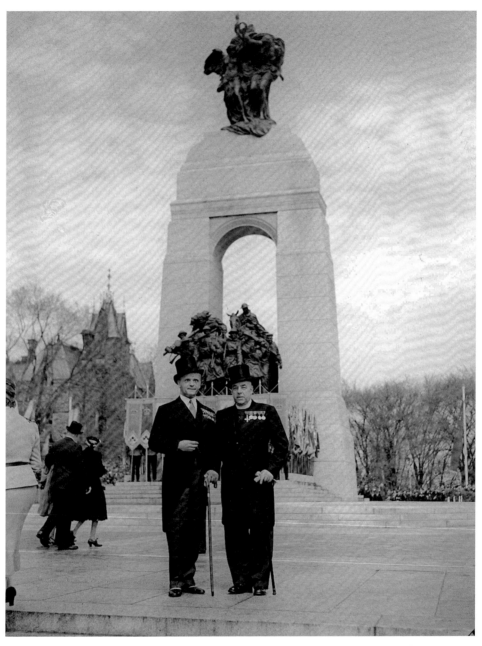

22 Edwin Baker with his close friend Lieutenant-Colonel the Reverend Sydney "Padre" Lambert, head of the Amputations Association of the Great War and SAPA's honorary president, at the unveiling of the National War Memorial in Ottawa, 21 May 1939. *CNIB Archives*

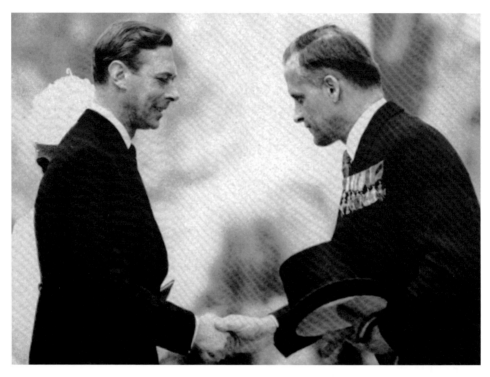

23 Edwin Baker shaking hands with King George VI on the occasion of the unveiling of the National War Memorial in Ottawa, 21 May 1939. *CNIB Archives*

Pensions: Fighting for What Was Owed

Historians Morton and Wright have bluntly noted that "the goal of civil re-establishment had always been to reduce Canada's responsibility for her returned soldiers."[129] In other words, the sooner repatriated wounded men were returned to gainful employment, the less Ottawa would have to spend to maintain them. By investing heavily in the repatriation process, Canada became the world leader in veterans' retraining and aftercare. The system was reasonably economical, since it generally worked to everyone's advantage.[130] Still, Canadian pension regulations in the postwar period were frequently complex, even Byzantine. Morton and Wright have termed the legislation and administration of Canadian military pensions "intricate, technical, and bewildering."[131]

The Department of Soldiers' Civil Re-establishment, these authors state, had "evolved into the cradle of Canada's welfare state," seeing to the needs of the largest group of Canadians for whose welfare the government had ever accepted responsibility. The 126,594 pensionable war wounded in 1922 included approximately 200 war blinded and 3,609 major amputees, some with multiple amputations. The DSCR supplied about a thousand glass eyes and twenty thousand orthopedic boots to veterans. Toronto's Christie Street Hospital was the DSCR's largest medical and rehabilitation facility, and many blinded soldiers benefitted from its services.[132]

Canadians did not begrudge government spending on programs for the war blinded, including their pensions. In 1920 the *Ottawa Citizen* opined that "everything that the state can do should surely be done to lighten such conditions of darkness in the lives of men who gave so much in the service of the state. The pension of a totally blinded man ... should be equivalent to a living wage." In a strongly worded editorial, the newspaper urged the government to immediately raise the war blinded's pensions from a maximum of $40 a month for a private to $60 (they rose to $50 not long after) and to significantly boost the allowance for attendants from the annual maximum of $300.[133]

Notwithstanding occasional administrative problems with the pension system and some uncharitable decisions on the part of the pension commissioners, there appeared to be relatively few complaints among the war blinded. Harris Turner wrote Baker after the war, "I am honestly of the opinion that the Government has dealt very decently with us blind gentlemen."[134] But some men fell between the cracks. T.D. Anderson, who had served in the Canadian Field Artillery and later the Canadian Army Medical Corps during the war, lost his eyesight and developed other health problems in the immediate postwar period. Despite the fact that the Board of Pension Commissioners had deemed his blindness unattributable to war service and found him ineligible for a disability pension, in 1919 Anderson trained at Pearson Hall but proved "unsuccessful." Though hospitalized under the auspices of the DSCR, by 1923 he had become hopelessly destitute and, according to D.J. McDougall, who sought to obtain help for Anderson from the Canadian Patriotic Fund, was "subject to only desultory assistance from other individuals and organizations." Married with a child, Anderson had no employment prospects. "The man's condition is lamentable," wrote McDougall.[135] But there was always the CNIB and, from 1922, SAPA, to assist in such cases, if only to the limits of their sometimes meagre resources.

There were many cases like Anderson's outside of the war-blinded community. In 1922 Ottawa appointed the Royal Commission on Pensions (the Ralston Commission) to review the entire pension program. Only about 5 percent of Canadian pensioners obtained the full disability allotment established by the legislation. In fact, 80 percent of those receiving a pension for disabilities attributable in whole or in part to military service received less than half of the maximum allowable for full disability cases, while most actually obtained 20 percent or less.[136] The Dominion Veterans Alliance (grouping together the major Canadian veterans' groups) ensured that veterans drawn from a number of special-interest categories presented briefs to the commissioners as the latter travelled the country. Among these were amputees, soldier-settlers, victims of tuberculosis, and the war blinded.[137]

SAPA rapidly became an organized, persuasive lobby group directly or indirectly affecting the fortunes of all pensioned and some non-pensioned veterans and their widows through the legislative precedents it was urging. In January 1923, SAPA's executive sought input from all its members to assist in the preparation of a brief to present before the Ralston Commission when it visited Toronto. Following a "thorough" discussion of the issues facing the war blinded, the executive decided that SAPA would mainly raise the matter of pension "stabilization," that is, transforming cost-of-living bonuses on pensions into permanent pension increases, and guaranteeing the permanency of pensions. Baker and McDougall would represent SAPA at the Commission hearing and plead the organization's case.[138] At SAPA's first AGM, in February 1923, the twenty-six members present agreed that the war blinded would co-ordinate their efforts with those of the Amputations Association prior to submitting their brief to the Commission; co-operation among Canada's permanently disabled veterans was deemed critical to a successful presentation.[139]

Raising the maximum attendance allowance was also a major concern for the war blinded, and SAPA made strong representations to the Ralston Commission on this issue. Away from the home or while travelling, the war blinded frequently needed aides and, in the absence of friends or family members, such people had to be hired. As a minimum, in the early months after being re-established in their homes, veterans frequently required assistance at meal times and needed someone to read to them, since almost no newspapers or magazines were available in Braille. The SAPA deputation made it clear to the commissioners that the attendants needed to be intelligent and, in the words of the SAPA minutes, "have the ability to read and write." The $300 per annum that Ottawa granted to eligible war blinded for this purpose was hopelessly insufficient; $25 a month could not retain a useful person. (Bed-ridden, helpless veterans received a greater allowance.) Baker had been petitioning the Board of Pension Commissioners since at least 1920 (while he was still at the DSCR) to increase this base amount. SAPA insisted to the commission that the allowance should be enshrined as permanent. SAPA also sought to broaden the pension eligibility for blinded soldiers' widows. Recognizing the complexities of these issues, SAPA established a standing committee dealing with pensions and re-establishment. Baker, McDougall, and Alexander Viets became its first members; they were a capable trio.[140] As a veterans' advocacy group, SAPA had no intention of remaining passive or relying on the CNIB to pressure Ottawa.

In September 1924, SAPA made it clear in a statement issued to the Ralston Commission that "no man who had suffered total loss of earning power while serving his country should suffer hardship." SAPA argued that blindness exacted a mental toll and that any measure of success in life was owed in large part to the intelligence and the powers of concentration of the blinded themselves. But many war-blinded veterans failed "to make good in the real sense of the word when faced with the continual mental strain necessary in the accomplishment of real work under such handicaps."[141] Ottawa failed to take the psychologically debilitating nature of blindness into account when determining pension allotments and benefits. Many war-blinded veterans were not up to the extraordinarily difficult task of constantly coping with their disability *and* working full-time. Of the 171 "totally disabled" war blinded in 1924, something like 40 percent could not count on stable income from their occupations, whereas a further 20 percent required "continual attention and assistance to keep going at anything worthwhile."[142]

Accordingly, meaningful and permanent federal pensions were essential to protect those who, despite retraining, would never earn a sufficient income to properly enjoy life's benefits. SAPA also pointed out that blindness was expensive: the war blinded paid for many services that the sighted took for granted. One example was life insurance: companies charged more to those with disabilities, hindering the veterans' ability to purchase life insurance to protect their families against financial ruin.[143] What of Whaley Austin, totally blind, with his left arm amputated just below the shoulder, shattered jaw requiring bone grafts, and a piece of skull missing? His poultry farming training at St. Dunstan's proved unsuccessful and his "mental capacity renders him incapable of taking up any profitable form of occupation." George A. Lyon, married with four children, was totally blind from a brain tumour discovered while he was on active service overseas. He was unable to retrain and incapable of work. B.F. Storey, perhaps Canada's only First World War-blinded prisoner of war in Germany, had both eyes removed in the course of medical treatment while incarcerated and "never recovered from his experiences." Despite a year's training at Pearson Hall, he could not succeed in any occupation and suffered domestic problems as well. These veterans all needed the stability offered by a reasonable disability pension.[144]

SAPA's Special Permanent Committee on Pensions and Re-establishment debated all pertinent issues SAPA members raised but insisted that "no representations except those of an absolutely reasonable character" should be made to Ottawa. The results of this moderate and realistic approach were that the DSCR and the BPC appeared more willing to accommodate the group's demands.[145] Baker wrote Ernest Scammell, the DSCR's secretary and assistant deputy minister, that he and McDougall had represented SAPA before the Ralston Commission and that one of Baker's roles had been to "prevent any wrong impression being given concerning the DSCR." In fact, the SAPA delegates reported to the Commission that, on the whole, blinded soldiers were satisfied with the treatment and retraining that they had received. "This, in view of the many criticisms which are being constantly put forward by ex-soldiers suffering from other forms of disability is very gratifying," stated the DSCR's 1923 Report.[146] That the war blinded did not constitute a large segment of the veteran population in Canada, and that satisfying their specific needs did not cost Ottawa a great deal, facilitated the spirit of co-operation that existed on both sides. Moreover, Baker's knowledge of the inner workings of the DSCR contributed to this harmonious working relationship; SAPA did not push harder than would be pro-ductive. On 29 September 1924, Baker and representatives from the Amputations Association met with officials from the BPC to discuss attendance allowance and, in March 1925, Ottawa raised this from $25 to $40 monthly, retroactive to November 1924. SAPA had adopted a wise strategy and a winning formula.[147]

Finally, on 27 June 1925, Parliament enacted a guaranteed Class 1 total disability pension of $900 yearly ($75 monthly), replacing the previous system based on a minimum monthly pension of $50 plus various bonus schemes normally amounting to another $25. Though not especially financially generous, this decision covered the whole of SAPA's membership. SAPA's Special Permanent Committee's report remarked that the success of the pensioners' three-year struggle "should relieve worry which has been present in the minds of many blinded soldiers with regard to the future."[148] In 1924 SAPA joined forces with the AA and the Canadian Pensioners' Association (re-named the War Pensioners of Canada after the Second World War) in petitioning the federal government on a variety of pension issues, but especially in support of non-pensioned widows, described as "widows of pensioners who married after the appearance of the dis-ability," and who were thus ineligible to receive a widow's pension.[149] Veterans' matrimony might have been inhibited in some cases since it was known that a widow would receive no survivors' benefits from the state because she had married an already disabled soldier. In 1928 SAPA and the AA secured an amendment to the Pension Act granting allowances in some cases for widows of soldiers who married after their husbands' disabilities had taken place. As usual, according to SAPA sources, there had been an "unqualified spirit of co-operation" between the two groups on this file.[150]

Formed of disabled but capable and active veterans, SAPA and the AA had much in common. In fact, several SAPA members were also amputees, Bill Dies being probably the best known. In Britain, about a hundred First World War St. Dunstaners were also amputees, including three who had lost both hands.[151] It was obvious that each group of disabled ex-servicemen could support the other on the issue of pension adjustments and claims. In fact, under Baker's guidance SAPA immediately allied itself with the AA and other veterans' groups seeking improved legislation from Ottawa and presented joint or complementary briefs to numerous Parliamentary committees and other government bodies. As Harry Coyle, a SAPA member blinded during the Second World War, put it in 1957, SAPA took on an important role in raising the "stature and dignity of the Canadian blind" and "for many years the blinded soldiers of this country were very prominent in the work of securing much needed consideration for disabled ex-servicemen and women and their dependants."[152] This was SAPA's true raison d'être. In the 1950s, even Harvey Lynes recalled that SAPA was founded mainly to further the war blinded's interests in pension legislation and government-sponsored vocational training opportunities. "It was felt that as an organization we would be heard and listened to," he stated, "and it would provide us with an opportunity to do what we could in the interests of the civilian blinded."[153] Coyle noted that "although the relationship between the Institute and the Club was intricate, the Institute dealt mainly in the training of the war blinded and the administration of aftercare while the Club determined its policies toward pensions and veterans' affairs."[154] And so SAPA developed its own niche, and with Baker shaping its direction, the group became a powerful voice for legislative improvement on veterans' issues.

One of the most vexing and frequently disappointing aspects of the soldiers' pension experiences was arguing the issue of attributability – that blindness or severe reduction in vision was the direct or indirect result of wartime service, including injury, disease, or exposure to harmful climates and working conditions. The number of Canadian veterans citing service conditions as having caused their postwar blindness grew throughout the interwar period. For example, in 1929 SAPA took on four new members, all in Ontario, as a result of medically documented war service-related deterioration in their vision.[155] The situation mirrored that in Britain, where men continued to be admitted to St. Dunstan's long after the cessation of hostilities. Some 25 percent of First World War St. Dunstaners' blindness was caused by disease contracted during the war – frequently a more difficult case to prove with British pension authorities. According to a 1929 report in a British newspaper, some eight hundred men had become blind as a result of worsening war injuries or other service-related causes since the Armistice.[156]

Moreover, in Canada, as in Britain, some men had joined the colours with existing eye diseases or defects, often undetected, that were greatly exacerbated by service conditions. Since these men should probably not have been accepted for service in the first place, it was unfair to reject a pension claim on the grounds that the eye condition leading to blindness or near-blindness predated wartime service. Some of the men thus affected were hardly young: British-born Private Digance, from Ottawa, enlisted in the Canadian Railway Corps in 1917 at the age of fifty-four after forty-eight years as a farmhand and labourer. He served overseas and was discharged in February 1918 as a result of failing vision. He later attended retraining at Pearson Hall, though it was obvious that his condition predated his service and that he should never have been enlisted. Private Foley, also from Ottawa, enlisted in 1916 at the age of forty-three, saw service in England, and was discharged in 1917 as legally blind.[157]

In general, Ottawa acted fairly on pensions. Morton and Wright even describe Ernest Scammell, Walter Segsworth, and "other framers of civil re-establishment" as "careful and far-sighted planners."[158] But it was mainly as a result of veterans' advocacy that military pensions, access to retraining facilities, and medical benefits became established as rights and not charity, as permanent and not temporary measures. "Without Eddie Baker, Sydney Lambert, and their organizations of blind and maimed veterans, all sightless and amputee Canadians would have faced a longer and more difficult struggle against tradition and prejudice," these historians wrote. All Canadians could share in their successes.[159]

SAPA's creation had resulted from the need for a CNIB veterans' sub-group to look after the special needs of its membership. But many among the war blinded sensed a closer bond to blind Canadian civilians than to non-disabled veterans. They weren't the only pensioned veterans feeling that they alone were best able to articulate their views and deal independently with the DSCR. Following years of bitter factionalism in the Canadian veterans' community, in 1926 the Canadian Legion of the British Empire Service League came into existence through the merging of several veterans' organizations. But the Amputations Association, for example, while broadly supporting the notion of a united veterans' front, rejected union with the Legion until the latter organization had shown itself conversant with and sensitive to the needs of AA members. The amputees believed that their relatively modest membership of nearly 1,500 would prevent disabled soldiers' interests being properly secured and protected by the much larger integrated organization. Nevertheless, the Legion's establishment of a special Tuberculous Veterans Section in October 1926 induced the Tuberculous Veterans Association to surrender its charter and merge its 4,000 members with the Legion. By 1930, the Legion's membership had grown to about 70,000 members.[160] Other smaller groups, such as SAPA, the Army and Navy Veterans in Canada, and the Canadian Pensioners' Association of the Great War remained unconvinced and rejected folding their operations into the Legion. Still, nothing prevented SAPA members from also belonging to the Legion or other veterans' groups, and many availed themselves of the opportunity.

The situation was far different in Britain, where St. Dunstan's was not, strictly speaking, a veterans' organization. There, Ian Fraser increasingly saw St. Dunstan's best interests furthered in closer co-operation with other veterans' associations, not only those concerned with disabled veterans but also the British Legion, of which he eventually became head. In fact, the British Legion and St. Dunstan's exchanged members on each other's councils and, for a time in the interwar period, the Legion delegate was himself a St. Dunstaner, revealing a very close working relationship.[161] This was never the case in Canada, notwithstanding SAPA's occasional co-operative ventures with the Legion.

In July 1929, St. Dunstan's Ian Fraser convened the eleven-day British Empire Blinded Soldiers' Conference in London to discuss aftercare. Edwin Baker helped arrange this gathering, which included only high-level participants, about ten in all, from Britain, Canada, Australia, New Zealand, and South Africa. Baker and Alexander Viets, among the first Canadian St. Dunstaners, attended as the Canadian representatives. The men discussed the progress of St. Dunstaners overseas, reviewed the usefulness of the professional courses, such as massage, shorthand, and typewriting, taught at St. Dunstan's and elsewhere, and re-evaluated the handicrafts taught, including mat making, boot repairing, basketry, and carpentry. The agenda was wide ranging, and the delegates also compared the financial assistance and programs offered by the British and Dominion governments, discussed fundraising possibilities, and compared employment experiences and prospects for graduates. All were concerned by the growing incidence of delayed blindness among veterans and the resources necessary for retraining and assisting with pension claims. The delegates were warmly received in London. Lady Pearson hosted them at a luncheon, and the Prince of Wales welcomed them at St. James Palace, chatting with each delegate individually. They also attended a royal garden party at Buckingham Palace and toured the St. Dunstan's poultry farm, the annex at Brighton, and the National Institute for the Blind.[162]

It had been more than a decade since the war had ended and all participants were anxious to learn from the experiences of others and strengthen their own training and aftercare programs. What none could anticipate, of course, was the catastrophic decade ahead in which economic collapse and social malaise would render the needs of the aging war disabled more acute than ever. The war blinded, and all Canadian veterans, needed to close ranks.

3 The Years of Struggle, 1930-39

Wars end, wounds heal, but blindness remains.

– Lord Lonsdale

The 1930s were dismal years for Canada. The Great Depression, beginning at the end of 1929, wreaked havoc with the economy. Unemployment rose to unprecedented levels while poverty and despair gripped millions of Canadians. Historians have appropriately termed this decade "the Dirty Thirties." Of all Western industrialized nations, Canada was perhaps the hardest hit and the nation in which the Depression lasted the longest. It was caused by a combination of factors, including commodity over-production, over-investment, under-consumption, strict international trade barriers, and inept government fiscal policy. The darkest year was 1933. That winter, the unemployment rate stood at a staggering 32 percent, while 20 percent of all Canadians depended on some form of charitable relief. Despite assuming some responsibility for the nation's disabled veterans, Canada had not yet implemented anything even approaching a welfare state. During this dismal period, some people no doubt had their lives shortened by health problems linked to poverty;

among them were First World War disabled veterans, including the war blinded.

Canada's status as an international actor changed significantly in the interwar period. Constitutionally, Britain's Balfour Report of 1926 followed by the Statute of Westminster in 1931 made Canada an independent nation with the right of discretion in matters of war and peace – a power that it had lacked in 1914. The British Empire had evolved into the British Commonwealth of Nations, in which member states voluntarily remained bound by allegiance to the same monarch. British foreign policy nevertheless heavily influenced all members of the Commonwealth. As the world lurched from crisis to crisis throughout the 1930s, it grew increasingly obvious to all but the most hopeful observers that the First World War, supposedly the "war to end all wars," would prove only the opening round of a continuing conflict with Germany.

The activities of the Sir Arthur Pearson Club of War Blinded Soldiers and Sailors provide a measure of the trials and successes of Canada's war blinded in the 1930s. SAPA matured as an organization, became more effective, and took on a higher profile in the veterans' community and with federal authorities. It also successfully prodded the government into maintaining and even improving pension allotments to its members, to all veterans, and to their survivors – despite the desperate economic times. Its fluctuating membership reflected the high mortality rate of the war blinded and also the fact that dozens of veterans who had suffered some vision loss or eye damage during the war became progressively more blind as the decade wore on and eventually joined SAPA. Edwin Baker's influence on the organization is everywhere to be found. He was a remarkable administrator and an energetic, devoted worker on behalf of the war blinded. SAPA's story is very much his own, as the organization developed into a responsible, moderate, and patriotic advocacy group.

Business as Usual

By 1930, SAPA was a small, active, and stable organization, intimately tied to the Canadian National Institute for the Blind (CNIB) and responsive to the needs of its membership. Working in conjunction with the institute's aftercare programs, SAPA's leaders, especially Edwin Baker, were devoted to ameliorating the condition of financially insecure or ailing members. The members of SAPA's Executive Committee, including its regional representatives, changed infrequently during the 1930s. Those changes that did occur at the organization's annual general meetings were generally sanctified without votes, with prearranged nominations and dutiful expressions of unanimity being the norm from the members present, most from Ontario. Baker, the club's industrious secretary and guiding force, was always returned by acclamation. While he more or less carried the organization, the old guard remained nominally at the helm: Alexander Viets was president from 1931 to 1933, succeeded by Bill Dies. In 1936, J. Harvey Lynes, who had helped found SAPA in 1922, became president for the next eight years. Lynes had generated some controversy in the group a decade earlier, but this was water under the bridge and he proved a good team player during the difficult years of Depression and war.

Throughout the 1930s, SAPA's meetings and proceedings continued in a friendly, informal atmosphere, with frequent expressions of sympathy for those ill or bereaved, congratulations extended on members' successes, greetings to kindred organizations, and heartfelt thanks to all those who assisted Canada's war blinded. All seemed harmonious and even familial. There are no hints of significant doctrinal or procedural divisions among the men. When there were general, or national, reunions the war blinded gathered in far greater numbers, often sixty or more, and accordingly were present for the coincident annual general meetings. These strong showings validated decisions taken and symbolized the men's unity.

The highlight of each September's AGM was undoubtedly Baker's very full report on the previous year's activities and his knowledgeable rendering of relevant modifications to pension legislation and other matters of interest to the blinded veterans. The SAPA members appreciated Baker, and the organization's minutes record frequent references to, for example, his "untiring efforts on behalf of his fellow members."[1] Of course, all war-blinded veterans were also CNIB clients and, as we have seen, some took up leadership roles within the institute, Baker foremost among them. As the managing director of the CNIB, Baker's imprint was everywhere in the institute's policies, public profile, and programs. He was also the principal author of the CNIB's annual reports.

One section in those publications close to Baker's heart was the annual summation of blinded soldiers' activities, in which he strove to make clear the importance of the war blinded to the institute and the fraternal feeling linking the Canadian war blinded to the civilian blind. In 1936 Baker wrote that the national office of the CNIB "kept closely in touch" with SAPA and that "ever since the establishment of the Institute, its pleasant association with the Sir Arthur Pearson Club has been one of its features and the bond between the two organizations seems to grow stronger as the years pass by." In 1939, Baker noted that the very name of the CNIB's well-known headquarters, Pearson Hall, had an obvious association with the war blinded and that "the club rooms of the SAPC are maintained in the Head Office building and are the scene of many a happy social gathering of the members and their friends."[2] The war blinded had become the institute's most publicly recognizable members and, along with Baker's presence and tutelage, afforded the CNIB a strong veneer of public service and sacrifice. The war blinded thus assumed dual roles as high-profile, patriotic veterans and disabled civilians.

Although SAPA was far from healthy financially, it did not seem to matter. SAPA's meagre bank balances, normally less than $100, and often far less, were usually spent on gifts, flowers, cards, and charitable donations, since most of SAPA's operating expenses were absorbed by the CNIB, itself subsidized by the Department of Pensions and National Health for aftercare costs incurred on behalf of the war blinded. In 1933 there was almost no movement in the bank account and no disbursements for the entire year, the balance being $8.45. This dropped to exactly 80 cents by September 1934.[3] Although SAPA never publicly raised funds, even in the midst of a worsening economic catastrophe appreciative Canadians continued to remember the war blinded. In 1931 the organizers of a Remembrance Day collection in Wakefield, Quebec, sent the small proceeds to Pearson Hall for the use of the war-blinded veterans. In 1934, a Mrs. Seymour bequeathed the comparatively large sum of $1,000 to "the home for blinded soldiers." In response to some suspicious executors' questions as to what place this was, exactly, Baker submitted a "statement of facts" confirming that the generous Mrs. Seymour could have intended only the CNIB's Pearson Hall.[4]

The donated money was not SAPA's, strictly speaking, but it directly benefited SAPA members by helping pay for social activities, being used for emergency loans, or simply being spent to improve the war blinded's comfort and surroundings. While the government had accepted the principle of responsibility for the men's retraining, perpetual aftercare, and reasonable needs, the poignancy of their war wounds was kept before the public. To this extent, the war blinded inspired a convergence of views among Canadians about the memory of the war's tragic and lasting effects on the nation's citizens. Even as many Canadians sought to forget the war, the existence of the sightless but independent-minded veterans obliged them to remember.

Sometimes the blinded and maimed depended on others, notwithstanding their own considerable achievements in retraining and rehabilitation. The female Voluntary Aid Detachment workers (VADs) giving their time at Pearson Hall were essential to improving the men's lives, and were key to SAPA's success as a beneficial social organization as well as a veterans' advocacy group. As they had since the end of the First World War, throughout the 1930s these women cared for those war blinded in need or distress, assisted in numerous tasks with which the men might have had difficulty, and, along with the Pearson Hall House Committee, organized frequent social and recreational activities. This work served to maintain a positive ambiance within the organization and contributed to fraternal feelings among members. If they needed friendship and companionship to help them succeed in life, they could find it; not all veterans could say the same. The VADs also visited the homes of all SAPA members in the Toronto area, no doubt to relieve loneliness, in some cases, but also to ensure that the men were getting on satisfactorily. They also regularly visited hospitalized members. Even the friendless among the war blinded could count on some practical help – with outings or shopping, for example.

Thanks to these women, SAPA members benefitted from a surprisingly robust social calendar. In a typical year there would be numerous members' activities, including the AGM, special events, and commemorative occasions at Pearson Hall and the Christie Street Hospital. There were, annually, an Easter dance and a June garden party at Pearson Hall, organized by the House Committee. Remembrance Day was also solemnly marked and then celebrated with an Armistice dance, and the year ended with the SAPA Christmas dinner at Pearson Hall. The 1935 Christmas dinner was attended by twenty-two members plus their wives or escorts, a strong showing indicative of the group's intense sense of belonging; these men needed each other.[5]

The House Committee was distinct from the VAD contingent, most of whose members had been formally trained as nursing auxiliaries by the St. John Ambulance. Still, some women had overlapping affiliations and roles. The House Committee ensured the building's upkeep and arranged for donations of needed furnishings or appliances. In 1938, for example, its members procured two rugs, some chairs, plants and shrubs, and an "electric sweeper." Since Pearson Hall housed CNIB offices and other facilities, these items and improvements were not for the exclusive benefit of the war blinded, though the latter's social events were central features of the House Committee's annual work.[6]

In some cases the VADs were perhaps as critical to the war blinded's survival as government pensions and employment training. Their efforts did no go unrecognized: at the 1931 AGM the VADs were thanked "amid the hearty cheers of the packed meeting."[7] Writing in the 1939 CNIB Annual Report, Baker noted that, from the beginning, the VADs, of whom there were then about nineteen attached to Pearson Hall, "have co-operated with members in a spirit of friendly comradeship," and he even went so far as to state that they were "largely responsible for the continuation" of SAPA.[8] Sometimes the veterans played the role of benefactor: Baker noted that "new ground was broken when the members of [SAPA] gave a dinner and dance to the VADs on the evening of March 6, 1937. The shock of being entertained after twenty years of providing entertainment did not prove fatal to any of the guests."[9] The war blinded held the VADs and House Committee members in very high esteem and this important act of repaying years of kindnesses and courtesies became a near-annual affair.

The VADs certainly were faithful: a photo in the CNIB's 1939 annual report shows seven original Pearson Hall VADs still "intimately" connected to the affairs of SAPA. Among those pictured was the venerable Clara Sutherland, the long-serving House Committee convenor.[10] Through the efforts of such devoted volunteers, too long and perhaps still mainly in the shadows, the lives of many of Canada's war blinded veterans were materially improved.

On the other hand, some of the blinded veterans were quite capable of outdoor activities without need of the VADs, or any other, assistance. Harris Turner, for example, was possessed of an excellent golf drive. He would tee his ball and place the driver immediately behind it. After repositioning himself without moving the club, he would hit the ball cleanly, regularly driving it 150 yards. His caddy would assist him upon their departure from the tee. Several Canadian veterans competed in the World Blind Golf Championships, which began in the 1920s. Following the Second World War a British St. Dunstaner recorded the remarkable score of 82. Another former St. Dunstaner, A. Glasspool, of Montreal, was trained as a boot-repairer. But, since so many Montrealers wore rubber overshoes during the winter and business lagged, he decided to shut his shop for the season and turn his attention to tobogganing and skating.[11] That was the St. Dunstan's spirit in action.

The International Fraternity of the War Blinded

Being war blinded meant belonging to a group that transcended national boundaries. Sightless veterans across the world bonded in a shared understanding of their experiences. In the 1930s, Canada's war blinded maintained close links with other veterans' groups in Canada and also with war-blinded groups across the world, especially British and Commonwealth organizations. Following the Second World War, these groups would even coalesce into an international organization. Almost every year a representative from one of the Commonwealth organizations visited Pearson Hall; alternatively, a SAPA member, usually Edwin Baker, travelled abroad, usually to Britain, to strengthen fraternal relations and obtain the latest information on the war blinded's lot and achievements in other nations.

A procession of high-profile war-blinded visitors dropped by Pearson Hall throughout the 1930s. In early May 1931, Ian Fraser, St. Dunstan's head, and Clutha Mackenzie, head of New Zealand's Jubilee Institute for the Blind, visited. Fraser, a member of Parliament, high-ranking British Legion official, and probably Britain's most famous blinded veteran, visited Canada several times before the decade was over. Baker and Fraser built up a strong working relationship and frequently exchanged correspondence and information, assisting each other whenever they could. Pearson Hall, although the CNIB's general headquarters, had also gained a reputation as a veterans' readaptation centre. The impressive training complex available to blinded veterans and civilians included annexes and nearby buildings purchased by the CNIB. Canada's war blinded were certainly "on the map," no doubt helped by Baker's strong presence. For example, on 5 September 1931, Earl Jellicoe, of Battle of Jutland fame, made a point of visiting Pearson Hall, where eighteen SAPA members were on hand to greet the celebrated admiral.[12]

Curiously, in 1934 no SAPA representative was able to attend Sir Ian Fraser's (he was knighted that year) Empire Blinded Soldiers' Conference, held in Australia on the eve of the general British Empire Service League (BESL) conference at which Fraser would represent the British Legion. On his way to Australia, Fraser, accompanied by his wife, visited Canada, arriving in Toronto on 30 August. During his whirlwind twenty-four-hour visit, he again visited Pearson Hall, inspected the CNIB facilities and its exhibit at the Canadian National Exhibition, and enjoyed a dinner in his honour at the Royal York Hotel organized by SAPA and the CNIB and attended by twenty-five Toronto-area blinded soldiers plus escorts. Fraser referred to the evening as a "delightful party," presided over by Bill Dies, who was joined by Baker and Lewis Wood, nominal head of the CNIB, in officially welcoming Fraser. "It was just like one of our most cheerful reunions in Britain, with the exception," Fraser wrote in the *St. Dunstan's Review*, "that we had not met our Canadian friends for so many years."[13]

Fraser left Toronto for western Canada on 31 August, with stops in Winnipeg, Regina, Calgary, Banff, and Vancouver. Everywhere, he met CNIB representatives and SAPA members. On 11 September, while in Vancouver, Fraser was treated to an excursion on the yacht of Colonel Victor Spencer, who, along with Brigadier Victor Odlum and Canadian St. Dunstaner and local CNIB aftercare officer M.C. Robinson, organized a tea in honour of all British Columbia blinded soldiers.[14] Paying tribute to the work of the CNIB, and recalling its wartime origins, Fraser noted that "St. Dunstan's can legitimately take pride in this outstanding Canadian development, for it arose out of the St. Dunstan's spirit."[15]

From 19 to 25 October 1936, SAPA and Pearson Hall hosted Alan Nichols, a blinded and armless British St. Dunstaner on an extended solo visit to the United States and Canada. Nichols symbolized the independence of action instilled at St. Dunstan's. While in Toronto, Nichols, something of an inspiration to the war disabled, addressed a number of social and veterans' groups and visited the Christie Street Hospital. Nichols's vibrant account of his time at Pearson Hall was published in the *St. Dunstan's Review:* "Toronto is English, comparatively speaking, after leaving the U.S.A., and I found Pearson Hall a relief after hotel life ... I can never find words to describe meeting chaps like ... Dies, Williamson, Turner, Baker and a dozen or so more of the old boys whom I had been in 'dock' with at St. Dunstan's ... All the boys were particularly well and you can imagine my surprise when they threw a luncheon party at Pearson Hall the day before I returned to New York ... Suffice it to say I want to remember that day for a very long time."[16] A year later, Captain Perrin, of the Australian Blinded Soldiers' Association, visited Pearson Hall to a warm welcome. Amicable relations existed between the Australians and Canadians and the correspondence between the two groups, fraternal in tone, concerned matters of mutual interest to the Empire's war blinded.[17] But distance made their meetings infrequent.

Edwin Baker, too, was busy. Besides his time-consuming duties as managing director of the CNIB, in 1932 and 1933 he visited St. Dunstan's, in the latter year attending the annual war-blinded's officers' dinner. In 1933, while in London for a BESL conference, at which he also represented the Amputations Association, Baker attended a luncheon of St. Dunstan's-trained masseurs, including two Canadians. He then discussed with Fraser those Canadian war blinded and their families living in Britain, some of whom had suffered a diminished standard of living as a result of deteriorating health and the weak economy. For example, SAPA member T.E. Scotland had died just days before Baker's visit, leaving a widow and children in Glasgow. Baker wished to know what would become of them and whether St. Dunstan's could help until he secured a pension for Scotland's widow, something he succeeded in doing in 1934. Baker also met with the Prince of Wales, the future Edward VIII, who hosted the BESL delegates.[18]

One event at mid-decade symbolized the close bond the Commonwealth's war-blinded felt for their original benefactor, Sir Arthur Pearson. Lady Ethel Pearson, his widow, arranged for the College of Heralds in London to design a special St. Dunstan's standard, which was unveiled at St. Dunstan's on 9 December 1934, the thirteenth anniversary of Pearson's death. It bore the St. Dunstan's (and SAPA) crest of a lighted torch. Lady Pearson earlier had dispatched copies of the standard to the blinded veterans' associations in Canada, Australia, New Zealand, and South Africa, where similar solemn unveilings took place on the same date. At Pearson Hall, following a memorial service for Pearson at which Baker's close collaborator, Sydney Lambert, officiated, the St. Dunstan's standard was dedicated in the SAPA members' club room for permanent display in a case secured to the wall.[19] Whether they had attended St. Dunstan's or been trained at Pearson Hall, all of Canada's war-blinded veterans had been exposed to the famed "St. Dunstan's spirit," and the standard reflected this shared experience and the social and personal successes that flowed therefrom.

Dr. Charles Dickson nearly always attended the SAPA AGMs. As SAPA's honorary patron since its inception, he often spoke with eloquence on the achievements of the nation's war blinded and their inspiring presence within the CNIB. Dickson was highly regarded by the men and was always given the honour of speaking last before the AGMs adjourned. In 1931 he gave an inspiring speech on the ideals for which SAPA stood and showed those present "by his exhortation to greater achievements, that he is still the warrior who has done such a great unselfish work in the cause of the blind, both soldier and civilian."[20] Dickson passed away on 9 July 1938, in his eightieth year. He had been "the only civilian ever honoured with an official position" in SAPA and, in Baker's words, had been a "fine gentleman and fast friend" to all the club's members.[21] The veterans, too, were aging and a surprising number died relatively young during this decade.

Attrition and Fluctuating Membership

The Great Depression proved tough on veterans, especially those whose position in the labour market was not firmly rooted. By 1932, the average age of Canadian Expeditionary Force veterans was already forty-four. They were often prematurely aged, in poor health, and all-too-frequently jobless. Even worse, some employers hesitated to hire veterans for fear of a public backlash if they should be let go.[22] Blinded veterans, too, had difficulty finding and retaining employment. In the face of government spending retrenchments, even hard-won pensions and entitlements appeared at risk.

The debilitating effects of the war remained a constant in the lives of many Canadian veterans, especially those who had been wounded. Large numbers of these men experienced ongoing pain, recurring health problems, frustration, discouragement, and a lowered quality of life. Added to this for Canada's war blinded was the greater likelihood of accident and mischance; for them, early mortality accelerated during the 1930s. Already by 1924, ten blinded veterans had died and by 1928 the number stood at eighteen. W.W. Hitchon, so successful in postwar life as an executive with Massey-Harris, died prematurely in 1928, and George Eades had died on Armistice Day 1927 in Reading, England. Nine years to the day earlier, Eades had proudly carried the St. Dunstan's flag in an Armistice parade in London.[23]

The grim harvest of the war blinded continued at a rate seemingly above the norm for Canadian veterans and blinded Canadians generally. At SAPA's tenth AGM in September 1931, four deaths were reported for the previous year. A year later, six more had died. Ronald Macdonald of North Sydney, Nova Scotia, was referred to the CNIB for aftercare in May 1932 and died in July, being both a new and deceased SAPA member in the same year. By September 1933, a further four had passed away, including two of the few French-Canadian members, O. Vézina of Ottawa and L. Marquis from Quebec. J.B.A. Renault and F.C. Dupuis had recently predeceased them. This brought to thirty-three the number of deaths since 1918, which represented about 17 percent of the known war blinded. Sixteen more would die before the decade was over, or more than a quarter of the total in about twenty years. Many left behind widows and children, often without means.[24]

Some of the members' stories are instructive. James Key, from Toronto, became a member of SAPA in 1936. He had suffered severe mustard gas burns at Arras in 1918 while serving in the 1st Battalion. He received a 100 percent disability pension in addition to attendance allowance. "This man was so badly burned with mustard gas," reported Baker, "that his vision has deteriorated to the point where he can perceive hand movements only. In addition he must keep his whole body and limbs bandaged daily. This is a permanent condition which will not improve, and the ability to perceive hand movements is not expected to continue very long." Married with three children, Key died in October 1937.[25] W.J. Chiswell of Verdun, Quebec, blinded by trench fever while serving with the 87th Battalion, died in 1937 at the age of fifty. Montrealer A.A. Bibeau, who had been blinded by a gunshot wound while serving in the 72nd Battalion, died the same year. Abel Knight, wounded at Ypres in May 1915 while serving with the Princess Patricia's Canadian Light Infantry, died in England, where he lived, in February 1938. Major H. Watts, one of the highest-ranking SAPA members, died in Victoria in May of the same year.[26]

Edwin Baker and other SAPA members became concerned. Why were so many dying? Was there a correlation between the kind of wounds they had suffered and their shortened life expectancy? Although some of the deceased had been in their fifties and sixties, Frank Atkinson being sixty-three at the time of his death in 1931 and W.M. Moore fifty-seven when he died in 1923, most war blinded dying in the interwar period were only in their thirties or forties. While most died in Canada, four died in Britain and one in the United States. One passed away in a psychiatric hospital in Manitoba and another at the Christie Street Hospital in Toronto.[27] It was difficult to establish a pattern. In 1933 Baker noted simply and caustically in the CNIB Annual Report that "the majority of [them] died prematurely." The CNIB and SAPA investigated each case to ensure that the men's families obtained what was owing them in terms of pensions and other survivors' benefits.[28] It was all that was left to do. While the ranks of the original SAPA members were thinning quickly, additional cases of war blindedness emerged throughout the 1920s and 1930s, tragically adding to the organization's and the CNIB's case files.

The Sir Arthur Pearson Club of War Blinded Soldiers and Sailors maintained strict membership criteria that, in practice, were linked to the Department of Pensions and National Health (DPNH) definitions of war blindedness and postwar blindness attributable to wartime service. These definitions dictated the government's disability rating levels and pension allotment. But SAPA's broader desire to help visually impaired veterans, some of whom did not fit the legislated and pensionable definitions, also drove membership policy to some extent. The situation was delicate and sometimes confusing. War blindedness, in all its tragedy, was also a badge of identity for members of the closely knit SAPA family; the sanctity of the sacrifice that bound them could not be diluted. Something of a hierarchy existed in the war-blinded community, with those having suffered combat wounds at the apex: there was neither doubt as to the nature of these men's sacrifice nor nagging questions concerning eligibility, attributability, or degree of blindness. Both SAPA and the department had to remain vigilant and avoid setting precedents by offering training and after-care services, not to mention pensions and allowances, to veterans unable to satisfy the eligibility requirements.

According to Baker, citing a 1925 Department of Soldiers' Civil Re-establishment (DSCR) ruling, veterans were eligible for CNIB after-care services if they were pensionable to any degree on account of blindness and had been granted an attendance allowance. They were also eligible if they were pensionable owing to 80 percent or more blindness but not in receipt of an attendance allowance.[29] These were the "official" war blinded and SAPA membership followed these lines. However, it was sometimes difficult to determine exactly who was a veritable blinded soldier, since some veterans' vision improved or deteriorated over time and, as Baker put it, "Some who had been sent to Pearson Hall for training were found to be far from blind while others were obviously not eligible but anxious to be included in the ranks of blinded soldiers."[30] Notwithstanding this, SAPA accorded membership privileges in the postwar period to veterans to whom the Board of Pension Commissioners had granted war-blinded status, "it being felt that ... such decisions should be in the hands of the Pension authorities who had full information on file including service qualifications."

Sometimes, the issue of membership eligibility obliged intro-spection. A 1934 application for SAPA membership by J.W. Miller, who was undoubtedly blind, instigated a lengthy and emotive dis-cussion in the Executive Committee and among members at large. The Executive Committee did not meet often in the early 1930s, but this issue forced a number of gatherings, including two general meetings of the Toronto-area members to obtain more input. Miller's wartime service overseas was very brief and his blindness had occurred following his return to Canada. Yet he had been trained at Pearson Hall and even participated in several blinded soldiers' activities while his pension claims were under review. In the end, the BPC attributed his postwar blindness to causes other than war service. However, he did obtain a 5 percent disability pension due to deafness and, given his blindness, was also awarded attendance allowance. Technically, since his pension was not on account of his blindness, he was ineligible for department-mandated aftercare and SAPA membership since he was a blind veteran and not a war-blinded one.[31] But Miller had, by and large, become part of the war-blinded community. Was membership to be based on social acceptance or the experience of war?

At an April 1934 special general meeting (though not an AGM) called to debate the question of membership, Baker presented the official interpretation of the membership clauses and noted that SAPA's policy of following government practice for membership eligibility had never been voted on or adopted by the resolution of any SAPA committee or general meeting; the practice was merely a convention. The much-discussed question for the sixteen SAPA members present was whether there should be an amendment to the SAPA constitution specifying the conditions of membership. In the end, those present empowered the Executive Committee to act in what its members felt would be the best interests of SAPA and the war blinded.[32] Baker had made up his mind on Miller's case: "It is felt that under no possible interpretation of membership by-laws in the [SAPA] Constitution, Executive Minutes or Ruling of the Department, can this application for full membership be granted."[33] As a compromise, SAPA offered Miller associate membership (a category which did not yet officially exist); as such, he would continue to be invited to SAPA functions. At a second general meeting the next month, the eighteen members present agreed that the membership rules needed to be enforced in the future but without specifically linking membership to DPNH aftercare policy.[34] In other words, the war blinded reserved for themselves ultimate authority in deciding who would join their organization.

Yet SAPA's membership continued to fluctuate, with the high mortality rates being offset by the addition of new members suffering service-attributed delayed blindness. There had been some 2,600 eye injuries in the Canadian Expeditionary Force (CEF), and some of these eventually led to total vision loss in one and then both eyes. This was attributable blindness, though establishing it before the BPC was another matter. Other men who had been completely blind since the war or immediately afterward had originally been denied pensions because the DSCR at that time assessed the cause of their handicap as preceding or not resulting from military service. Subsequent information, sometimes twenty years later, showing the aggravating nature of onerous service conditions, obliged the department to assume at least some responsibility for the men's blindness and provide a disability pension. These veterans were then considered war blinded.

Once these men became known to SAPA, normally as a result of their being made eligible for CNIB training and aftercare services, they were automatically welcomed as SAPA members and the organization contacted them to this effect. For example, fourteen new members, including two former officers, were announced at the SAPA AGM of September 1931.[35] More veterans became eligible for membership in almost every year of the 1930s. In 1938, four new members were added, including Nursing Sister Florence Leamy of Montreal (one of the very few female war blinded in either world war). James Saunders, of Kingston, had served with the CEF in France and suffered severe eye damage during the Halifax Explosion in December 1917 while serving with the Royal Canadian Navy. Within twenty years his eyesight had deteriorated to the point where he could see only hand movements. Edward Wheaton, a veteran of the 26th Battalion, had suffered such severe mustard gas burning that his eyes finally had to be enucleated. Harold Ellison had served with the Princess Patricia's Canadian Light Infantry and lost an eye in 1916, returned to active service and, twenty years later, could no longer see from his remaining eye. On the other hand, in 1938, E.S. Palmer was struck from the SAPA membership rolls after treatment improved his vision.[36]

One blinded veteran, Charles Davey, formerly of the Royal Newfoundland Regiment, had lost an eye in action and lost the use of his remaining eye in a boiler explosion while working aboard a merchant vessel during the war. Beginning in 1934, the CNIB assisted Davey with rehabilitation training and other services and, two years later, Newfoundland's blinded soldiers were made associate members of SAPA.[37] Of course, they would become full members following Newfoundland's entry into Confederation in 1949.

Like SAPA, despite a high death rate in the early postwar years, St. Dunstan's experienced membership growth as a result of soldiers' war wounds worsening to the point of causing blindness. Eighty new cases were admitted in the three years ending in March 1934, bringing to more than 2,000 the number of war blinded treated there, compared to the 1,300 known to St. Dunstan's at the cessation of hostilities in 1918. Of nineteen new cases admitted to St. Dunstan's in 1934, for example, five resulted from the lingering effects of mustard gas.[38]

Although membership in SAPA almost always meant a veteran was pensionable as disabled, it did not automatically follow that the vision loss would be permanent or even that the pensions would always be there.

The Continuing Pension Struggle

Throughout the interwar period, SAPA worked informally with other veterans' groups to press the federal government for improvements to pension legislation or, in some cases, to prevent or repeal increasingly restrictive pension policy. SAPA especially supported the Amputations Association's petitions and resolutions and often followed the AA's lead on critical pension matters related to disabled veterans, such as attendance allowance. Attendance allowance was granted all blinded soldiers without useful sight – those with light perception only and those "dark blind." Ottawa also provided this assistance to pensioned veterans whose blindness was not attributable to war service. These men were ineligible for SAPA membership.[39] However, complete blindness from any cause made veterans eligible for membership in the AA, and the ties between the two groups were exceptionally close.[40]

Captain the Reverend Sydney Lambert, the British-born president of the Amputations Association, had joined Alberta's 50th Battalion as a private and lost his left leg at the thigh in action in 1916.[41] Like Baker, Lambert was one of Canada's most recognizable veterans. He almost always attended the SAPA AGMs, at which he unfailingly expressed strong praise for the organization and its advocacy work, especially Baker's, on behalf of all veterans' causes. At the 1931 AGM, Lambert, almost universally referred to as "Padre" Lambert, was elected honorary president of SAPA in a motion carried "with much enthusiasm" by the sixty-eight members present that reunion year. Reciprocally, Baker served on the Dominion Executive of the AA. Lambert also normally officiated during the nomination and election of officers and was a very popular figure in SAPA circles. That year, as mentioned in Chapter 2, the AA convention was held at the same time as the SAPA national reunion in Toronto.

In fact, so intertwined had these two groups become that James W. Doiron, a member of SAPA's executive and a leg amputee, could not attend the SAPA AGM, being tied up with AA work. SAPA stalwart Bill Dies was an arm amputee, and he and Doiron worked closely with Lambert to forge a common disabled veterans' agenda, especially in dealing with the federal government.[42] Of the approximately two hundred official Canadian war blinded of the First World War, three had lost one arm each: Bill Dies, Whaley Austin, from Huntsville, Ontario, and S.W. Johnston, from the Montreal area. Johnston and Dies were also normally members of the SAPA executive.[43] In 1937 eleven SAPA members, including virtually the entire executive, attended the AA convention in Saint John, New Brunswick.[44]

These harmonious relations worked to mutual advantage when dealing with a succession of parsimonious governments, or in seeking to coalesce varied, and sometimes bickering, veterans' organizations into a common front. Without a firm, united veterans' voice, the federal government could more easily delay or disregard their demands. Baker, a former DSCR official, admitted that it had proven difficult for Ottawa to move forward on pension matters given the multiple, and occasionally conflicting, demands of various veterans' groups. Before the end of 1931, a new group had been established to pressure the federal government to maintain pension levels: the Associated Veterans Organizations of Canada, which connected in common cause the Canadian Legion, the Army and Navy Veterans in Canada, the Amputations Association, the Canadian Pensioners' Association, and SAPA. With the mere adoption of a joint agenda, Baker claimed that "more was accomplished ... than in ten years previously" in terms of influencing the government on pension issues.[45]

The issue of widows' pensions was of great importance to SAPA, as it was to the AA. The men wanted assurances that, in the event of their demise, especially given the early mortality of so many of them, their survivors would have at least some guaranteed income in difficult economic times. Both groups sought an amendment to the Pension Act, which automatically denied continuing pensions to survivors unless the veteran's death was directly attributable to the cause of the disability, including blindness.[46] This was not always easy for widows to establish, and many who had depended on their husbands' disability pensions found themselves in straitened circumstances. Moreover, women who married already disabled veterans were ineligible for survivors' benefits. This policy did little to advance the matrimonial prospects of disabled veterans.

In 1930, veterans made some important gains, including the reinstatement of some commuted pensions and the granting of pensions to widows who had married disabled veterans prior to that year – which extended benefits to seven hundred widows previously excluded. The War Veterans' Allowance Act (WVAA) also significantly improved the lot of many war-blinded Canadians by accepting broader pensionable claims based on the "aggravation" of existing health conditions while on active service. The WVAA even accepted the notion that general service could be debilitating in the long term, explaining many veterans' premature aging and physical and mental "burn-out" while still in their forties or fifties. The years of exertion and privation at the front had caught up to many, and by September 1939, twenty-three thousand veterans had qualified for the allowance. In fact, the WVAA constituted a form of welfare for exhausted, unemployed, or unemployable veterans who were not otherwise eligible for pensions.[47]

SAPA continued to agitate for changes on behalf of non-pensioned widows, specifically wanting "widows of blinded soldiers [to] be eligible for widows' pensions irrespective of the ... cause of the soldier's death."[48] Finally, in 1936, Baker reported to the SAPA AGM that the Pension Act had been amended: the widow of any blinded soldier in receipt of at least an 80 percent disability pension, married prior to 1930, and dying from whatever cause, would automatically be entitled to a pension. Baker thereupon made a careful check of SAPA's records and noted that of thirty-five known widows of blinded men, eight were not receiving any pensions. All these cases were reviewed for eligibility.[49]

In 1933, Tom Bowman, president of the Canadian Pensioners' Association, attended the SAPA AGM and heaped effusive praise on SAPA for its feisty defence of veterans' entitlements. According to the SAPA minutes, Bowman "voiced his appreciation of the untiring efforts being made by the ... Club on behalf of disabled soldiers, pointing out this formed a very great stimulus to other organizations

whose memberships have suffered less in the service of their country."[50] SAPA's relatively small size was no measure of its, and Baker's,
influence.

In the spring of 1932, prompted by continuing pressure from
the Associated Veterans, the federal government decided to investigate the whole issue of veterans' pensions. One result of the study
was Bill 78, effective 1 October 1933, which abolished the Board of
Pension Commissioners and created a Canadian Pension Commission
(CPC) instead. This bill also inserted a clause in the Pension Act that
forbade changing the basis of a veteran's pension from "incurred on
service" to "aggravated on service" without a full review of the veteran's file. Such a change in status reduced the amount of the pension
for which Ottawa would be responsible, making the veteran only
"partially pensionable."The automatic file review would at least eliminate the possibility of a veteran's income being diminished by the
stroke of a bureaucratic pen. Given the nature of their wounds, however, most SAPA members received 100 percent disability pensions
and full attendance allowances. According to the DPNH, in 1934, 109
war blinded were fully pensioned with attendance allowance, 7 received less than 100 percent pensions as well as attendance allowance, and 37 others, who were blind between 80 and 100 percent,
received pensions varying from 10 to 100 percent, but did not qualify
for the allowance. All were eligible for federally funded aftercare.[51]

Some pension downgrading took place despite protests by the
Associated Veterans. For example, in 1933, four blinded soldiers who
for years had been receiving 100 percent disability pensions were
reduced to 20 percent in three cases and 10 percent in one, because
their vision had improved. Shortly thereafter another blinded soldier
was similarly downgraded. "These cases are under investigation and
no effort will be spared in ensuring just consideration of their claims,"
wrote Baker.[52] This was no idle boast. Within a year, SAPA, in co-
operation with other veterans' groups, was able to successfully argue
for the reinstatement of the five blinded veterans' pensions, at least

pending the submission to the commission of "special evidence" to prove their entitlement.[53] This was the first step in a lengthy process but it reaffirmed SAPA's raison d'être. By 1936 Baker had achieved partial success: two men were maintained at 100 percent disability rates and one was dropped to 40 percent. SAPA then lobbied success-fully to raise his pension to 60 percent. The other two cases were lost, with one man deemed "not sufficiently blind to warrant considera-tion as a blinded soldier."[54] Baker also obtained full disability pensions for SAPA members Richard Graham, W. Lamont, and J.D. McNeill. Graham had lost one eye during the war and had subsequently lost the vision in the other as a result of sympathetic blindness. He and Baker fought a three-year battle with pension authorities.[55]

The desperate government of Prime Minister R.B. Bennett, seeking to cut costs at the height of the Depression, wished to claw back as much as possible from the formidable expense of veterans' pensions. In March 1933, Ottawa even tried to cut pensions to veter-ans employed by the federal government. Seven war blinded, hun-dreds of war amputees, and thousands of other veterans would have been adversely affected. The Associated Veterans protested vigor-ously and the government backed down.[56] Meanwhile, the federal government had begun to dismiss pensioned veterans, including disabled veterans, from its employ on the dubious grounds that their pensions alone provided sufficient income. In 1932 the DPNH, pursu-ing this policy, incensed Baker by seeking to oblige the CNIB to dis-charge blinded veteran W. Jones from the CNIB's broom-making workshop in Toronto. His annual salary of $1,215 was at least partial-ly, and indirectly, being subsidized by Ottawa through its aftercare payments on his behalf. "If we discharge a blinded soldier on the grounds that he has sufficient pension to maintain him and without regard to the desirability of his being employed rather than idle, we would not have public opinion solidly behind us," argued Baker to the department. Ottawa threatened to withhold the CNIB's aftercare payments; Baker countered with the threat to launch a public appeal for funds on behalf of blinded soldiers' aftercare, something the original CNIB agreement with the federal government forbade. "You will readily understand," wrote Baker to the DPNH's A.M. Wright, "that an appeal on behalf of blind soldiers would readily net considerably more money than we have ever received from the Government of Canada for blinded soldiers' aftercare." The department did not argue the point, nor did it want a public battle with the blinded veterans. The compromise reached was that Jones could stay, but no additional pensioned war-blinded soldiers would be hired. Baker fought hard for the war blinded but never went so far as to damage the generally harmonious relations existing between the CNIB and the DPNH.[57]

The DPNH had also notified James Rawlinson, by then the departmental representative at Canada House, London, that he was to lose his position effective 31 August 1933. Furious, Baker immediately sought "reinstatement or transfer to some other department." Again, doggedness paid off: after a lengthy battle pitting senior departmental officials against Baker, Rawlinson was reinstated in his old job in 1934.[58] Because the disabled veterans represented patriotic wartime service and sacrifice and symbolized war's horrors, tampering with their pensions or employment prospects, even in depressionary times, could be fraught with political danger.

In March 1934, in a show of veterans' solidarity, the Amputations Association and the Legion held simultaneous conventions in Ottawa, with some joint functions. The Associated Veterans also met in Ottawa that year, and the entire SAPA executive, plus Alexander Viets and Harvey Lynes, attended the conference as delegates.[59] Several SAPA members also were accredited to the AA convention. The AA held a memorial service in the ballroom of the Chateau Laurier with the vice-regal couple, the Earl and Countess of Bessborough, in attendance, as were Prime Minister R.B. Bennett, William Lyon Mackenzie King, the Liberal leader of the Opposition, J.S. Woodsworth, leader of the Co-operative Commonwealth Federation, and a "very large number of prominent persons." SAPA, Legion, and Army and Navy Veterans representatives were also present. Their Excellencies then met with all the amputees and blinded soldiers.[60] In something of a publicity stunt, the veterans also marched to Parliament Hill in an ice storm. Among their number were many disabled veterans being manoeuvred in wheelchairs or hobbling on crutches through the sleet. The image was indelible. Later that week a delegation of veterans visited the prime minister and members of the cabinet to argue against any reduction in pensions, which the veterans felt were an entitlement unrelated to the men's ability to earn additional income. The Bennett government shelved its plans to curtail the men's incomes.[61]

Decades later, Brigadier James Melville, a former DPNH and Department of Veterans Affairs official, head of the CPC, and subsequently an honorary SAPA member, also noted, from the perspective of a government official, the very close and effective relationship between the AA and SAPA. Melville was present at many meetings of the Parliamentary Committee on Veterans Affairs and recalled how the "War Amps Storm Troopers," a veterans' delegation led by Sydney Lambert, Edwin Baker, and leg amputee Dick Myers of the War Amps, proved a formidable force in dealing with parliamentarians on pension issues. According to Melville, "Syd never held back his punches. If he had a point to raise he ... often would call on Eddie to present part of the brief which had been well prepared. If the Padre thought that proceedings were lagging he would call for a song from the Amps delegation and lead off [to the tune of the derisive Canadian First World War song 'Sam Hughes's Army']:

> We are the Amputations
> We are the Amps you know
> We cannot shoot, we cannot fight
> What bloody good are we?"

The parliamentarians normally yielded to these well-rehearsed theatrics. This trio was ably supported in the years before and after the Second World War by other high-profile veterans, including SAPA members Harvey Lynes and Bill Dies, Curly Christian, Canada's only quadruple amputee from the First World War, Edmonton's Madeline Jeffrey, Canada's only female amputee, Jack Counsell, a Second World War veteran and member of the Paraplegics Association, and Andy Hall of Regina, a double-arm amputee who graduated with a law degree from the University of Saskatchewan.[62]

At the November 1934 SAPA AGM, Baker was upbeat: "There has been no change in the basic scale of pension rates. This danger, which at one time appeared very imminent, now seems to be safely passed." He further felt that the recent creation of the Canadian Pension Commission had served to "humanize" the system. Mr. Justice Fawcett Taylor was the CPC's chairman, and Brigadier Harold F. Macdonald – himself, tellingly, a member of the Amputations Association – served as his chief assistant.[63] Things were looking up, after much struggle.

One issue of particular concern to Canada's war blinded community was the department's timely provision of artificial eyes. Of the 118 blinded soldiers resident in Canada in 1934, approximately 40 required fittings for both eyes and 50 for a single eye. Some 1,500 other veterans also needed artificial eyes. During and immediately after the First World War, these men (Baker among them) sometimes experienced difficulty in obtaining or replacing artificial eyes in Canada. Those who had been to St. Dunstan's normally were able to obtain excellent fits in London, and many obtained spare sets. Those returning to Canada without benefit of St. Dunstan's training had mixed results in obtaining glass eyes, especially if they had also suffered any damage to their eye sockets. Those who had suffered disfigurement in the area of the eyes frequently suffered ongoing discomfort, save for a few who travelled to New York for proper fittings of custom, handmade eyes.[64] Glass eyes did not last indefinitely; secretions from the eye sockets corroded the glass, often within a year. The corrosion was rough and perceptible to the touch. If worn in this state, the eyes could cause serious irritation, inflame the eyelids, and form heavy amounts of mucous. Extreme cold or hot temperatures also caused discomfort and could damage the eyes. Over time, small perforations could occur, and some eyes splintered or shattered, damaging the surrounding sockets.[65]

It was not until 1920 that the Department of Soldiers' Civil Re-establishment retained the services of a proper eye maker, Clifford Taylor, who nevertheless needed special training for the task of treating the war blinded. After several years of "conscientious effort, ability and experience," according to Baker, Taylor's expertise had become "second to none in the world" and SAPA members reciprocated with complete confidence in his skills.[66] However, Taylor was based at the Christie Street Hospital in Toronto, whereas the SAPA membership was scattered across Canada. Accordingly, during the 1923 and 1926 war-blinded reunions in Toronto, attendees from outside the region availed themselves of Taylor's services. The DSCR later furnished Taylor with travelling service equipment and sent him on periodic visits to eastern and western Canada to fit the men with replacement eyes. However, in 1933 the DPNH, the successor department to the DSCR, abruptly cancelled Taylor's scheduled trips, presumably as a result of fiscal restraint. He had not been west since 1929 or east since 1930.[67]

Many of the war blinded needed special fittings to ensure comfort, safety, and proper appearance, and, even though Taylor had created three basic eye models that met the requirements of many, he often needed to examine the men in person. The SAPA delegates attending the AA convention in March 1934 reaffirmed the need for the DPNH to provide these services and insisted that personal contact with Taylor was necessary for proper and effective eye fittings.[68] Baker sent a lengthy memorandum to the department outlining the situation. Ottawa proved attentive, and that year the DPNH authorized

Taylor to resume his trips to western and eastern Canada to meet with the war blinded individually.

Moreover, the DPNH took an important step toward the prevention of blindness in veterans by agreeing that glass eyes would be furnished not only to blinded soldiers but also to veterans who had lost one eye, in an attempt to forestall "trouble" with the remaining eye. This made financial sense to Ottawa, since sympathetic blindness attributable to wartime injuries was one of the primary causes in the growth of war blindedness in the interwar period. In addition, wherever warranted, protective goggles, eye camouflaging, and corrective lenses would be provided to blinded veterans, including those having lost a single eye, free of cost and as a matter of right.[69] In fact, SAPA believed that eye replacements were a routine aftercare service that should have been handled by the CNIB in the first place, using DPNH funds.

The persistent Baker, possessed of expert knowledge of pension issues and veterans' affairs generally, repeatedly proved his worth to the war-blinded community. Despite the veterans' Depression-fuelled fears and their battles against downward pension adjustments, the 1930s were not nearly as bad as forecast.

The War Blinded and Veterans' Unity

In the late 1920s and early 1930s, there were a number of calls within the veterans' community for greater "unity" among the disparate veterans' organizations in order to more successfully militate for better pensions and entitlements. Yet the smaller, special-interest veterans' groups, like SAPA, had never felt that their members' needs would be met by being absorbed into a broader organization, such as the Canadian Legion. So long as these small groups, the most prominent being the Amputations Association, SAPA, the Army and Navy Veterans in Canada, and the Canadian Pensioners' Association, did not attack or compete with the Legion, co-operation was possible. But even the

Legion itself was wracked by factionalism at this time and disillusionment gripped many veterans. The Legion was also experiencing
grave financial difficulties and a stagnant membership; it seemed
to lack leadership and a dynamic action plan.[70]

The government, press, and ordinary Canadians could not help
but notice that Canada's veterans could not find a unified voice, especially given that some discontented veterans, within and without
the Legion, voiced increasingly radical political ideas and social solutions. Perhaps the Legion was too moderate in its dealings with Ottawa? There was an attempt at veterans' unity in 1930 but, while
supportive of the concept, the SAPA AGM passed a motion that year
that "nothing should be done prejudicial to the relationship between
this Club and the Amputations Association," the latter group being
occasionally at odds with the Legion. Not all veterans got along, and
SAPA had to make some choices, the obvious one being to maintain
its firm alliance with the AA. Some years later, Baker noted that SAPA
members "value the interest which the AA has always taken in our
Association and reciprocate to the best of our ability in supporting
their legislative and other activities since our interests are so closely
allied with theirs." In fact, so close were the ties between Baker and
Lambert, and between their respective organizations, that, for SAPA,
collaborating with the AA had become a matter of "established
policy."[71] Participating in the Associated Veterans Organizations of
Canada, an umbrella group of like-minded institutions formed for
the purpose of demonstrating solidarity before federal authorities,
was as far as SAPA was willing to go.

In August 1934, SAPA members attended the Canadian Corps
Reunion in Toronto, held at the famed Canadian National Exhibition
in conjunction with the city's centenary celebrations. SAPA had
moved back by one month the date of its local reunion so that members could also attend the grander veterans' gathering, which was
organized according to service in wartime units. The organizing
committee, made up of representatives from several veterans'

organizations, provided special bus transportation to the thirty blinded veterans who took part. "All who attended enjoyed the re- markable demonstrations of the old Canadian Corps spirit," wrote Baker. Several blinded soldiers attended their individual unit dinners but most chose to dine together at Pearson Hall, where the House Committee had, as usual, made all the arrangements.[72] This implied a greater commonality with the similarly afflicted than with wartime comrades, suggesting in this instance that postwar veterans' experi- ences supplanted wartime soldiers' bonds.

Still, SAPA sought the friendship of all groups, and relations with the Legion were generally amicable and co-operative. For ex- ample, in 1934 the SAPA AGM expressed thanks to Colonel W.H. Scarth, secretary of the Legion's Ontario Command, for his "thought- ful consideration ... and many kindnesses."[73] Moreover, representatives of the Legion sometimes addressed the SAPA AGMs and, in 1938, Baker could note the friendly relations existing between the two veterans' groups.[74] Many SAPA members had also joined the Legion. Besides, the formidable Baker was well connected with the Legion's leaders and ordinary members, was frequently taken into their confi- dences, and engaged in voluminous correspondence with Legion officials. He benefitted from virtually a standing invitation to any Legion activity, commemorative event, anniversary dinner, or public gathering.[75] Baker, in his report to the 1935 AGM, noted that SAPA "has enjoyed the friendliest relationship and the fullest possible co-operation" of all veterans' organizations.[76]

SAPA's representations to the 1936 Parliamentary Committee dealing with veterans' affairs were, as usual, delivered in association with the AA. This relationship was rock-solid, but Baker noted at the 1936 AGM that "some difficulties were experienced as a result of rela- tionships existing between other organizations."[77] SAPA sought scru- pulously to avoid the fractious internecine rivalry among Canadian veterans' groups. For example, when the contentious and firebrand Canadian Corps Association (CCA), founded in 1934 to rival the more

moderate Canadian Legion, invited SAPA to send a delegate to the
planning committee for its July 1938 convention in Toronto, considerable discussion, perhaps consternation, ensued among SAPA's
Executive Committee members. Matters had become extremely political and bitter between the Legion and the CCA, which were actively competing for members and funds, and the war blinded sought
to avoid becoming ensnared in the conflict. SAPA demurred until
learning which other veterans' organizations (i.e., the AA) would be
participating at the CCA convention. In the meantime, to preserve
peace for the upcoming SAPA Christmas dinner at Pearson Hall,
representatives from all of the major groups, save the CCA, were
invited to attend.[78] By this action, SAPA seemed more inclined to
the Canadian Legion's point of view.

The issue of how to deal with the CCA was delicate. The intense
rivalry between the CCA and the Legion had deteriorated to the
point where all major veterans' organizations were publicly stating
their opinions about the CCA in the press. Although SAPA president
Harvey Lynes had tentatively been appointed a SAPA delegate to the
CCA reunion committee, he had not attended the committee's January 1938 meeting and "was doubtful of the advisability of doing so"
in the future. SAPA wrote to the CCA to explain in a friendly manner
that the war-blinded's participation was "contingent upon general
representation and co-operation of all veteran organizations." This
included the Legion. Since it was clear from recent incendiary comments reported in the press that this would be impossible, SAPA
elected not to participate in the CCA's deliberations. However, SAPA
officially encouraged its members to attend the CCA convention as
part of any unit reunions that might be organized, and SAPA distrib-
uted literature about the upcoming event. In addition, the war blinded held a local (Toronto area) reunion at the same time as the CCA's
1938 convention, so that the war blinded might attend both events
if desired.[79] The SAPA executive thus tried to strike a careful balance.

Despite these precautions, SAPA very nearly became directly embroiled in the Legion-CCA feud. In 1938, two Executive Committee meetings on the matter took place within nine days, the second to deal with a letter received from the Ontario Command of the Legion on the subject of SAPA's position in the dispute. SAPA replied that it "did not wish to take part in any controversy, nor should the name of the Club be used either by the Corps or the Legion" in the public debate between the two groups.[80] Wishing to appear strictly neutral, and also perhaps to broker a reconciliation for the good of all veterans, SAPA invited representatives from all veterans' groups, including the CCA, to its 1939 Christmas dinner.[81] It is unclear who actually attended. The quarrels besetting the veterans' community were of great concern, but could not be allowed to distract SAPA from pursuing its own objectives. Even the momentous 1936 reunion of CEF veterans and their families on the hallowed site of Vimy Ridge, in northern France, had not moved the veterans to common ground.

The Vimy Pilgrimage

Following the First World War, Britain, Australia, and the United States organized official pilgrimages to the battlefields and the memorials located there dedicated to their war dead. Canada, which had suffered about as many battle deaths as Australia or the United States, was a bit slower off the mark. Yet, when a national pilgrimage was finally undertaken in 1936, the impressive spectacle powerfully symbolized the bonds existing between Canada's war dead, its surviving veterans, and a grateful nation.[82]

At the SAPA AGM of 5 September 1930, the possibility was raised of the war blinded's participation in a large-scale Canadian veterans' pilgrimage to France, to coincide with the inauguration, still years away, of the massive Canadian national war memorial at

Vimy Ridge, in April 1917, the site of one of the Canadian Corps' most impressive victories. Although the veterans' community in general had been publicly discussing the prospect of a European pilgrimage tour, little concrete planning had taken place thus far. Within a year the dismal and worsening economic crisis forced a postponement. SAPA had intended to participate as a joint venture with the Amputations Association, but many of the amputee pensioners felt that they could not afford the trip. SAPA's leaders believed strongly that the nation's war blinded should be represented in any future endeavour and agreed that the organization would assist any of its own members wishing to attend as individuals.[83] But as the Depression deepened, talks stagnated and plans were shelved.

In August 1934, the Canadian Legion, in co-operation with federal authorities, took the pilgrimage project in hand. It had long been the Legion's idea that a Canadian pilgrimage would coincide with the unveiling of the Vimy memorial and that a series of lesser events in France, Belgium, and Britain commemorating important Canadian feats of arms would also take place. Seeking to embrace all veterans and veterans' groups, the Legion formed a National Pilgrimage Committee that included representatives from several other ex-servicemen's organizations. The purpose of the committee was to organize a trip to Vimy by as many Canadian veterans and their immediate family members as wished to go. Ben W. Allen, of the Legion's Dominion Command, served as the full-time main organizer of the pilgrimage. The Legion invited Edwin Baker, as one of Canada's best-known and universally respected veterans, to join the National Pilgrimage Committee as a SAPA representative. The Amputations Association and other groups of disabled or pensioned veterans were also represented. Given his public profile and administrative skills, Baker would be a key figure on this committee and also served as the chief organizer for the contingent of war-blinded veterans.[84]

In August 1935, Baker wrote to every member of SAPA asking them to consider participating in the pilgrimage, noting that this voyage would likely be the "only opportunity most" members would have of returning to the battlefields at the very modest cost of $160 per person, accommodations included. To encourage them, Baker also reminded members that a reunion of Canadian and other St. Dunstaners was in the offing. The CNIB, with assistance from the DPNH, committed to funding any Canadian war-blinded pilgrim's travel expenses to Montreal, the port of departure. As late as October, Baker hoped that thirty SAPA members would take part in the pilgrimage, though this proved optimistic. By January 1936 only ten had registered – a not inconsiderable number from a small base of members, especially taking into account the nature of their handicap and the limited resources of most.[85]

Baker wanted the war blinded to travel together on the same ship, berthed in close proximity in accommodations "suitable" for the travelling blind. This way the men could be assured of the greatest safety and least inconvenience and also be available to support one another. Some among the prospective blinded pilgrims were concerned about the travel arrangements, but Baker saw to everything – though not without effort and perseverance.[86] As late as April 1936, the Legion's Allen was unconvinced that so many blinded veterans should travel across the Atlantic in a single group, apparently fearing for their safety should the ship suffer disaster. A testy Baker made it plain to Allen that there were no special risks and that, quite the contrary, in the event of an emergency, a blind person is "less apt to be affected than a general passenger; this has been demonstrated time and again on land in cases of fire." Baker strongly reiterated the war blinded's desire to travel as a body and made only a single concession: that no more than three or four be assigned to the same lifeboat.[87] This sort of misunderstanding of the abilities and needs of the war blinded reinforced the rationale for having formed and maintained a war blinded's veterans' organization separate from the Legion. In early July pilgrimage organizers assigned the war blinded, as a body, to the passenger liner *Antonia*, which departed Montreal on 16 July.[88]

At the September 1936 SAPA AGM, Baker submitted a very detailed report of the activities of Canada's war blinded on the 1936 Vimy Pilgrimage. Fourteen participated among a group of more than eight thousand Canadian veterans and their families travelling from North America and Britain. Baker and his wife did not accompany the main group since, as a member of the planning committee, he was required to travel with the advance party. He and Jesse departed on 3 July from Montreal in company with his close friend, Padre Lambert, and his wife. Nine SAPA members, most from Ontario, travelled with the main pilgrimage party and all but one brought their wives. SAPA stalwart Bill Dies could not attend at the last minute due to illness in his family. Two other Canadian war-blinded veterans travelled separately to England and then to Vimy, while another two blinded CEF veterans resident in Britain also attended.[89]

During the ceremony, on 26 July, the fourteen Canadian war blinded were, according to Baker's report, the first group of veterans to be greeted by King Edward VIII. One Toronto newspaper reported that the king spoke to each man individually and asked where they came from, apparently at the instigation of Curly Christian, Canada's only surviving quadrilateral amputee, who sought to introduce his "blind pals" to the monarch.[90] The blinded men placed a commemorative wreath at the base of the Vimy Memorial and also at the Tomb of the Unknown Soldier in Paris, the tomb of Marshal Foch in Paris, the Unknown Soldier's Grave in Brussels, and at the Menin Gate in Ypres. The wreaths were stylized torches with maple leaf flames and ribbons inscribed, "Blinded Soldiers of Canada."[91] While in Paris, Baker also paid a fraternal visit to Monsieur Scapini, the president of the French war blinded's association, the Union des Aveugles de guerre.

The blinded veterans then returned to London with the main pilgrimage party. On 31 July, St. Dunstan's arranged a special reunion of the Canadian war blinded in the British Medical Association Hall on Tavistock Square, not far from St. Dunstan's offices in Regent's Park. The twelve blinded soldiers who had travelled from Canada were joined by twenty-four resident in the United Kingdom and one in Belgium. Sir Neville Pearson (son of Arthur) and Sir Ian and Lady Fraser greeted them as they arrived, and a luncheon for all thirty-seven men was arranged to which was also invited Vincent Massey, Canadian high commissioner in London. There were also present four Australian, one South African, and one New Zealand war-blinded veterans. This prompted Massey to quip in his remarks that the assembly reminded him of an imperial conference. The Commonwealth veterans renewed many old acquaintances from St. Dunstan's days. That evening a number of war blinded accepted the invitation of the French government, tendered to all Canadian pilgrims, to spend five days in France as guests of the French Republic. Those availing themselves of this opportunity included ten Canadian war blinded and their wives or escorts, though Baker was not among them.[92]

The Canadian war-blinded community was well represented at Vimy, and Baker had been one of the highest-profile veterans there. The men had assumed pride of place at the ceremony and a grateful nation seemingly had not forgotten them. Canada's war blinded were proud of their war service and throughout the dark years of the Depression remained true to the ideals for which it was rendered.

The 1930s brought richly deserved honours to the loyal Edwin Baker for his work on behalf of Canada's veteran and civilian blind. In 1935 he received the Order of the British Empire in the King's New Year's Honours List, and in 1939 he received an honorary doctorate of law from Queen's University, his alma mater.[93] The previous year, Minister of National Defence Ian Mackenzie wrote Baker, whom he knew well, that he was promoting the latter to the rank of honorary lieutenant colonel, a "pleasant surprise" for which Baker was deeply appreciative. The announcement was gazetted 19 February 1938. Subsequently, for other than his intimates, he was normally referred to as Colonel Baker.[94]

Notwithstanding some disillusioning postwar experiences, SAPA remained a proudly patriotic, even conservative institution. Like other Canadian veterans' groups, SAPA adopted a robustly patriotic stance as the international situation deteriorated in the late 1930s. At SAPA's September 1938 AGM, held during the war scare resulting from the Czech crisis, members present passed a resolution "in support of any policy of adequate defence ... to safeguard the interests of Canada and permit effective co-operation with the Empire forces where such is vitally necessary for the preservation of Empire security."[95] The old soldiers, who knew first-hand the horrors a new war would surely bring, did not question the righteousness of Britain's, and Canada's, cause.

But before war broke out, the nation's war blinded had yet another opportunity to display their loyalty and rub shoulders with the monarch (since December 1936, George VI). As a sign of Baker's prominent profile in the veterans' community, the Department of National Defence invited him to serve on the committee arranging the May 1939 visit of the king and queen to Canada, with special reference to their unveiling of the National War Memorial in Ottawa. Baker, representing Canada's war-blinded servicemen, met the king at the unveiling ceremony. The Department of Pensions and National Health transmitted to SAPA George VI's appreciation for the role blinded soldiers had played in welcoming the royal couple to Canada. Baker mailed copies of the message to each blinded soldier.[96]

On 1 September 1939, the day Germany invaded Poland, launching the Second World War, the SAPA Executive Committee cancelled the reunion slated for mid-September, "in view of the existing crisis." The upcoming AGM was postponed until further notice and expressions of support were sent to the federal government and to the king.[97] Nine days later Canada was at war once again. At that time there were 157 living former members of the Canadian forces who had been blinded during the First World War or as a result of their wartime service. Of these, 118 lived in Canada, 34 in Britain, 4 in the United States, and 1 in Belgium.[98] The Second World War meant these survivors would be joined by an even greater number who would pay a similarly terrible price in the defence of the realm.

4 Rehabilitating the Blinded Casualties of the Second World War, 1939-50

One of the Department's greatest responsibilities is the rehabilitation of those who have incurred disability in the defence of their country.

– Walter S. Woods, Deputy Minister,
Department of Veterans Affairs

On 10 September 1939, Canada, acting in its own right, declared war on Germany. Although not with wild enthusiasm as in 1914, Canadians went to the aid of Britain with grim determination. From a population of nearly twelve million in 1945, slightly more than one million Canadians donned uniforms during the conflict. Overseas, following tragedy at Hong Kong and disaster at Dieppe, Canada's army fought in Sicily and on the Italian mainland and participated in the invasion of Normandy and the campaign to liberate northwest Europe until victory in 1945. The Royal Canadian Navy grew fifty-fold, enrolling nearly 100,000 and playing an important role in winning the Battle of the Atlantic. From a meagre force of largely obsolete aircraft in 1939, the Royal Canadian Air Force (RCAF), which enlisted almost 250,000 men and women during the war, played a major role in the Allies' gaining of air superiority in

Europe and in mounting devastating bomber raids against enemy targets.

These military contributions helped win the war, but the cost was high: more than forty-two thousand Canadians lost their lives, and another fifty-five thousand were wounded. Hundreds of thousands of veterans returned after the cessation of hostilities to a confident country, able and willing to extend to these men and women comprehensive civil re-establishment programs. But long before the shooting stopped, a regular stream of wounded military personnel returned to Canada to obtain medical care, and, if disabled, to be retrained to continue productive lives. So it was with the country's war-blinded veterans, whose disabilities were severe but who successfully reintegrated into civil life.

The Canadian National Institute for the Blind (CNIB), using funds made available by the Department of Pensions and National Health (DPNH), and, from October 1944, the Department of Veterans Affairs, organized a complete retraining regimen for the returning war blinded, including arranging for their accommodation in Toronto and delivering a full range of aftercare services. This model of public and private co-operation built on the foundations of the First World War experience and benefitted from the existence of the well-established fraternal veterans' organization, the Sir Arthur Pearson Association of War Blinded (as it was renamed in 1942, or SAPA). Edwin Albert Baker, the CNIB's managing director and SAPA's secretary-treasurer, was, throughout this period, the catalyst for ensuring that the institute provided the returning men with the immediate care, subsequent training, and postwar employment opportunities to which they were entitled.

Planning for Success

From the outbreak of the Second World War, the CNIB reprised its role as provider of rehabilitation training, employment placement, and perpetual aftercare for Canada's new generation of war blinded. The institute, SAPA, and the DPNH worked together to put in place a comprehensive re-establishment program. St. Dunstan's, too, remained important in the lives of many of Canada's Second World War blinded veterans.

Sensing the approach of war, in November 1938, St. Dunstan's had made an offer to representatives of Britain's War Office, Admiralty, Air Ministry, and Ministry of Pensions to replicate its services from the First World War and assume responsibility for the care and training of Britain's war blinded, including members of the auxiliary services. This offer was "gratefully accepted." Sir Ian Fraser also offered the use of St. Dunstan's new headquarters and superb ophthalmologic centre at Ovingdean, a twelve-acre site near Brighton on Britain's south coast, where the latest treatment and surgical practices could be offered to two hundred patients.[1]

Fraser highlighted the critical importance of quickly transferring men from service hospitals to St. Dunstan's before they were discharged to civilian life. This had been possible during the First World War through an "informal understanding" with No. 2 London General Hospital, which served as a clearing house for eye cases. The British government agreed that all service personnel totally blind or "blind for all practical purposes" would be released to the care of St. Dunstan's "as soon as the patient is considered fit for travel." Fraser expected no payment for hospital expenses while a man remained in service. But, after a man's discharge to civilian life as a pensioner, he expected the Ministry of Pensions to "pay the standard fee as it would to any other hospital." If St. Dunstan's required funding for men experiencing lengthy periods of pre-discharge hospitalization, this would be negotiated at a future date.[2]

In November 1939, with the first Canadian troops shortly to be dispatched to Britain, Fraser sent Vincent Massey, Canada's high commissioner in London, a copy of St. Dunstan's agreement with the British government and made a nearly identical offer to assist the

Canadian war blinded. The only change Fraser wished the Canadian authorities to consider was that, given the likelihood of a longer delay between a Canadian soldier's arrival at Ovingdean and his discharge from military service (indeed, the Canadian government might not discharge its military personnel overseas), St. Dunstan's would ask for payment for their hospital treatment. However, St. Dunstan's would assume the costs of retraining following the men's hospitalization. Similar offers were made to all the dominions, though Fraser agreed that the existence of the CNIB and the uncommon zeal and devotion of Edwin Baker had made Canada easily the leader among the dominions in the care of the blind. Fraser recognized that Baker might wish to repatriate Canadians as soon as feasible and train them in Toronto; in fact, Fraser encouraged this practice. But he also noted that, during any "waiting periods" in Britain, the men should attend St. Dunstan's, where they would be better off than anywhere else. In fact, St. Dunstan's was preparing to establish new training facilities elsewhere in England.[3]

Massey forwarded a copy of the St. Dunstan's agreement and offer to Prime Minister William Lyon Mackenzie King, who also served as the secretary of state for external affairs. The file was passed to O.D. Skelton, the undersecretary of state for external affairs. There seemed to be no hurry in the matter; it was the period of the so-called Phoney War, following the occupation of Poland by the Germans but before the desperate days of the spring of 1940 when the Germans defeated France and occupied most of western Europe, imperilling Britain itself. Few Canadian troops had arrived in the British Isles by January 1940 and there had as yet been no Canadians blinded in service.

Skelton consulted officials at DPNH and the Department of National Defence (DND). R.E. Wodehouse, MD, a deputy minister at DPNH, recommended that Fraser's offer be accepted and further advised Skelton that any costs incurred for Canadian soldiers' hospitalization at St. Dunstan's would be paid by his department. But such was Baker's standing in government circles that before DND would concur in accepting Fraser's offer, departmental officials thought it best to consult with Baker. In fact, he was busy preparing his own brief to Ottawa. Wanting the war-blinded casualties of the current war to benefit from the St. Dunstan's experience he knew so well, Baker felt it was essential for any blinded Canadians to be concentrated at Ovingdean, where all British eye casualties were sent. Not surprisingly, Baker replied to DND that so "Canadian soldiers may receive the benefits of early, expert training in a suitable environment," they should be sent to St. Dunstan's at Ovingdean as soon as possible. Baker was strongly of the opinion that "the Canadian Government should take advantage of any reasonable plan" St. Dunstan's might offer rather than "attempt to set up special independent facilities."[4] Convalescing war-blinded soldiers should proceed to St. Dunstan's for preliminary training until their return to Canada or discharge in Britain. If discharged in Britain, the men should remain at St. Dunstan's for rehabilitation training as well. All servicemen discharged in Canada would receive benefits under the authority of the DPNH, including rehabilitation training at the CNIB.[5]

Armed with the concurrence of these two ministries, and assured of Baker's approval, Skelton replied to Massey that, as a matter of policy, Canadians should be sent, at least initially, to St. Dunstan's.[6] There would be no repeat of the confusion in this regard that had reigned during the First World War. Given the timing of Fraser's offer to Ottawa and the existence of Baker's very detailed plan of action, collusion between the two men to help convince a probably already-willing Canadian government to send its blinded soldiers to St. Dunstan's cannot be ruled out. In any event, the result was what was best for the men.

Since the outbreak of war, Baker had been in frequent contact with DPNH, DND, and St. Dunstan's to ascertain what arrangements were being made for the war blinded of the Second World War and pledging the CNIB's full assistance. His recommendation to stream any newly blinded casualties into the existing CNIB training and rehabilitation framework, honed by more than twenty years of experience, became the cornerstone of Ottawa's war-blinded rehabilitation policies. Baker had provided DPNH with the blueprint for rehabilitation and also for entering into an agreement with St. Dunstan's.

Baker expected a "radical change" from the post-1918 experiences of the repatriated Canadian war blinded.[7] The existence of the CNIB would make all the difference, especially given its extensive training facilities, experienced staff and volunteers, nationwide aftercare services, and successful job placement programs. Baker outlined his scheme to the DPNH in his 6 December 1939 memorandum, "Treatment and Care of Blinded Soldiers of the Present War." To begin with, a "carefully selected rehabilitated blinded soldier" from the earlier conflict should contact the newly blinded soldier at the earliest possible time. "Any soldier on first learning that he is definitely blind for life needs care that cannot be given by the ophthalmic surgeon, the doctor or nurse. His special need is for someone ... who, having passed the same way, can sympathize while at the same time reassure." Baker, who had benefitted from such a visit by Arthur Pearson in 1915, was convinced that this sort of initial contact had a "distinct therapeutic value and will actually influence if not hasten general recuperation."[8]

The St. Dunstan's facility at Ovingdean served the same function that the 2nd General Hospital at Chelsea had performed during the First World War. British forces suffered forty-three serious eye injuries in the first six months of the war, and by 1941 more than one hundred war-blinded men had passed through the facility. Owing to the threats of bombardment and even invasion following the German occupation of the French channel coast in June 1940, St. Dunstan's relocated its rehabilitation facilities, men's accommodations, and some medical facilities to the relative safety of Church Stretton in

Shropshire, northern England, where St. Dunstan's operated until the summer of 1946. In 1943 Sir Ian Fraser wrote that Church Stretton was "the St. Dunstan's of this war."[9]

St. Dunstan's, either at Ovingdean or Church Stretton, would provide wounded Canadians with immediate counsel and familiarization training in Braille, typewriting, and various handicrafts during their convalescence, until the men could be returned to Canada. These activities were not vocational training but rather were meant to "cultivate their manual dexterity and interest them in some absorbing hobby." However, Baker was adamant that if a soldier "is anxious to return home and desires a course available, or which can be provided, then he should be returned as soon as possible."[10] No one argued the point. If a soldier preferred training in Canada or if it became more advisable or convenient that his training be carried out in Canada, he would be repatriated and the CNIB would become responsible for his welfare, on behalf of DPNH.

Occupational rehabilitation training would be offered in Britain only in the event of a man being discharged overseas and deciding to take up permanent residency there, or if certain specialized training courses were not offered in Canada. Such cases proved very rare. The CNIB provided the full gamut of rehabilitation training in Toronto. At this early stage in the war, the educational and vocational courses were planned to include handicrafts such as broom making and leather working, business courses such as Braille shorthand, commercial typewriting, and the operation of concession stands and canteens, joinery, poultry keeping, and industrial work. Specialized courses might be offered to individuals exhibiting specific aptitudes. Thereafter, employment placement and aftercare services would be extended to the men. Baker noted that the CNIB and SAPA "have always regarded hospital [care,] training and aftercare service for Canadian soldiers blinded in war as the responsibility of Government" and that "in accordance with the policy followed since the last war ... it is expected that actual cost for training and aftercare will be met by the Government of Canada."[11] Still, where DPNH would not cover the expenses of "emergency or special services" that the CNIB deemed important to a blinded soldier's well-being and rehabilitation, the CNIB would find sufficient monies from its small but still active Blinded Soldiers' Fund, maintained through bequests and unsolicited donations.[12]

Baker worked hard to secure a workable system of immediate assistance and supervision in Canada for the returning war blinded. After the federal government accepted the St. Dunstan's offer, it was also understood that the CNIB would be informed and perhaps consulted about each such casualty. The CNIB worked out an arrangement with the Department of National Defence whereby a sighted escort in Britain would help the blinded to their point of embarkation for Canada, while DND informed the institute of their impending arrival so that the institute's representatives could meet them.[13] Baker also suggested to the Inter-Departmental Sub-Committee on Major Disabilities, of which he was a leading member, that since the war blinded were to be concentrated at Toronto's Christie Street Hospital, a blinded soldier and a Voluntary Aid Detachment worker (VAD) should visit them "for encouragement" and to provide small comforts and amenities. It was his view that, if medically feasible, the men should begin preliminary training at Pearson Hall even while on strength of the Christie Street Hospital.[14]

To 31 March 1940, no Canadian war blinded had yet been brought to Baker's attention, but he was aware that such casualties were "inevitable" in war. "The obligation which devolves upon the Institute," he wrote in 1940, "is to see that we are prepared to meet any demands the Government makes upon us for the provision of the necessary facilities. The Institute is prepared to fulfill any such obligation." In the absence of a formal agreement, and while still somewhat vague on details, the CNIB and DPNH had an "understanding" on the principle that "adequate provision will be made for the care and re-education of any soldiers who suffer loss of sight as a result of current hostilities." Moreover, the institute and SAPA were "in complete accord" and worked in tandem on matters pertaining to new blinded casualties' rehabilitation.[15]

Baker seemed quite clear on how rehabilitation should proceed. In October 1940, he wrote Ottawa's Inter-Departmental Subcommittee on Major Disabilities that "every Canadian soldier should be required to take one to three months general training. This training period will vary greatly depending on the intelligence, aptitude, outlook, physical condition and extent of preliminary training already received during the treatment and convalescent period." Of occupational training he wrote, "On completion of the general course, each blinded soldier, having been carefully studied as to characteristics, mental and physical, disabilities other than blindness, if any, [and] previous education and experience" was to be channelled toward a suitable line of work for which the CNIB would provide training. Although each man's interests would be taken into account, the chances of career success needed to be high. "In general," he wrote, "the policy of the Institute is to oppose training any individual ... for an occupation in which there may be no prospect of employment." The CNIB exhibited a deep understanding of the men's desires to be independent and to pursue their own interests, and would assist every step of the way so long as these goals remained realistic. "It is the definite purpose of the Institute," noted the 1944 CNIB Annual Report, "to encourage every blinded soldier to make full use of whatever abilities he possesses." Baker felt that those war-blinded veterans who might prefer to settle in their homes without benefit of full training lacked "imagination and ambition." On the other hand, the institute would be in a position to provide some sheltered workshops where some men with minimal physical abilities, or who suffered from psychological problems, could find employment under "considerate supervision."[16]

As heartened as Baker must have been early in the war by the seeming lack of Canadian war-blinded servicemen, so, too, must he have been frustrated by the slow pace at which formal arrangements were concluded between the CNIB and Ottawa for a rehabilitation scheme. He carefully shepherded his ideas through the Sub-committee on Major Disabilities, which endorsed all the points expressed in his December 1939 memorandum. Well organized, and highly respected by his colleagues on the committee, Baker submitted lengthy reports and suggestions for treating and caring for the war blinded at virtually each meeting and, in November 1940, the sub-committee accepted almost verbatim the plan he outlined in yet another lengthy memorandum of 26 October 1940.

But translating this acceptance into government action, such as an Order-in-Council, was another matter. In addition to a lack of urgency occasioned by the absence of blinded casualties, to October 1940 no firm agreement had been reached between DND and DPNH respecting the timing of the transfer of administrative responsibilities for casualties.[17] This slight turf war and budgetary issue to some extent delayed the conclusion of government agreements with outside agencies such as the CNIB. Finally, on 4 August 1942, the Canadian government passed Order-in-Council PC 6837, which formalized the DPNH's arrangements with the CNIB for the men's aftercare along the lines suggested by Baker and more or less in accordance with the system already in place. The agreement was signed by both parties six days later.[18] This was just in time, since the first few war-blinded casualties had begun to return to Canada.

In October 1942, at which time fewer than ten Canadians had been blinded and only a few had been repatriated to begin CNIB training, Baker reported that the agreement between the CNIB and the DPNH called for a monthly payment of forty-five dollars to the CNIB per man for room and board, plus additional costs pertaining to retraining, including instructional fees and equipment. Furthermore, for every man on the Blinded Soldier Register, Ottawa agreed to pay fifty dollars a year to the institute for aftercare, including staying in regular contact with the men, organizing social functions and reunions, and maintaining equipment. Half of this aftercare money would be turned over to the CNIB regional division in which the men resided, with each division clearly reporting the services it was providing.[19] After the war, the Department of Veterans Affairs (DVA) doubled the amount allotted to each man's aftercare.

Meanwhile, there were some important details to be worked out in Britain. On 31 August 1942, Baker and Fraser, who was spending several days in Toronto, proceeded to Ottawa to meet with Brigadier R.M. Gorssline, director general of medical services at DND, to make firm arrangements for the retraining of the Canadian war blinded at St. Dunstan's. Notwithstanding Ottawa's eager earlier acquiescence in sending Canadian casualties to St. Dunstan's, the costs and charge-back system for medical attention at the ophthalmologic hospital at Ovingdean still had not been established formally. Given that St. Dunstan's was extending its training benefits to Canadians, Baker and Fraser proposed at the meeting that the Canadian government extend the period for which it would pay hospital fees to cover the preliminary training period as well. Moreover, the CNIB sought an assurance from DND that all cases of serious eye wounds, even though the victim remained outside the definition of blindness, be reported as soon as possible to St. Dunstan's and the CNIB for "review" and to "follow the progress of selected cases, especially where there is an uncertain or bad prognosis."[20] Baker hoped that, if they were identified early, these men's eyesight might be saved. This was another example of his proactive approach in dealing with a slow-moving bureaucracy. Finally, in February 1943, Ross Millar, MD, assistant deputy minister (medical) at DPNH, wrote Gorssline that DPNH had made all necessary arrangements with St. Dunstan's and was "prepared by direct contract with St. Dunstan's to cover all the expenses necessary" until the men could return to Canada, when they would pass into the hands of the CNIB. Similar letters were written to Gorssline's counterparts in the air force and the navy.[21]

Despite some differences between the St. Dunstan's experience of the First World War and that of the Second, the St. Dunstan's
spirit had not changed. Walter Thornton, a British war-blinded veteran
of the Second World War, recalled that "the spirit of victory over
blindness is embodied in the lives of [St. Dunstan's] members. This is
a spirit you catch in savouring the comradeship of the St. Dunstan's
community life. During training the steps toward the cure become
apparent – acceptance, the support of others, attaining perspective,
and acquiring the practical skills of everyday life. There is no doubt
that you achieve these more readily in the company of your fellow-
blind, partly inspired by their example."[22] This is how it had been
under Pearson's tutorship during the earlier war. The blind learned
best from each other.

In May 1943, Lieutenant-General P.J. Montague, senior combatant officer at Canadian Military Headquarters, London, visited Church
Stretton and reported to Ottawa by telegram: "I was much impressed
with the efficiency of the organization [and] what to me seemed
incredible results and the happy courage of the men and women
patients ... Fullest co-operation exists between Canadian Military
Headquarters and Fraser. Cannot conceive of a better man to direct
this work."[23] Baker's planning had paid off; the system was working.
In April 1944, nine Canadians were in training at St. Dunstan's.[24]

Helping Beleaguered St. Dunstaners

When the Second World War broke out, St. Dunstan's Sir Ian Fraser
was worried about the strain it would impose on the Commonwealth's war-blinded veterans. Prophetically, he "thought of their
sons, now growing into manhood, many of whom would be sacrificed
in the war ... [and] these thoughts made me very sad." At least forty-
eight sons and daughters of SAPA members served during the war,
of whom five lost their lives and several others were wounded, as

their fathers had been. Harry Minnett, son of war-blinded veteran
A. Minnett, and Francis Taylor, son of T.H. Taylor, were both killed at
Dieppe during the ill-fated raid of 19 August 1942. Two other SAPA
members' boys were wounded there, with one, William Alexander
Ewener, winning the Military Cross. In October 1942, Edwin Baker
announced that SAPA would start an honour roll listing the names of
members' children on active service, including Baker's own two sons,
John and David. In April 1945, Baker and his wife, Jesse, received the
dreaded news that David, serving in the Far East in the Royal Navy's
Fleet Air Arm aboard the aircraft carrier HMS *Illustrious*, was killed in
action. Jesse took the news very hard, never fully recovering from
her sorrow, while a devastated Baker lost a beloved son he had
never seen.[25]

But despite the enormity of their families' sacrifices over two
world wars, patriotic sentiment remained strong among the Canadian war blinded. "Association members have every right to feel
proud," noted the SAPA section of the CNIB's 1943 annual report, "of
the contribution made in battle by their sons and we are inspired to
go forward on the home front." As early as April 1941, Harvey Lynes,
SAPA's president, had urged members to "continue serving as fully as
possible on Canada's war and home fronts, to invest if at all possible
in War Savings Certificates, to quash false rumours, and to be active
in community life."[26] Interviewed in the postwar period, Lynes recalled with brimming pride that "two highlights stand out in my
memory. First, the part we played in the Canadian welcome to Their
Majesties, the King and Queen, in 1939. Secondly, and certainly very
important, was the unselfish way in which our members gave of
their money and time during the war years 1939 to 1945, assisting
the national government in its war and victory bond efforts and
shipping food and much needed supplies to our counterparts in the
United Kingdom."[27] This last-mentioned initiative highlighted the
commitment of SAPA members in assisting bomb-ravaged Britain in

its hours of peril and also in seeking to improve the lives of their fellow war blinded overseas.

Following the defeat of France and the German occupation of most of western Europe in June 1940, Britain found itself in a desperate military and economic situation. Would it prove the next victim of the Nazi juggernaut? This appeared likely during the summer of 1940, as the Germans assembled invasion barges along the Channel coast and initiated a vicious air campaign against British military and civilian targets. The Blitz lasted in earnest until May 1941, and, for the remainder of the war, shortages of fuel, raw materials, and food were keenly felt by all elements of the population. Government-imposed rationing became severe. To make matters worse, Britain's overseas supply lines were also dangerously threatened by Germany's submarine offensives.

In this discouraging atmosphere, in April 1941, Sir Ian Fraser wrote SAPA in the hope that Canadian war-blinded veterans might assist their British counterparts by sending food supplies to supplement their meagre diets. Since SAPA already had shipped to St. Dunstan's a hundred-pound parcel of foodstuffs, purchased from the T. Eaton Company at a cost of fifty dollars, the Canadians invited the St. Dunstan's chairman to review its contents and suggest modifications for further shipments based on local needs. At the April 1941 SAPA AGM, Lynes "strongly urged" those present to consider the shipment of food to St. Dunstan's as an ongoing wartime assistance program, especially given the "very fine treatment" St. Dunstan's had provided Canadians during the First World War. Accordingly, SAPA members voted to initiate a continuous fundraising campaign among the war blinded, with Lynes suggesting that the members might donate one dollar each a month for this purpose.[28]

Given Britain's perilous plight, St. Dunstaners undoubtedly would be without life's small amenities, and even many basic food needs. That November SAPA's Executive Committee resolved to reduce SAPA's rather meagre bank account to a one dollar balance and borrow nearly eight hundred dollars from the CNIB to send a massive shipment of four thousand pounds of plum pudding, in family-sized packets, to St. Dunstan's in time for Christmas; each of the more than 1,700 British St. Dunstaners on aftercare, and those of the current war undergoing rehabilitation training, received a share. Moreover, SAPA requested that St. Dunstan's refrain from sending its annual Christmas present of one pound sterling to each of the Canadian war blinded for the duration of the war; St. Dunstan's needed the money more.[29]

In 1942 Lynes reported that "Canadian blinded ex-service men and women are going 'all out' in their efforts to assist Canada in its fight against world barbarism." They sold and bought War Savings Certificates and Victory Bonds, and most contributed to the Overseas Food Fund, "so that our much bombed and acutely rationed blinded ex-service men in the Mother Country may receive comforts and delicacies otherwise denied them."[30] The Canadian war blinded were obviously grateful to St. Dunstan's: on average sixty dollars a month was raised for the Food Fund (later renamed the Comforts Fund), and more than eight hundred dollars had been received by January 1942. But before the end of 1942, Britain's immediate food crisis had passed and even Fraser admitted when visiting Canada in October 1941 that St. Dunstaners "were not suffering any great hardship" at that moment. Despite this, Fraser eagerly accepted SAPA's standing offer of help if any pressing needs should arise. In the meantime, the fund grew to more than one thousand dollars, with regular amounts paid back to the CNIB for its November 1941 loan, the debt being settled in March 1943. SAPA resolved not to borrow any more money for the fund and, hearing little of the matter from Britain, in 1942 Baker contacted Fraser to determine St. Dunstan's needs. In the short term, using part of the $81.50 remaining in the fund, SAPA sent St. Dunstan's a bulk shipment of scarce razor blades. Seventy-six SAPA members had contributed thus far, of whom thirty-five gave one dollar a month.[31]

From September 1943 until the end of the war, SAPA sent hundred-pound parcels of varied goods, usually worth more than one hundred dollars, to St. Dunstan's every three or four months, with the Red Cross acting as the shipping authority. The first such parcel included razor blades, chocolates, and cigarette lighters, but, at St. Dunstan's urging, also such items as braces, belts, and garters, and even hot-water bottles, washcloths, and bobby pins. These were meant for all resident St. Dunstaners, not only the Canadians. Beginning in the summer of 1943, SAPA also sent to the three or four Canadians training at St. Dunstan's at any given time individual monthly packages of one thousand cigarettes and a food parcel containing, among other things, a one-pound fruit cake, twelve packages of chewing gum, chocolate bars, and tinned lobster.[32]

By January 1944, with the military situation much improved for the Allies and the sea lanes mainly cleared of German submarines, contributing to the St. Dunstan's Comforts Fund seemed less urgent. In the previous year 51 SAPA members had donated $787, a 40 percent participation rate from the 127 members.[33] But numerous consumer items and foodstuffs remained scarce in Britain for several years after the end of the war. In September 1945, a parcel costing $179 was sent with candies, pipes, sponge bags, hot water bottles, and other items "unobtainable" in Britain. The 160-pound parcel sent in April 1946 included candy, fruitcake, raisins, prunes, cheese, nuts, coffee, tea, orange and lemon juices, and tinned chicken and lobster.[34]

Nor did SAPA neglect the thirty-one war-blinded Canadian First World War veterans resident in Britain, all of whom were sent food parcels in time for Christmas 1946. Nine of the men responded to the generosity of their fellow war blinded with "deep appreciation." One wrote, "The contents are a great luxury to my family in these monotonous days of rationing. In fact, some of the tinned foodstuffs I haven't tasted for many years." Another said "I and my family are enjoying the contents immensely, which are all unobtainable here, and are considered luxuries." More food was sent for Christmas the following year.[35] Reflecting the shift toward assisting Canadian ex-servicemen, the St. Dunstan's Comforts Fund was changed in name to the Overseas Comforts Fund. But, despite the fact that Britain's postwar needs were as great as had been its wartime needs, the fund began "running low" in 1947. That year, following a special appeal, 61 SAPA members from a total of 198 contributed $521 for their comrades living in food-deprived Britain. In the previous year only 12 members had contributed.[36]

Still, the time came to wind down the fund. A shipment in the autumn of 1948 cost $60 more than monies on hand, and the SAPA executive began discussing the fund's future. From 8 May 1941 to 28 January 1949, the fund had collected an impressive $3,768 from SAPA members while various donations had swelled the total to $4,342. Most of the money was spent on food with less than $500 spent on cigarettes. At the January 1950 AGM, the fund was discontinued, the last shipment having taken place in December 1949.[37] In addition to displaying comradeship, this fund also represented the Canadian war blinded happily repaying a perceived debt.

The Canadian Blinded of the Second World War

In 1942 Baker noted the great difference between the returning men of the First and Second World Wars. He lamented the fact that during the earlier conflict some soldiers were returned to Canada without benefit of St. Dunstan's training and found that their country, "from the standpoint of knowledge of the problems of the blind, or the presence of any machinery to take care of the problems, was about as backward as any civilized community could be." Now, with the CNIB in full operation, Canada's war blinded could return with the utmost confidence that their training and billeting needs would be met. The institute was "equipped and prepared to handle, receive, re-educate and rehabilitate all the men who suffer loss of sight in this war."[38]

Baker recalled that although many returning First World War veterans with St. Dunstan's training "had been fitted for some occupation, many of them found that they were unsuited for the calling they had chosen and others failed to find the necessary encouragement that would have enabled them to become something more than pensioners." These disappointments were hard on morale, and some of the veterans "lost much of the zest and the thrill of accomplishment which makes life worth living." Baker wanted to make sure that it was not "going to be like that this time."[39] The CNIB had a nationwide organization, extensive experience, public sympathy, and complete governmental support. And it had anticipated the casualties. Baker's confidence, buttressed by careful planning and administration, would, in general, be proved correct.

In 1941 the CNIB and SAPA received word of the first reported Canadian war-blinded casualties. In April, Robert S. Hunter, from Amherst, Nova Scotia, was blinded in a German air attack in England. He insisted on returning to Canada, bypassing St. Dunstan's. Three other soldiers had suffered such severe loss of sight in earlier incidents that eventually they also came, as Baker noted, "within the definition of blindness and are now registered with the Institute."[40] They had not gone to St. Dunstan's because Canadian medical authorities did not believe their degree of vision loss warranted it. Back in Canada, however, their eyesight deteriorated sharply.

These men's blindings offer interesting vignettes about the eye's fragility and the varied means of losing one's sight while on active service – often without even being in the presence of the enemy. Corporal Denzil W. McLeod, from London, Ontario, married with a three-year-old daughter, was injured in a traffic accident while driving a military motorcycle during the short-lived Canadian military presence in France in June 1940. His eyesight deteriorated to the point where he was listed as 2/60 in each eye (6/60 being the definition of legal blindness). Following his occupational training in Toronto, McLeod managed one of the CNIB-operated cafeterias in a war plant, a job for which the institute trained several war blinded and civilian blind as well. Lieutenant Samuel Clarke, twenty-six, from Woodstock, New Brunswick, married with two children, and serving in the Carleton and York Regiment, was blinded in May 1940 by the accidental discharge of a blank cartridge in his face. He had perception of light in one eye and was listed as 3/60 in the other. The CNIB undertook his retraining, and by 1942 he was raising potatoes in his native province. In mid-1941 the third hospitalized man was "still in the process of adjusting himself to his new situation." These were the war's first blinded Canadians known to the CNIB, but they were not, in fact, the first. Only in the autumn of 1942 did the CNIB learn of a Native veteran named Ounjay who, while training, had been blinded by a blank cartridge fired in his face. He was discharged in January 1940 and returned to his home in Pictou, Nova Scotia, in receipt of a 100 percent disability pension from DPNH and an assessed vision of 4/60 and 5/60. For whatever reason, he had fallen through the cracks. He did not report to Toronto for training, though the CNIB looked after him locally.[41]

By January 1943, seven Second World War cases had been identified, while another five Canadian Expeditionary Force (CEF) cases had emerged in the previous year, continuing the trend of delayed blindness attributable to service conditions. The CNIB had already taken them in hand on an ad hoc basis. Thirty-seven-year-old Second World War veteran Harold VanKoughnet, married with three children, was looking to farm near Kingston, while Robert Hunter, referred to above, recently married, was expected in Toronto for training in early 1943. Meanwhile, news was received that R. Shortt had been blinded in a motorcycle accident. Although the blinded casualties were beginning to mount, even as late as March 1943, Baker reported that "the problem has not attained the proportions we once feared, but we realize that Canada's fighting forces have not as yet been generally engaged, and it has been, and still is, our policy to stand prepared for any eventuality."[42]

In fact, other Canadians had already been blinded in combat. On 19 August 1942, nearly five thousand Canadians participated in the ill-fated nine-hour raid on the German-held French port of Dieppe. Canadian casualties were extremely severe. Among the more than two thousand wounded were at least two blinded men: Lieutenant F.J.L. (Fred) Woodcock, 37, from Winona, Ontario, serving in the Royal Hamilton Light Infantry, the married father of a two year-old son, and Private Gordon Buchanan, from Prince Albert, Saskatchewan, serving in the South Saskatchewan Regiment. Woodcock was aboard a landing craft approaching the beach when it was struck by German fire and destroyed. One of the few survivors, Woodcock was also wounded in the shoulder and partly deafened, and was taken prisoner. Buchanan managed to return to England and, with only light perception in one eye and some guiding vision in the other, returned to Canada in February 1944 following his preliminary training at St. Dunstan's.[43]

Fred Woodcock was the only war-blinded Canadian held prisoner by the Germans. Yet the matter of blinded prisoners of war already had been considered by the federal government. On 5 January 1942, the Canadian high commissioner in London, Vincent Massey, informed Ottawa that in two days' time there would be held a meeting in London of the Imperial Prisoners of War Committee. One of the agenda items was blinded POWs. According to Massey, the "German Government is willing to arrange for British prisoners of war to be admitted to [the] Educational Institute for the Blind at Marbourg [sic] if blinded German prisoners of war in Great Britain and [the] Dominions would be given training in similar special establishments. At present [the] number of Imperial blinded prisoners of war in Germany is as follows: both eyes 16, one eye 53." The Canadian response was simple: Lieutenant-Colonel H.N. Straight, the commissioner of internment operations, wrote to the Department of External Affairs that the German "proposal is agreed to, and arrangements will be made if necessary – no blind prisoners of war in Canada at present."[44]

The Germans appeared to be as good as their word. In June 1942, a press report noted that "special privileges have been accorded by Nazi camp authorities to the handful of blind British prisoners in their hands. Some 30 blinded men have been brought together in one camp where the Nazis permit them to study reading, writing and type-writing in Braille. Equipment is supplied by the British Red Cross."[45] The report was accurate. Oswald Phipps, the fourth Marquess of Normanby, a young officer captured at Dunkirk, had sought to help the war blinded in his POW camp at Obermassfeldt in Thuringia. Moved by their condition, he persuaded the German authorities to relocate all the blinded prisoners together and, finding a Braille alphabet in a dictionary, he began to teach his fellow POWs Braille through a system of raised dots he created by pushing matchstick heads through pieces of cardboard. He also organized courses in typing, book-keeping, economics, and anatomy. The Germans helped with some teaching supplies and equipment and, in time, a blinded German officer arrived to more formally teach Braille, showing again that, in general, the fraternity of the war blinded knew no national boundaries.[46]

Sir Ian Fraser wrote encouragingly to each blinded POW and informed them of the retraining possibilities available at St. Dunstan's. After the war, he wrote, "I pictured these men as dejected and resigned, hopeless and helpless, just sitting around cursing their luck." He could not know that, already, Lord Normanby had gathered the first group of men and begun teaching them. "They had, in fact," wrote Fraser, "started a branch of St. Dunstan's in the heart of enemy territory." The British Red Cross served as a means for Normanby and Fraser to be in touch, and soon St. Dunstan's sent the blinded men typewriters, Braille writers, Braille magazines and books, tools, and Braille cards and games.[47] Normanby wrote Fraser, "I often wish that you could be with us to see our branch of St. Dunstan's ... Never will these men forget that they owe everything to St. Dunstan's, as indeed they do. So St. Dunstan's will also, I hope, be infused by their especial spirit, which in dark times of depression has not received the advantage of freedom and tuition which have helped their fellow St. Dunstaners at home."[48]

Among those benefitting from Lord Normanby's energetic devotion to the war blinded was Fred Woodcock, and the matter of blinded POWs took on added urgency in Canada as SAPA and the CNIB deeply interested themselves in Woodcock's case. While in March 1943, Baker was able to report to SAPA that St. Dunstan's had managed to send blinded British and Commonwealth POWs some Braille material, and to help arrange for some instruction, Woodcock's situation was not fully known. SAPA contributed comforts to the parcels Mrs. Woodcock sent her husband through the Red Cross.[49] In October 1943, after fourteen months' incarceration, Woodcock was repatriated along with the other British blinded POWs, via Sweden. They arrived at Church Stretton from the German POW hospital for eye casualties and blinded men at Kloster Haina. Lord Normanby was repatriated with "his" men and maintained an active role with St. Dunstan's for decades after the war. One British veteran recalled, "He did so much in helping us back on our feet. He saved us from a couple of years of useless waste of time."[50] Woodcock, who went on to a thirty-year career with the CNIB and was a key executive with SAPA for decades following the war, also sang Normanby's praises. For the blinded POWs, Normanby had been elevated to Pearson-like status.

The controversial issue of attributable blindness following the First World War had but a faint echo immediately after the Second. In 1945 pension authorities had a better grasp of war-related blindness and vision damage. This was due in no small part to more than twenty years of close co-operation between the Canadian National Institute for the Blind (CNIB) and SAPA and between these organizations and the federal government. Also, although men with existing eye defects were enlisted during the Second World War, subsequent evaluations weeded out many whose vision was insufficient for their

assigned tasks. According to William R. Feasby, the Canadian army's
legally blind official historian of the medical services, early in the war
medical officers' testing of recruits' vision was clearly "inadequate,"
and a "great many" soldiers had to be reclassified as to fitness for certain duties while some were discharged outright. On the other hand,
some men rejected with amblyopia or other lesser visual problems
could certainly have been enlisted or retained for useful service away
from front-line units.[51] Once on active service, Canadian troops benefitted from a much more extensive and sophisticated system for
treating eye wounds and diseases and preventing blindness than
they might have encountered as civilians or than their First World
War counterparts had known.

In July 1944, No. 6 Canadian General Hospital became oper-
ational in northwest Europe, and it served until after the end of hostilities. The hospital provided a full range of ophthalmologic services,
mainly using British equipment. Its mobile ophthalmic unit, trans-
ported in two trucks, could set up a full operating theatre in less than
two hours. Since ophthalmologists normally saw serious cases within
two hours of their wounding, and medical officers in front-line units
were trained in ophthalmic first aid, some wounded men were able
to escape partial or complete blindness. The use of penicillin, which
was unknown during the First World War, also prevented the spread
of infection and undoubtedly saved many men's eyes. Following
their operations, patients were normally evacuated to Britain by air
as soon as feasible. Evidently, the existence of this specialized ophthalmic unit was "a source of relief" to the troops, who greatly feared
eye injuries. By the end of the war, No. 6 Canadian General Hospital
was dealing with 25 percent of all eye casualties in the whole of British 21st Army Group; half the casualties treated were not Canadian.[52]

"Eye surgery in the field was almost always of the traumatic
variety," stated the official history of the Canadian Medical Services.
Complete loss of vision could occur without the eye being touched.
For example, minute pieces of high explosive could lodge in sensitive

places outside the eyeball, resulting in "extensive inter-ocular damage," including massive hemorrhaging. Enucleation often resulted. More positively, sympathetic blindness was rare during the Second World War, possibly due to the early treatment of the wounds with sulphonamide drugs and the availability of penicillin. Far fewer cases occurred among those losing a single eye than during the First World War. In addition, the prevalence of eye injuries and blindness in the RCAF was relatively low. One reason was that serious facial wounds or injuries occurring in the air, often accompanied by a crash or a long flight back to base, normally proved fatal. Still, facial burns could involve the loss of an eye or a deterioration in vision.[53]

From one world war to the next, there were some major differences in the causes of blindness. A study of the US war blinded has shown that during the First World War about two-thirds of these casualties were blinded by enemy action, especially by penetrating wounds caused by shell and grenade fragments. The remaining one-third suffered their blindness as a result of accidents, disease, or the wartime aggravation of pre-service visual impairments. During the Second World War, most shells and aerial bombs were encased with non-ferrous metals, significantly decreasing facial penetration wounds. However, much blindness occurred as the result of blast concussion, which caused internal eye damage, especially hemorrhaging. Another difference was in the greater use of contact-detonation land mines. In addition to blinding, these mines also frequently caused other disabilities, especially leg amputations.[54]

Notwithstanding large-scale Canadian participation in the invasion of Sicily in July 1943 and the subsequent campaign on the Italian mainland that began in September, that November Baker sent a memorandum to all SAPA members stating that "there have been so few blinded Canadian soldiers as a result of the present war that the problem of retraining them has not assumed serious proportions." It was a far cry from the large numbers of Canadians blinded in the corresponding period during the First World War. But as the number of war blinded was expected to increase, the CNIB realized it would no longer be acceptable to deal with each case individually and on an ad hoc basis.[55] Definite procedures would be demanded by the sheer volume of casualties, and the latter were on their way. SAPA's Executive Committee decided that "blinded soldiers of the present World War should be advised by letter, on their arrival in Canada, of training, equipment and supplies, and concessions to which they are entitled."[56] These benefits included SAPA membership, of course.

The surviving minutes of the meetings of SAPA's executive and, after January 1944, those from the CNIB's War-Blinded Training Committee, highlight the very immediate, personal, and direct engagement of the CNIB and SAPA in the care of the war's blinded casualties. For example, CNIB and SAPA officials frequently contacted or called upon the war blinded's next-of-kin. In March 1943, Charlemagne Dion, from Verdun, Quebec, serving in the Royal Canadian Corps of Signals, was blinded in a grenade accident while training in Britain and suffered the additional loss of his left hand, which was replaced by an artificial one. Baker called on Dion's father, who admitted that his wife "was very disturbed" by the severity of her son's wounds. Arrangements thereupon were made for SAPA and CNIB members in the Montreal area to visit Mrs. Dion and stay in contact "in an effort to reassure her." Lieutenant W.M. Robinson, exceptionally successful at St. Dunstan's, wished to return to Canada to pursue university studies. In the meantime, CNIB and SAPA members visited his parents, who returned the call by visiting the retraining facilities at Pearson Hall. Since the blinded Harold VanKoughnet wished to settle on a farm, but the Soldier Settlement Board was slow in setting up the process, the CNIB bought him a twelve-acre farm in Sydenham, Ontario, the purchase price to be repaid in due course by the Soldier Settlement Board. Robert Hunter hoped to buy a home in Amherst, Nova Scotia, and both SAPA and the CNIB pledged to assist him realize this goal.[57] These were services the government did not and was not obliged to provide, but Ottawa was no doubt content to allow its partnership with the CNIB to facilitate without public charge the homecomings and rehabilitation of the nation's blinded servicemen.

The blinded men of the Second World War took an early interest in the affairs of SAPA and the CNIB, even before the war had ended. Almost immediately upon his return to Canada in February 1944, Fred Woodcock became very active in both organizations. While in Canada he underwent operations on his shoulder and eyes, both leading to some improvement and facilitating his ability to work. He was promoted to captain in early 1944. Conductor[58] David Dorward, Royal Canadian Ordnance Corps, and Major Edward A. Dunlop, of the Queen's Own Rifles, were both twenty-four and from Pembroke, Ontario, when they were blinded in 1943. Dorward lost his sight in an artillery barrage in Sicily, while Dunlop was blinded in a grenade accident that caused numerous other wounds including the loss of part of his right hand. Dunlop, who retained some very slight vision in his right eye, attended St. Dunstan's. In January 1944, Dorward and Dion attended their first AGM and were elected to the SAPA Executive Committee though without holding any executive positions. Two other blinded men of the Second World War attended that AGM: J.A.O. Desjardins and Maurice Campeau, both from Montreal. While training in Canada, the latter had been injured in the turnover of his Universal carrier, a light tracked vehicle.[59]

For the year ending January 1944, Baker reported eight new cases of war-blinded Canadians and four more cases of delayed blindness from CEF veterans. By 31 March 1944, twenty-four Canadian military personnel were reported as having been blinded since the start of the war. The following table shows the annual progression in the number of Canadian war blinded known to the CNIB.[60] (The asterisked totals do not include those blinded at Hong Kong, who are discussed below.)

31 March 1940	0	31 March 1946	86*
31 March 1941	0	31 March 1947	93*
31 March 1942	4	31 March 1948	109*
31 March 1943	9	31 March 1949	124*
31 March 1944	24	31 March 1953	204
31 March 1945	63		

According to William R. Feasby, medical officer, official historian of the army's medical services in the war, and himself a war-blinded veteran of the Second World War, by 1953 "only" 204 men were rendered "economically" blind as a result of their wartime service: 187 in the army, 10 in the air force, and 7 in the navy. Of the total, 177 suffered their wound, injury, or illness outside of Canada and 27 in Canada. Of this number, 66 were taken prisoner at Hong Kong.[61]

SAPA's new memberships were outstripping the still-high mortality rates of First World War veterans. Not every man attended St. Dunstan's and some did not report to Pearson Hall, either. Wilfred L. Hamilton, from Saskatchewan, received his orientation training at home. Richard Randall, from Vancouver, was also home-taught and found employment in June 1943 at North Vancouver Ship Repairs. Some, like J.A.O. Desjardins and Gordon Buchanan, returned from preliminary training at St. Dunstan's and attended Pearson Hall for more extensive vocational and occupational training. This was the preferred process. Others required ongoing medical attention or sought leaves of absences. For example, Charlemagne Dion trained at St. Dunstan's, spent time in the Christie Street Hospital in Toronto, went on home leave, and returned to Pearson Hall for further training.[62]

Because in 1943 only a few war-blinded veterans required training or accommodation at the same time, it proved "difficult to set up any residence or training arrangements of a permanent character." By late 1943, however, three or more Canadian war-blinded

men required training simultaneously and other cases were anticipated in the near future.[63] This expected intake of trainees led to the
opening in early 1944 of Baker Hall (discussed below) as a dedicated
residence for the men in training at Pearson Hall. At the same time,
Pearson Hall became the War-Blinded Training Centre, with programs
administered by a committee of specially selected CNIB and SAPA
members.

Even as late as 1944, the CNIB felt obliged to frequently remind
and strongly counsel the government that Canadian casualties in the
European theatre be admitted to St. Dunstan's "as soon as they can
be moved" to obtain the best ophthalmologic care available and to
begin their preliminary training.[64] This adjustment training, whether
at St. Dunstan's or Pearson Hall, familiarized trainees with looking
after their own washing, shaving, tooth brushing, nail clipping, shoe
polishing, and brushing of clothing, as well as maintaining hand-
writing skills. According to Baker, "One of our principal objects in this
training is to develop normal social contacts free from embarrassment,
normal habits in the home, and independence."[65] This first phase of
the men's habituation to blindness served three main purposes. It
gave them the opportunity to engage in social and recreational activities, facilitating their social reintegration. It built confidence and
allowed each individual to mix with others in the same predicament,
share ideas and information, and learn just how capable and productive blinded people could be. Finally, it allowed for a thorough
assessment of each individual's interests, strengths, and weaknesses,
and assisted a rehabilitation or training committee to direct them to
the most appropriate employment prospects.[66]

Once back at home, every man's situation was different. "A
properly adjusted case ... soon reaches an understanding with members of the family," wrote Baker in 1944 to a concerned army chaplain.
However, in cases where "independence of the individual is not so
apparent, or the over-sympathetic attitude of the wife or mother of

the family is about to break down his independence, we take a hand in advising and administering the limited maximum needs. We find there is much merit in allowing the individual himself to prove his independence to his family." Sometimes, CNIB aftercare officers or field secretaries made "special efforts to adjust the outlook of the mother or wife, since otherwise the man will either surrender to what he considers the inevitable and allow himself to be served to an undue extent, or he will be irritated by the constant interference with his efforts to take care of matters for himself."[67] There was no mention of indulgent fathers or brothers.

"Already in this war," continued Baker, "I have found the families of the newly blinded much better acquainted with the capabilities of the blind, and more ready to accept the idea that the son or husband will be able to carry on ... than was ever the case during the first Great War. This I believe is in part due to the widespread education which we have been carrying on for a good many years past in stressing the capabilities of the blind rather than their frustrations and inhibitions."[68] The enormous growth in the positive public profile of the civilian blind – in no small way owing to the efforts of the war blinded from the First World War – facilitated the acceptance and reintegration of the war blinded of the Second World War.

Some men lost their vision due to illness. RCAF Warrant Officer Ronald Somers, barely out of his teens, suffered quickly deteriorating eyesight to the point of blindness while stationed in Britain. Retro-bulbar neuritis left him with vision of 1/60 in each eye and a dark spot obstructing his central vision. After a time at Christie Street Hospital, he entered the CNIB training stream in March 1944. Herbert V. Anderson, Royal Canadian Naval Volunteer Reserve, from Winnipeg, was blinded by a brain tumour. G.J. Barrett, a marine engineer serving as a stoker petty officer in the Royal Canadian Naval Reserve, lost his vision as a result of high blood pressure and hypertension incurred while engaged in active operations at sea. Anne Michielin, from Edmonton, served in the Canadian Women's Army Corps and developed bilateral macular degeneration while on active service. Five decades later she would become president of SAPA.[69]

The gruelling ten-week campaign in Normandy, beginning with the D-Day invasion of 6 June 1944, led to a sudden increase in the incidence of combat-related blindness. Pearson Hall soon reverted to its post-1918 use as a busy retraining centre with most of the second floor, parts of others, and an annex building devoted to that task. When Ian Mackenzie, the minister of pensions and national health, visited on 9 September 1944, Baker, his old friend, claimed that the minister had been "very pleased with [the] arrangements for the war blinded."[70] He should have been; these exertions were among the largest undertakings the CNIB had embarked upon since its founding in 1918.

In December 1944, eight war-blinded men arrived at Halifax aboard the hospital ship *Lady Nelson*. Their example serves to show the system as it worked upon the war-blinded's arrival on Canadian shores. Each had taken preliminary training at St. Dunstan's and, upon repatriation, was granted thirty days' home leave. Following their leave they were transferred to Military District 2 (Toronto) and discharged from military service. The CNIB district offices across Canada were directed to assist with the men's timely arrival in Toronto. They were then taken on strength of the Christie Street Hospital, administered by the Department of Veterans Affairs, set up in October 1944, which assumed formal responsibility for them. Their care was entrusted to the CNIB, occasionally as outpatients, and they entered the training stream at Pearson Hall for additional adjustment training followed by specific vocational instruction. As soon as possible, they took up residence at Baker Hall.[71]

Five other men recuperating in Toronto's Christie Street Hospital in the summer of 1944 were under review for possible reclassification as war blinded, while several other severely wounded and blinded men died after returning to Canada and before being discharged to the care of the CNIB. Most war-blinded cases requiring ongoing or recurring medical attention were grouped together in Christie Street Hospital's Ward 229, offering at least six beds, where the duty nurses had received special training and instructions for dealing with the needs of the blind. VADs were on duty for two hours each day while a sighted person was always on hand at meal times. The CNIB sent the men a talking-book machine and a radio for use in the ward, and also chocolates, cigarettes, Braille playing cards, cribbage boards, and other distractions. Members of the Pearson Hall House Committee, especially its convenor, Clara Sutherland, visited the hospitalized men on a regular basis. These visits could be important and moving experiences for all concerned. In November 1943 Sutherland wrote, "We feel that nothing is too good for these men who have gone through such terrible experiences, and who have to face living in a dark world the rest of their lives – they are so young! They are facing their new life so bravely, even so cheerfully, [and] are an inspiration to us who have suffered so little."[72]

Elizabeth Rusk, the CNIB's Braille and handicrafts teacher, already extremely busy training the war-blinded veterans, also visited the men at Christie Street Hospital to read to them or write letters on their behalf. The women of the House Committee saw many sad sights. As Sutherland put it in 1944, "The work we are privileged to do here is full of interest – of hopefulness, and of sadness too, as the men hover between hope and despair for their eyesight, between life and death. Their courage in facing the future cannot but fill one with admiration."[73] The women viewed visiting the hospitalized blinded soldiers as a priority. "Many of these men come as strangers to the city," wrote Sutherland, and "the committee tries to provide a friendly atmosphere for these lonely lads, so far from their homes and families in their time of suffering." Following surgeries or other medical procedures, the women would write the men's families to "relieve anxiety as soon as possible." By 1946 more than ninety men had been visited regularly, as often as five or six times a week, by VADs, House Committee members, or frequent visitors Sutherland

and Rusk. Not all were blinded, but all had serious eye wounds or severe loss of sight, and many suffered from "pain and depressing boredom." In November 1946, Sutherland resigned her convenorship of the Pearson Hall House Committee after eighteen years at the helm to devote her time to hospital visits. The veterans were appreciative and many, like Fred Woodcock, decades later fondly remembered Clara Sutherland's devotion to them. In June 1947, she was made an honorary vice-president of SAPA.[74]

The war blinded's inspired approach to rehabilitation apparently exerted a "heartening" effect on other wounded soldiers at the hospital. Lewis Wood, the CNIB's president, wrote in 1945 that "it is very plain that these young war veterans are already wielding a very stimulating influence in the whole field of Canadian rehabilitation."[75] They served as an example to other wounded men, but also to government, which clearly saw the advantage of specialized, focussed rehabilitation programs undertaken by experts in the field.

The War-Blinded Training Committee and Employment Placement

On 7 January 1944, SAPA's First World War veterans, in collaboration with the CNIB's rehabilitation and employment-placement experts, set up the War-Blinded Training Committee (WBTC) within the CNIB. This committee, struck to organize the training and civil re-establishment of the Second World War blinded, met weekly during the war and once or twice a month thereafter until its disbandment in 1950. No veterans were to be retrained in any measure by any CNIB department without the WBTC's authorization. Drawing on the best talent available within the CNIB and SAPA organizations, the committee members weighed each blinded veteran's case carefully and individually. Often, the committee arranged for individualized training and rehabilitation services, and it unfailingly proved accommodating, generous, and understanding toward the men, even the occasionally difficult physically maimed, emotionally unstable, and psychologically scarred veterans. The WBTC siphoned off a great deal of the CNIB's staff time and material resources but, because of its considered and dedicated approach, it would prove one of the most important elements in the successful re-establishment of Canada's war-blinded veterans.

The WBTC's membership included such SAPA-CNIB stalwarts as Harris Turner (chairman), Edwin Baker, Bill Dies, Alexander Viets, L.G. Williamson, a long-time SAPA member and future president, Dr. S.A. Saunders, Pearson Hall's rehabilitation specialist, Arthur V. Weir, who managed the employment-placement program, Elizabeth Rusk, and various other CNIB department heads. Once the Baker Hall residence opened in March 1944, Elsinore Burns, the head of the House Committee, attended most WBTC meetings. The purpose of the committee was to ensure that a proper training program was in place to prepare the veterans for life without sight and to assist them to secure employment. Another goal was to systematize the ongoing review of each trainee's progress and to make recommendations as to training adjustments or future needs "to give the soldiers the best chance for social and occupational adjustment." The CNIB and SAPA agreed that a further objective was "to utilize to the fullest extent the experience of blinded soldiers of the first war ... in order that the rehabilitation of blinded soldiers of this war may be most complete and thorough."[76] The chairman of the committee prepared monthly reports on each trainee, and the program in general, for the CNIB council and especially Baker, the institute's managing director. Baker was the main point of contact with the DPNH and was responsible for the overall rehabilitation program and the blinded veterans' well-being.[77]

Along with Baker, S.A. Saunders, who obtained a PhD from the University of Toronto in 1933, was a key influence in the men's success. An expert in the rehabilitation of the disabled, and blind himself, he had long experience working at the CNIB. In 1946 the

Toronto Daily Star noted that Saunders was responsible for the "semi-miraculous" work the CNIB was doing in "making new men of the war's blind."[78] Saunders explained that the objectives of rehabilitation were to "equip each veteran with the tools ... to cope; ... to train him in the art of substituting touch and hearing for the sense of sight; ... to enable him to handle himself under all social conditions in such a manner as to make his blindness least conspicuous; to assist him to accept his blindness philosophically; [and] to guide him in his choice of occupation."[79]

By November 1944, Pearson Hall and its adjacent training annex were crowded with war-blinded veterans. The men trained there five days a week from 9:00 to 4:30 daily, with lunch in the cafeteria and classroom instruction. Eventually they took over the entire second floor when some CNIB departments moved to nearby buildings and properties.[80] To men who had not already received blindness familiarization training at St. Dunstan's, the CNIB taught typing and Braille (which could take six months to master) and, since "nearly every person who goes blind experiences difficulty with spelling," they were given spelling lessons as well. Handicrafts training and carpentry sharpened their sense of touch, facilitated manual dexterity and mastering spatial relations, and boosted self-confidence. Self-navigation was taught by a blinded First World War veteran, who instructed those of the Second World War on the use of the white cane in getting aboard public transportation and in and out of buildings. Languages, math, and history were also taught. Instruction in academic subjects was given out orally, with readers acquainting the students with the literature on the subject. A current-events course honed the blinded veterans' all-important listening skills.[81] While the men took preliminary training, the WBTC members closely monitored their progress and aptitudes so as to channel them toward appropriate vocational training.

Some men were anxious and impatient to begin their new lives. For example, Charlemagne Dion, who had also lost a hand, had to be

reminded on several occasions following poor results that typing
and Braille skills were important to his future and that vocational
training could not begin until they were mastered. The eager, ebulli-
ent Dion, who also had had his ups and downs at St. Dunstan's, required "intense supervision" and admitted that he had "wasted time"
in not taking preliminary training seriously enough. Eventually, he
did very well. On the other hand, Maurice Campeau impressed Baker
right away, despite a very serious head injury that necessitated
eighteen months in hospital. Success was often a question of
personality and attitude.[82]

Baker applied gentle pressure on the men to succeed and
measured success by the level of a casualty's complete social reintegration, including employment. He must have been pleased with the
first group of graduates. Of eighteen men who had completed training to 31 March 1945, four had settled on small farms, two worked in
war industry, three operated concession stands in federal buildings,
two owned their own commercial businesses, one worked as a personnel officer with a private firm, one worked at DVA, one sold insurance, and another worked as a field secretary for the CNIB. This left
only three unemployed. On the same date, twenty-three more men
were in training, with more either in hospital, at St. Dunstan's, or returned to Canada and on leave.[83]

In fact, so successful had the CNIB rehabilitation program become that in May 1944 Ian Fraser suggested that Canadians arriving
at St. Dunstan's would henceforth be encouraged to return home as
quickly as possible. And why not? Canada had its own version of St.
Dunstan's. Certainly Bill Dies believed that "no time should be lost"
in repatriating the men and getting them started on a new career
in Canada. Nevertheless, in November 1944 there were still fifteen
Canadians either in training at Church Stretton or in St. Dunstan's-
administered medical facilities. Approximately seventy-five Canadians
attended St. Dunstan's during the Second World War, to their great
benefit.[84]

The CNIB's training was designed to take advantage of the men's aptitudes and skills. "Unless they are ... given every opportunity to develop their personalities and their talents, their war injuries can become irreparable disasters," wrote Baker. Various special arrangements, sometimes with other organizations, assisted with training in such diverse activities as agriculture and poultry farming (at the Ontario Agricultural College), physiotherapy, salesmanship, and public speaking. Many war-blinded veterans took music lessons, and at least six underwent upholstery training at the Ryerson Institute.[85]

One of the most common forms of occupation available to Canada's war blinded was managing a concession stand, or kiosk, selling newspapers, cigarettes, soft drinks, chocolate bars, and other confections. "Stand training" was a specialty of the CNIB and was directed by D.R. Strong, who, along with Saunders, was responsible for assessing a man's suitability for the job, ensuring proper placement, and providing ongoing support. The stands were located in public spaces such as train stations, post-office buildings, and hospitals, and were nominally operated by the CNIB. The veteran-managers, many occasionally benefitting from war-blinded trainees as assistants, were paid employees of the institute. In 1944 they earned a minimum of twenty dollars a week, often more, normally for a six-day week. This was not a high wage, but it provided a reasonable standard of living when combined with a disability pension.

As early as 1940, Ottawa began awarding rent-free space for concession stands in federal buildings to blinded soldiers in the first instance over other veterans. In the spring of 1944, an Order-in-Council formally reserved these spaces for them for the duration of the war, plus six months thereafter. The majority were in larger urban centres; Toronto, Ottawa, other Ontario cities, and Montreal provided most of the early opportunities. For example, in November 1944, J.A.O. Desjardins operated a stand at the post office building at Place d'Armes in Montreal, while Charlemagne Dion's stand in the building housing the Toronto DVA offices was doing well. Many provincial and municipal buildings housed CNIB concession stands in their lobbies as did several large businesses and office buildings. Sometimes the kiosks were outdoors, and a few were independently run by the veterans as their own businesses. While some made stand operation a career, other veterans used the experience as a stepping stone to other commercial or business opportunities. In March 1946, twelve veterans were operating stands with many others in training to do so.[86]

By early 1945, a number of men wished to pursue their education and three, including Maurice Campeau, were completing the requirements for high school matriculation prior to entering university.[87] Three veterans, Harry Coyle, David Ferguson, and Mervyn Carlton, were enrolled at Victoria College, University of Toronto, with the wives of the latter two also attending and taking notes for them. Carlton had guiding vision and was a former POW at Hong Kong. They took their exams through dictation.[88] Up to June 1947, the blinded veterans seeking to enter university were prepared by the Ontario Training and Re-establishment Institute in Toronto. When that institution closed, the CNIB took over the responsibility for tutoring the war blinded and hired two trained teachers to carry on this work from Pearson Hall's War-Blinded Training Centre.[89] By June 1950, five men had graduated university, most in social work, including two who had entered graduate studies programs. Two more were still undergraduates, and several others would follow.[90]

Ottawa proved generous with those seeking to further their education, especially with specialized vocational courses that could be arranged or administered by the CNIB. Priority for approval and payment of tuition, instructors' fees, Braille material and tools, and other related costs, on the recommendation of the CNIB, went to courses preparing veterans for employment with the institute or in industry. Moreover, the one-to-three-month course on concession-stand management was paid by DPNH, and later DVA.[91]

Individual Experiences

Many of the blinded men's stories demonstrate the long-term effects and trauma of being severely wounded and are emblematic of Canadian disabled veterans' reintegration into civilian life, including some of the mechanics of the men's medical treatment, rehabilitation training, and employment opportunities. But, in many cases, they also represent the overcoming of adversity sufficiently to carry on in life. When written in their own words, their experiences are especially evocative.

David Dorward was born in Dartmouth, Nova Scotia, but lived in Ontario at the time of his enlistment in the Royal Canadian Ordnance Corps. In the summer of 1943, he was twenty-three, had married his wife, Ellie, in Britain, and was the father of a baby girl, when he was knocked unconscious in action in Sicily by a shell explosion. "After an indefinite period of time, I came to and didn't seem to be badly hurt. My head was pounding, I couldn't walk straight, and I was badly shaken up, but nothing seemed to be broken and there was no blood," he wrote years later. The medical officer gave him "a cursory check, some headache pills, and told me to sleep it off." The next morning, he awoke to "excruciating" pain in his head, had lost his sense of balance, and suffered from "badly blurred" vision. Examined that day at a British hospital in Catania, it was discovered he had a hairline skull fracture, a concussion, and almost certainly a permanent loss of vision. Bandages were applied and "from this point on, I saw nothing ... I depended on what I was told, and what I heard or in some way sensed."[92] Dorward described the period immediately following this devastating news as "nightmare weeks," during which he was in a "state of shock and confusion." "I had entered a dream world," he recalled, "haunted by distorted, unhappy thoughts." To add insult to his injuries, he learned that the shell had been an errant Allied artillery shell landing short. He became very depressed. "Many of my thoughts at that time elude me. I was a mass of sensitivity, feeling rather than thinking; I was engulfed by an emotional state, constantly close to despair and breakdown. The smallest kindness brought tears to my eyes; a slight rebuff, unreasonable annoyance."[93]

A Canadian ophthalmologist told Dorward some time later that although his eyes had suffered permanent damage, some sight might yet return. But, not having been sent to St. Dunstan's or exposed to a more positive view of his future, aboard the hospital ship returning him to Canada he wondered how he would make a living following his discharge. After training at Pearson Hall, Dorward successfully operated a small business in Pembroke, Ontario, selling confectionaries and some handicrafts made by the CNIB "Blindcraft" program. He hired a "sighted girl" with retail experience to assist with the running of the shop. Dorward later described himself as "reasonably successful in the competitive world of business," even authoring several business manuals. By October 1945, his vision had improved to 6/60 and 6/36, which was "to the point which brings him outside our category," noted the WBTC minutes. His disability pension was reduced to 60 percent, but he found work at the atomic energy installation at Chalk River, Ontario. Four decades later, he would be the SAPA president.[94]

In August 1944, Sergeant Barney Danson, serving in Normandy with the Queen's Own Rifles, was hit in a German *Nebelwerfer* ("Moaning Minnie") mortar barrage that he described as "a whining, whistling, groaning, ear-splitting roar." "I felt as if someone had taken a baseball bat or a sledgehammer, wound up, and hit me in the left eye," he wrote. "There was a momentary pause and blood started to gush out of my mouth like Niagara. I could feel my strength draining rapidly." A shard of steel had entered his temple behind his eye, severed the optic nerve, and detached the retina. He had been in France barely a week.[95] Danson would go on to be a Liberal cabinet minister in the 1970s; he joined SAPA in 2002 after his vision had nearly completely failed in his remaining eye.

In September 1944, Neil Hamilton, serving in the RCAF as an instructor, was aboard a training flight over Britain, following extensive air operations in the Mediterranean. All was proceeding smoothly when "suddenly, my world changed ... forever. As I pointed to one of the instruments, my eyes went blurry. There was no pain or discomfort, but all I could see was black dots and then blood. I realized my eyes were haemorrhaging." Shortly thereafter specialists in Birmingham, England, informed him that the hemorrhaging might have been caused by the altitude, but they were not sure. What was known was that he would be permanently and seriously visually impaired. His left eye was next to useless. "I had completed my tour, had nearly finished instructing, and was almost ready to go home on regular leave ... for this to happen now – it came as quite a jolt. I broke down [in] tears." He had less than 10 percent vision in both eyes: "I could distinguish light and shapes, but mostly it was like peering into a London fog." Taken off flying operations, he stayed in the air force for a time by bluffing his way through. He was even promoted to flying officer. After returning to Canada and experiencing some additional serious health problems, he took rehabilitation training and embarked on a successful career as a CNIB field secretary, liaison officer, and administrator in Saskatchewan and Alberta.[96]

John Windsor, from Listowel, Alberta, served in the Lord Strathcona's Horse and suffered grievous facial wounds when the Sherman tank he commanded in Italy was struck by a German anti-tank shell at the Melfa River crossing in 1944. Windsor was "plunged into darkness." "I knew right away what the trouble was," he wrote. "This was not the blackness of unconsciousness, nor the blackness of death ... I was blind ... trapped forever in this awful night. I slumped forward in the turret, hands rubbing at my eyes, trying to brush away the veil, trying to see something, anything, that would tell me it wasn't true."[97] Windsor, married overseas and with a baby daughter, began his road to rehabilitation at St. Dunstan's. "The real secret of [St. Dunstan's] success," wrote Windsor in his memoirs, "was [its] ability to somehow transform us from bitter, frightened, dispirited creatures into confident men and women sure that we could go out into the world, even though we had something of a handicap."[98] Windsor trained as a personnel manager but experienced difficulty finding work in this field in Canada. At Baker's invitation, Windsor, depressed, went to stay at Baker Hall and look for work in Toronto. Woodcock accompanied him for interviews with some personnel departments, but the task seemed fruitless. Baker felt that Windsor remained "in need of re-adjustment and recuperation." Eventually he joined the staff of the CNIB, though not before he had become disenchanted with his rehabilitation experience.[99]

In the immediate postwar period, the Toronto press was full of accounts of the progress and successes of the dozens of war-blinded veterans training and working in that city. One remarkable story featured two best friends from Alberta, Ronald Hewlett and Fred Koenig. Nicknamed "Mutt and Jeff" by their fellows due to their great disparity in height, both served in the 6th Field Park, Royal Canadian Engineers, and, shockingly, both were blinded in separate incidents. Sergeant Koenig lost his sight and most of his fingers following an anti-tank mine explosion in which his comrades thought he had been killed. "Fred was blown ... into the air – just like a doll," recalled Hewlett. "His face and hands seemed to be in tatters. All his clothing was gone except for a bit around his neck." Hewlett had returned to Canada following service overseas and was blinded by a grenade exploding in his face during a training accident at Petawawa, Ontario. They renewed their friendship while training at Pearson Hall. Hewlett went on to become a field secretary for the CNIB while Koenig became a concession stand operator.[100]

Trooper Rolland Pilon was blinded while serving with the Sherbrooke Fusiliers when the Sherman tank in which he was a crewman was struck by a German shell at the Albert Canal in Belgium. He obtained his preliminary training at St. Dunstan's and, following vocational training at Pearson Hall, became a master weaver on a loom and also found work as a concession stand operator. Harold Bartlett, blinded in action, returned to his old job at Trail Smelters in British Columbia, handling and smoothing lead sheets. After one month of refamiliarization, he was able to regain the work speed he possessed prior to his enlistment. No wonder, according to SAPA president L.G. Williamson, who had visited the firm, "the company [was] most anxious for him to go back to his old job." Similarly, in 1948 J.M. Reid also found work at Trail Smelters and appeared "very happily rehabilitated." Bartlett had no doubt proved to his superiors what a motivated and properly trained blinded veteran could do.[101]

Norman Daniel was only nineteen in February 1945 when he was blinded after stepping on a land mine in the Netherlands while serving with New Brunswick's North Shore Regiment.[102] He was among Canada's youngest servicemen to lose his eyesight during the war. He returned to his hometown, Verdun, Quebec, in the winter of 1946. A popular star athlete, he was well-connected in local circles, and community-minded individuals established a trust fund so that he might further his physiotherapy training at St. Dunstan's. The Daniel Fund gave poignant symbolic expression to the wartime sacrifices of his city. Contributions were deposited in charity boxes displayed in many local businesses. Benefit concerts and sporting events were organized to finance the fund. For example, the Montreal Canadiens fastball team played a Verdun all-star team, collecting $200 for the Daniel Fund. Included in the Canadiens' line-up were Toe Blake, Butch Bouchard, Bill Durnan, Elmer Lach, Kenny Reardon, and Maurice "Rocket" Richard. By the end of June 1946, the fund had swelled to $3,500. In 1948 Daniel, highly successful at St. Dunstan's, returned to the Montreal area a qualified physiotherapist and established a practice.[103]

One especially tragic group of war-blinded Canadian veterans were sixty-six men who suffered near or total blindness while prisoners of the Japanese following the battle for Hong Kong in December 1941. The men, nearly all from the Winnipeg Grenadiers and the

Royal Rifles of Canada, a Quebec regiment, developed blindness mainly as a result of avitaminosis and diphtheria, brought on by near-starvation diets and malnourishment, poor or non-existent medical care, and the generally brutal conditions prevailing in Japanese POW camps.

The Hong Kong veterans constituted the greatest single bloc of war-blinded men and, repatriated together, they entered the CNIB's training stream in 1946 and 1947, helping to keep the War-Blinded Training Centre and Baker Hall operating at full rhythm. By early 1948, DVA and the CNIB had identified thirty-nine blinded Hong Kong veterans, but each year's new tally eclipsed the previous year's anticipated total. In addition to their blindness, many of the skeletal former prisoners remained "far from well," according to S.A. Saunders, and frequently suffered from "shattered physiques." Although most retained at least some sight, recovery was a slow process and many could begin rehabilitation training in Toronto only months or even years after their return to Canada.[104] The numerous war-blinded Hong Kong veterans who had suffered the ravages of pellagra or beriberi also suffered impairment of their sense of touch, making it difficult, if not impossible, to learn Braille or even to type properly. These veterans could take up to twice as long to train.[105] Many others, not sufficiently visually impaired to qualify as war blinded in the immediate postwar period, nevertheless suffered the ill effects of their incarceration the whole of their lives, becoming pensioned members of SAPA decades later.

Bill Mayne, from the farming community of Pilot Mound, Manitoba, enlisted in the Winnipeg Grenadiers in 1939. Along with more than 1,600 other Canadians, he was captured by the Japanese when Hong Kong surrendered on Christmas Day 1941. In March 1943, he detected a serious deterioration in his eyesight that worsened sharply over a matter of days to the point where he had enormous difficulty seeing. He was among a growing number of Canadian POWs permanently losing their vision due to vitamin deficiencies. Their

Japanese captors were fully aware of what was happening but, Mayne recalled years later, they did "absolutely nothing" to prevent the men's blindness. Repatriated in September 1945, Mayne learned that he had about 5 percent useful vision in both eyes. Like many Hong Kong veterans who suffered from beriberi, a vitamin deficiency, Mayne developed a lack of sensitivity in his fingers, making Braille difficult to learn, though this condition improved with time. He could not successfully return to farming on a full-time basis and, in 1946, reported for training at Pearson Hall.[106] The WBTC described Mayne as "very keen" and Baker admitted to being "very favourably impressed."[107] Mayne, who graduated with a BA from the University of Toronto, would go on to a highly successful twenty-five-year career with the CNIB and was a key SAPA official for the next six decades.

The CNIB also monitored the cases of some men, most of them veterans of Hong Kong, with "badly defective vision" who had not been categorized as war blinded. Baker wanted no veterans to "fall through the cracks" and presumably wished to ensure that a case for war-service attributability could be made in the event of their eventually becoming blind.[108]

Some men did not report to Toronto for training. Charles Glump, an American serving in the Canadian Army, was blinded while serving as an instructor at Camp Borden. The CNIB agreed to home-teach him in Hamilton. Likewise H.W. Van Norden, from Nova Scotia, refused training. Young RCAF veteran Ronald Somers was slated to take over his father's shoe business in Tillsonburg, Ontario, and took preliminary training only. A.C. Thomas abandoned his training in September 1948 "on account of family problems" and returned to Winnipeg. Others refused to take woodworking or handicraft training, insisting on proceeding with vocational training. The kind-hearted but firm Fred Woodcock, blinded at Dieppe and, from March 1945, the War-Blinded Training Committee's liaison officer with the men in training, would interview the men and seek to iron out any differences in an encouraging manner. This became Woodcock's full-time job that

August. It extended to visiting the men's families to explain medical conditions, training opportunities, and lifestyle options available to the blinded men and to arrange for aftercare.[109] For example, Woodcock visited the Brantford, Ontario, family of Elmer Terrill, blinded and a leg amputee, and "found the family in a greatly distressed state of mind, but before leaving had managed to give them a brighter outlook." Moreover, the CNIB and SAPA sent encouraging letters to the men's families reporting on their progress. As evidence that there was life and ability after blindness, the letters indicated that they were typed by the CNIB's blind stenographers.[110] The CNIB's 1948 annual report described Woodcock's role as a "special representative to assist and advise his fellow blinded servicemen with the innumerable problems of re-establishment."[111] He was kept very busy for the next two decades and beyond.

Others hit bumps along the road to recovery. In 1946 Robert S. Hunter, among the first war-blinded veterans of the war, was unemployed and "living in the coloured section" of Amherst, Nova Scotia. The CNIB's earlier plan to assist him purchase a home does not appear to have worked out, and the local CNIB office hoped to find him some sort of industrial work and better housing. Eventually he returned to Toronto for training in the operation of a concession stand, though Baker believed that an industrial job was probably more suitable. Still, the WBTC felt that Hunter was "deserving of every consideration as a badly wounded case with multiple disabilities."[112] On the other hand, Kenneth Thompson consistently displayed erratic and disagreeable behaviour while in training and in residence at Baker Hall. This included drinking, overspending, not repaying loans, and impolite behaviour. He was withdrawn from concession stand training as a result of his "instability" and poor attitude with customers. Jean St. Jean, from Montreal, was also a difficult case. He had no interest in training seriously or of finding work and proved a great bother to Baker and others. In 1948 he was admitted to the psychiatric ward of Sunnybrook Hospital "in order more or less to give his family a rest from him," according to the WBTC minutes. Both Thompson and St. Jean remained unemployed, and probably unemployable, in 1950.[113]

Some blinded veterans had difficulty leaving the shelter the program offered. In 1946 the committee decided that naval veteran Herbert Anderson had "spent long enough at the Training Centre to make the most of his talents and condition" and should "very definitely ... terminate his training." According to the WBTC minutes, Baker felt that "the improvement in Mr. Anderson since he had first come to Toronto was a feather in the cap of the training committee and the house committee at Baker Hall, as the doctors who had examined [him] had never expected him to be other than a bed-ridden invalid." But after returning home to Winnipeg, Anderson longed to return to Baker Hall. The real world could be a daunting prospect for the returned men, even for those, unlike Anderson, who were not so badly off. In December 1948, Herbert Anderson died in Winnipeg's Deer Lodge Hospital, only several weeks following a visit from Baker.[114]

In 1944 the Department of Veterans Affairs established its Casualty Rehabilitation Section, the purpose of which was to train disabled veterans and help them find employment and become responsible for their economic well-being. Walter S. Woods, the deputy minister with whom Edwin Baker enjoyed a warm relationship, wrote that "one of the Department's greatest responsibilities is the rehabilitation of those who have incurred disability in the defence of their country."[115] Woods hoped to employ in this unit disabled Second World War veterans who had overcome their disabilities to lead productive lives. The DVA-appointed district casualty rehabilitation officers also were often drawn from the ranks of the war disabled to serve as "examples of successful rehabilitation."[116]

The first supervisor of the section, and one of its organizers, was Major Edward A. Dunlop, a Second World War blinded veteran with a badly mangled right hand. Dunlop was a St. Dunstan's and Pearson Hall graduate, and a member of SAPA. In the summer of 1944, he had married Dorothy Tupper from Toronto, a VAD who had been working at St. Dunstan's while Dunlop was in residence. While there, this especially hard-working veteran mastered one-handed typing, Braille typing, and Braille shorthand. Dunlop epitomized Woods's view that "a man who has been seriously disabled and who has regained control, as it were, and mastered the ordinary functions of life despite his disability can, by his mental attitude and his physical mastery of handicaps be a tremendous inspiration to others." In fact, Dunlop had earned the George Medal for courage in trying to save men from the effects of an accidental grenade explosion, having lost his own vision and hand in the same catastrophe. He became committed to the issue of war-related disability, studied sociology at the graduate level, and headed DVA's Casualty Rehabilitation Section "in a highly competent manner" until he left in 1948 to head the Canadian Arthritis and Rheumatism Society.[117]

Dunlop believed that the disabled had to be integrated fully into society and the labour market, and not be pigeon-holed. He felt that to slot these veterans into preconceived occupational ghettoes, such as elevator operation for amputees, "condemn[ed] many thousands of persons to jobs ... below their proper level of attainment." In other words, under his direction, the Casualty Rehabilitation Section intended to offer the disabled a chance to realize their personal goals.[118] In this respect, he carried the St. Dunstan's philosophy to his work and undoubtedly used the CNIB-SAPA rehabilitation organization as a model to be emulated. Certainly Woods felt that the relationship between the CNIB and DVA worked especially well and that the successful rehabilitation of the war blinded stood as testimony to the value of careful planning, building on success, and instilling into disabled veterans a positive spirit to assist with their social reintegration.[119] In September 1945, Dunlop was appointed the DVA's representative to the CNIB's national council and attended a meeting

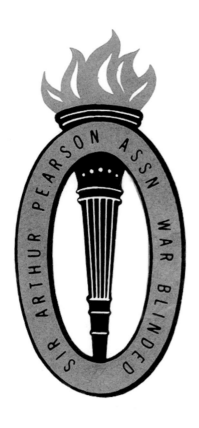

24 The official crest of the Sir Arthur Pearson Association of War Blinded, which took on this abbreviated name in 1942. The torch symbolizes way-finding in the future and is a link to St. Dunstan's. *SAPA Archives*

25 This remarkable German photograph shows Lieutenant Fred Woodcock (centre), of the Royal Hamilton Light Infantry, not long after being severely wounded, blinded, and captured during the Dieppe Raid, 19 August 1942. *LAC*

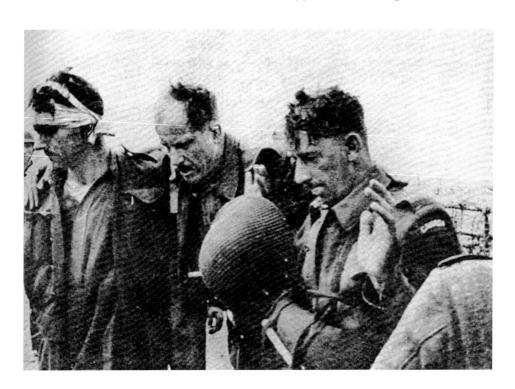

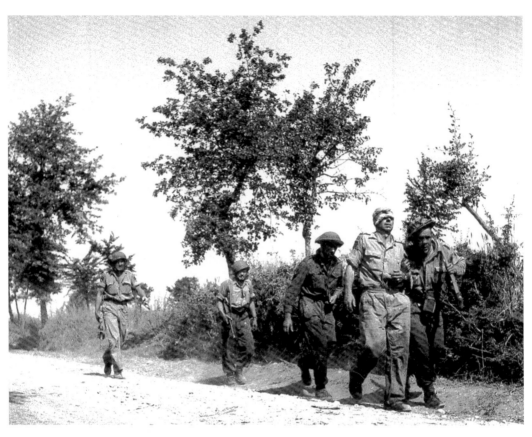

26 Canadian soldier with eye wounds suffered in Italy in May 1944. *LAC, PA-136311*

27 Lieutenant-Colonel Edwin Albert Baker, OBE, MC, Croix de Guerre, c. 1942, by which time he had become nationally and internationally prominent for his work on behalf of the Canadian civilian blind and war-blinded veterans. *CNIB Archives*

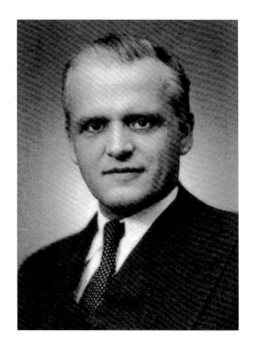

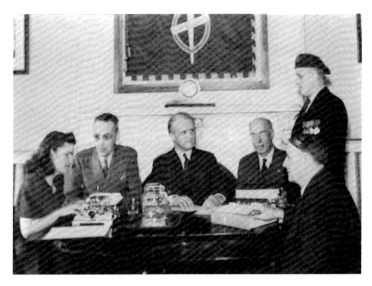

28 SAPA First World War veterans and executive members meet in 1941 to plan the CNIB-SAPA rehabilitation program of the Second World War. From left, Braille stenographer Mary Edwards, SAPA president J. Harvey Lynes, Edwin Baker, Alexander Viets, Bill Dies (standing), and Harris Turner. *CNIB Archives*

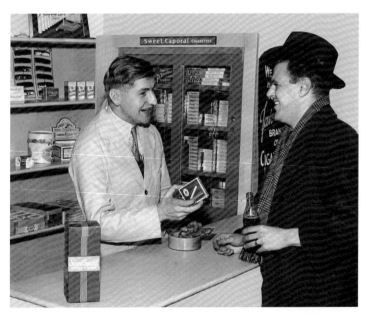

29 Blinded veteran J.J. Doucet, severely wounded in Italy during the Second World War, at his stand in the Dominion Public Building, Toronto, c. 1946. Many blinded veterans trained with the CNIB as stand managers, and the government awarded them rent-free space in federal buildings. *CNIB Archives*

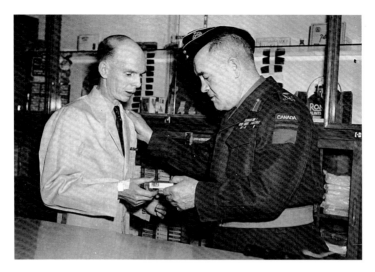

30 Gordon Buchanan, blinded at Dieppe in 1942 while serving with the South Saskatchewan Regiment, operated a stand at a federal building in Toronto. Here he sells an item to Major-General A.E. Potts, the District Officer Commanding, Military District No. 2 (Toronto), c. 1944. *CNIB Archives*

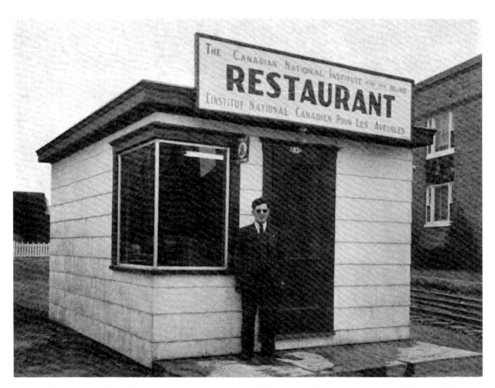

31 Fernand Cinq-Mars lost an arm and his sight in the Second World War. Following his re-establishment training with the CNIB, he operated this refreshment stand in Sherbrooke, Quebec, c. 1946. *CNIB Archives*

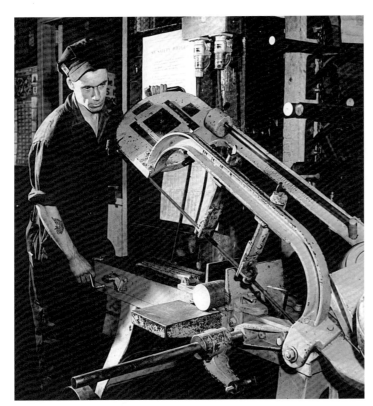

32 Following rehabilitation training, Richard Randall, a naval veteran of the Second World War, successfully operated a steel-cutting saw in a Vancouver ship-yard, c. 1943. *CNIB Archives*

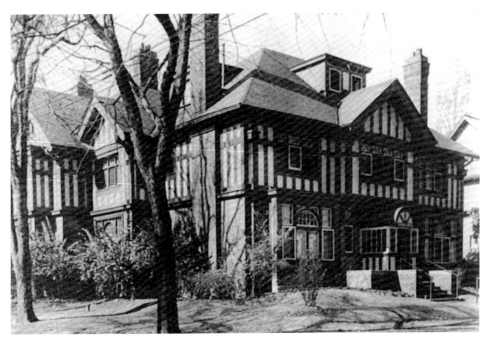

33 From 1944 to 1950, Baker Hall, 78 Admiral Road, Toronto, served as a residence and social centre for war-blinded veterans. Virtually all shared fond memories of their time there. *CNIB Archives*

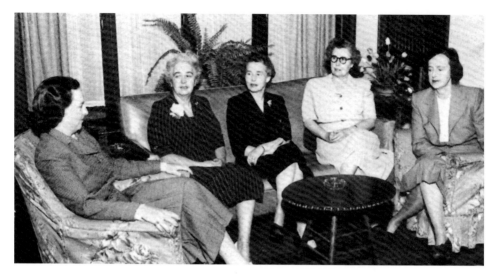

34 The Baker Hall House Committee, c. 1945, was made up of diligent, giving, and extremely capable women who organized the proper functioning of the facility and who also acted as friends and confidantes to the men in residence, many of whom needed occasional bolstering and reassurance. From left: Mrs. Geoffrey Boone, Mrs. A.M Sutherland, Mrs. H.E. Cochran, Miss Elsinore C. Burns, and Mrs. Chester Russell. *CNIB Archives*

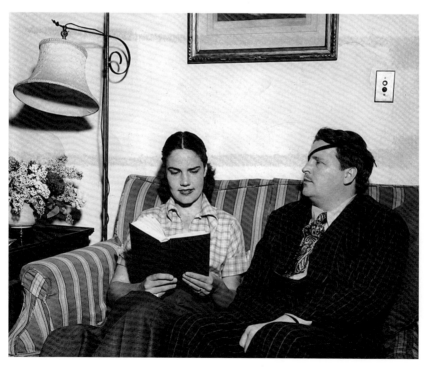

35 Mrs. G. Gibson of the Toronto Junior league helped war-blinded veteran Harry Coyle earn his BA at the University of Toronto by reading to him almost daily at Baker Hall, c. 1946. *CNIB Archives*

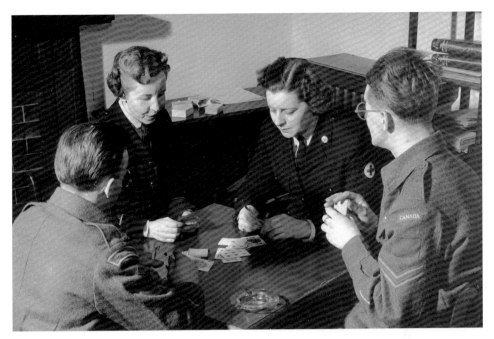

36 From left to right, blinded soldier Rolly Dolbeck, Royal Canadian Army Service Corps, Voluntary Aid Detachment workers (VADs) Laurie Bentley and Joan Burke, and Georges Bertrand, blinded in Normandy in 1944, using Braille playing cards, Baker Hall, c. 1945. *CNIB Archives*

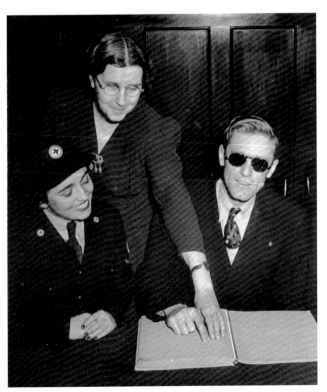

37 Maurice Campeau, from Montreal, learning Braille at Pearson Hall from long-time CNIB teacher Elizabeth Rusk and VAD Margaret Yorick, c. 1945. *CNIB Archives*

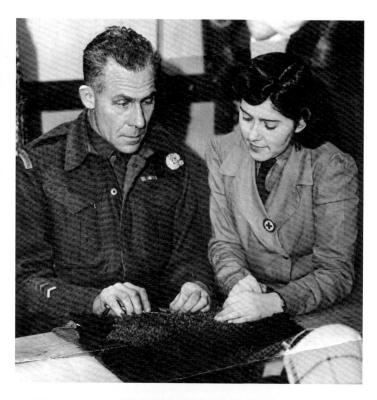

38 Russell Rose, a veteran of both world wars, was blinded in Italy by a mine blast while serving with the Royal Canadian Engineers. Here he is learning some handicrafts to improve manual dexterity at the St. Dunstan's wartime location of Church Stretton, Shropshire, c. 1945. *CNIB Archives*

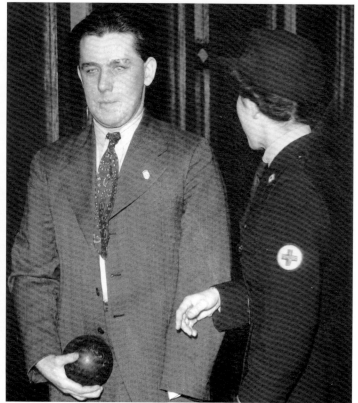

39 Charlemagne Dion, a one-armed, war-blinded veteran on a bowling excursion with a VAD, c. 1945. The VADs took the "boys" shopping and also accompanied them to social and recreational events. *CNIB Archives*

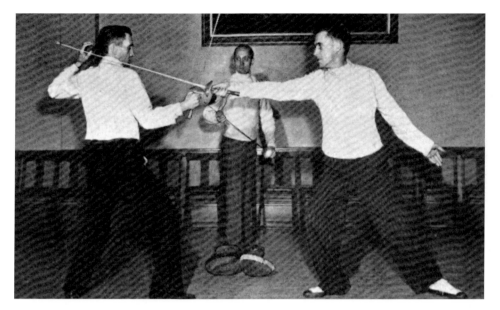

40 Richard Randall, left, and H.V. Teasdale practice at a blind fencing class in Vancouver, 1946. *CNIB Archives*

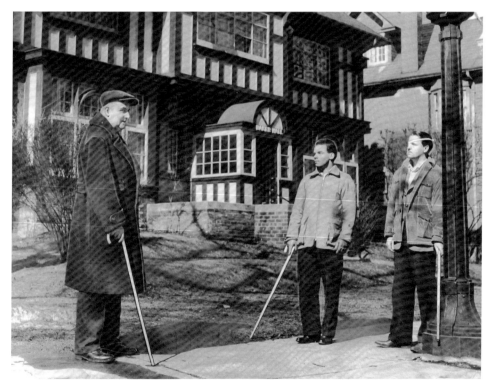

41 David Ferguson and Harry Coyle, at right, learn self-navigation with a white cane from Earl Green, a First World War blinded veteran, Baker Hall, February 1947. *CNIB Archives*

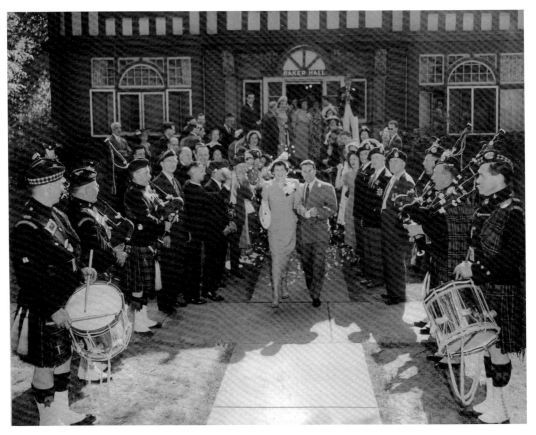

42 Wedding of T.J. Hunter at Baker Hall, June 1949. Twenty-one war-blinded veterans married VADs, volunteers, CNIB employees, or other women whom they met at Baker Hall. *CNIB Archives*

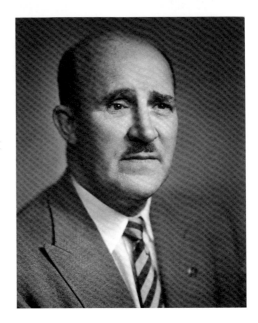

43 F.J.L. (Fred) Woodcock (1905-98) was blinded at Dieppe in 1942, and served as the CNIB's aftercare officer from 1945 until his retirement in 1970. A long-time executive of SAPA and the National Council of Veteran Associations, he devoted his life to furthering the causes of blinded veterans. *CNIB Archives*

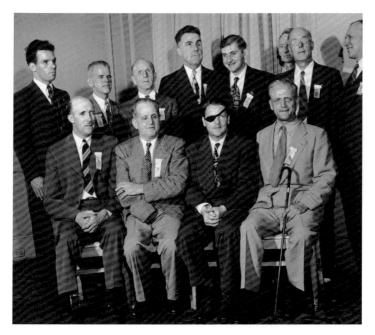

44 The 1947-48 SAPA Executive Committee contained members from both world wars and symbolized the beginning of a smooth, fraternal transition from one generation of leaders to another. Front row from left, Fred Woodcock, Bill Dies, Harry Coyle, and Edwin Baker; back row from left, David Ferguson, A.R. Mallory, Charles Hornsby, E.A. Howes, J.J. Doucet, A. Foster, Alexander Viets, and Guy Foster. *CNIB Archives*

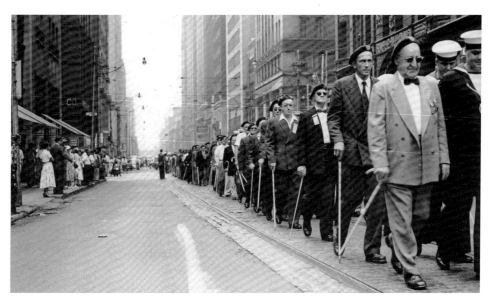

45 In a stirring and poignant moment, on 18 June 1957, during SAPA's fifth general reunion, more than 150 Canadian war-blinded veterans marched on Toronto's Bay Street to lay a wreath at the cenotaph. *CNIB Archives*

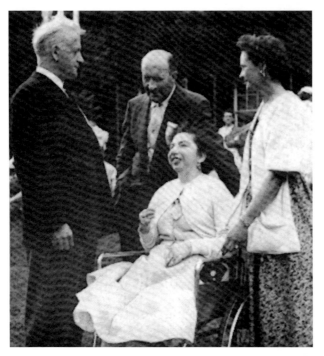

46 Ruth Slater was one of two female members of SAPA attending the 1957 reunion in Toronto. Surrounding her are, from left, Edwin Baker, Fred Woodcock, and Helen Van Brabant, Slater's guide. *CNIB Archives*

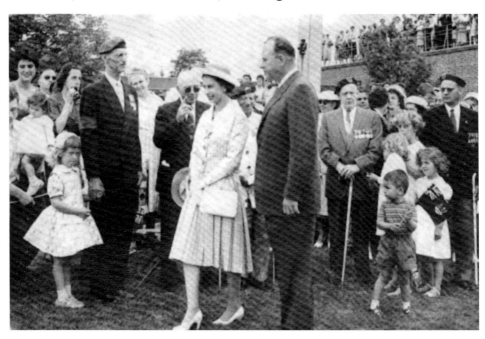

47 Queen Elizabeth II, escorted by CNIB president Ralph Misener, meets SAPA members from both world wars during a 1959 visit to Bakerwood, the institute's Toronto headquarters. *CNIB Archives*

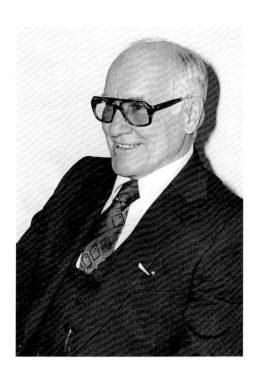

48   William (Bill) Mayne (1916-)
on the occasion of his retirement
from the CNIB, 22 December 1978.
Serving with the Winnipeg Grenadiers, Mayne was captured by
the Japanese at Hong Kong in
December 1941 and suffered near-
total vision loss due to avitaminosis
— the result of near-starvation
conditions. He has been a stalwart
member of SAPA for more than six
decades. *CNIB Archives*

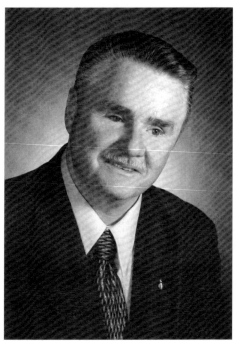

49   In July 1989, Jim Sanders
(1947-), the CNIB aftercare
director, became the new SAPA
executive director, a position he
would hold for more than twenty
years. Although Sanders was not a
veteran, he proved a prescient
choice. *CNIB Archives*

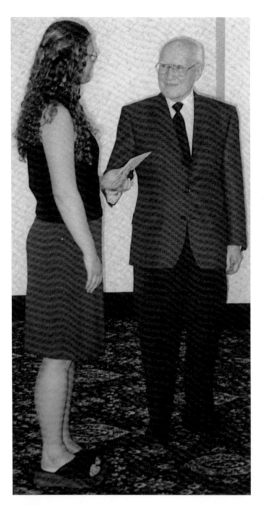

50 Bill Mayne, acting as president of the F.J.L. Woodcock/ SAPA Scholarship Foundation, presents an award to Jennifer Challenger of Omemee, Ontario, May 2001. *SAPA Archives*

51 The SAPA Lounge at the CNIB headquarters at 1929 Bayview Avenue, Toronto. *SAPA Archives*

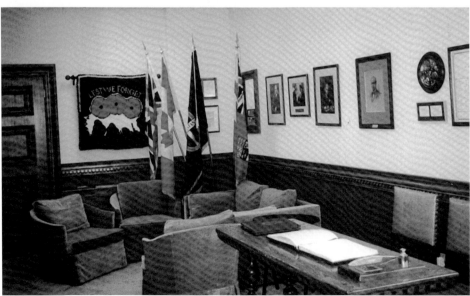

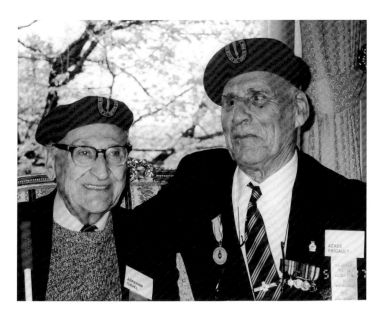

52   Abraham Israel and Azade Frigault at the 1997
SAPA reunion in Aurora, Ontario. *SAPA Archives*

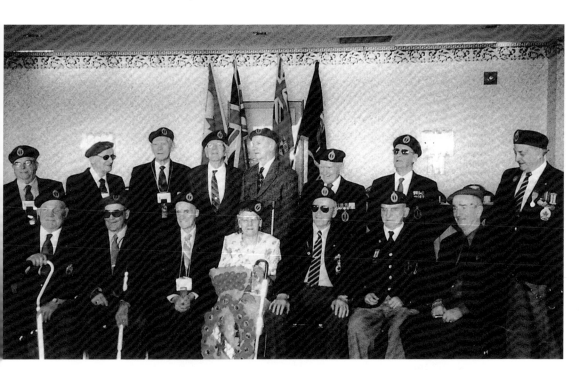

53   Fifteen of the sixteen SAPA members who attended the final reunion
in Belleville, Ontario, in May 2001. SAPA president Anne Michielin, front row
centre, was the first woman to hold the position. She oversaw the winding
down of the organization. Bill Mayne is in the back row, third from right.
SAPA Archives

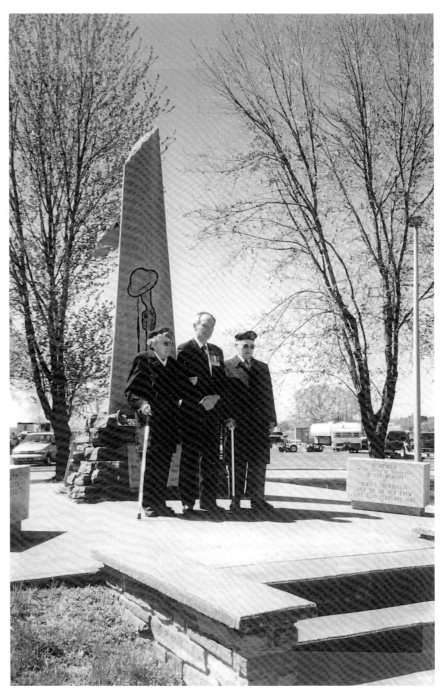

54 SAPA president Anne Michielin and vice-president Bill Mayne flank VAC Deputy Minister Larry Murray at the cenotaph in Trenton, Ontario, May 2001. *SAPA Archives*

of the CNIB's War-Blinded Training Committee, where he was warmly welcomed. According to the minutes, Dunlop "expressed the wish that all casualties could be handled as efficiently as the war blinded are looked after by the Institute."[120]

By the late 1940s, the DVA-CNIB-SAPA relationship was working well. Like its predecessor ministries, the Department of Veterans Affairs agreed that where non-governmental facilities existed that could best serve the needs of the veteran in need of rehabilitation, then arrangements would be made to have these available to veterans. As Woods pointed out, "An outstanding illustration of this is in the case of the Canadian National Institute for the Blind."[121] The CNIB enjoyed a solid reputation and a high profile with the authorities and with the public as a non-governmental agency partnering with Ottawa in the business of re-establishing disabled veterans.

In 1949 the institute and the department concluded another bilateral agreement to provide perpetual care to blinded veterans. As usual, the department assumed financial responsibility for initial training, occupational training, residence costs, and the various activities required to assist veterans in their "general adjustments to sightless life." Further, DVA paid the CNIB one hundred dollars annually per man on the aftercare roll, double the early wartime allotment. Personal equipment, such as typewriters, talking-book machines, and tools, and repairs to these, were also paid for by the department. These provisions had been incrementally gained by Baker, SAPA, and the CNIB throughout the interwar years. The post-1918 experiences certainly facilitated agreement on what was needed during and after the Second World War. Several years later, Woods was firmly of the opinion that the terms of the DVA-CNIB agreement "have been faithfully observed by both parties to the great advantage of the blinded veteran."[122]

While the men needed and obtained special training and rehabilitation facilities during and following the war, by 1944 they also needed a place to stay. And it was in residence, together, that they developed social re-establishment skills and gained the confidence needed to carry on.

Baker Hall

At a September 1943 CNIB council meeting, two war-blinded members, also prominent in the affairs of SAPA, took the lead in proposing that a suitable building be acquired as soon as possible to serve as a residence and perhaps light-training centre for war-blinded veterans of the Second World War. Several men had already been trained at Pearson Hall, and others were about to begin. With Canadians in sustained ground combat in Italy by that time, a lengthening list of war-blinded soldiers was inevitable. But finding appropriate accommodations in crowded wartime Toronto for newly blinded men was no easy task. Some new trainees were living in boarding houses or at the YMCA, looked after by the VADs and the Pearson Hall House Committee.[123] The obvious solution was for the CNIB to establish its own residence.

On the motion of Alexander Viets and T.E. Perrett, a CNIB Residence and Training Centre Committee was struck with Viets as chairman, made up of CNIB president Lewis Wood, general manager Arthur V. Weir, a fixture at the CNIB since the 1920s, Edwin Baker, Grace Worts, Baker's long-time assistant, Harris Turner, and two members of the CNIB's Women's Auxiliary. They had to move quickly before the CNIB's training commitment outstripped the organization's ability to house the disabled men. Pearson Hall, which the federal government had originally provided to the CNIB as a residence, would be too expensive to convert back to that purpose again and, besides, was desperately needed as an administrative and training centre. Financial assistance was required and, using the sympathetic press, the CNIB publicized its urgent quest in the hope that a suitable property might be donated by a local philanthropist.[124]

In less than two weeks, committee members visited seven prospective properties from among twenty-eight proposals received, though none was deemed immediately suitable. In the event that none could be found or donated, Lady Virginia Kemp, widow of industrialist and former minister of militia and defence Sir Edward Kemp, strong supporter of war charities and patron of the arts, offered to purchase a property for up to fifteen thousand dollars as a donation to the CNIB. Kemp had been a CNIB volunteer since 1927, when she joined the Women's Auxiliary in Toronto, and served as its president from 1934 to 1945. In 1939 she became a CNIB vice-president. Before the end of October, Wood reported that a spacious home, about one and a half miles from Pearson Hall, had passed a professional inspection and seemed ideal.

Recognizing the importance of the experiences of war-blinded veterans of the First World War in guiding decisions to be taken on behalf of those of the current war, Wood sought SAPA's official input before rendering a final decision. Moreover, although Wood felt certain that DPNH would be "agreeable" to the purchase plan, and would continue to pay the CNIB for the men's room and board, he worried that so large a house for so few war blinded (to that date) might raise the eyebrows of those interested in how the institute disposed of its funds. But Baker felt that this sort of criticism would be easier to deal with than that which might be raised if the CNIB and SAPA, after four years of war, were found to be unprepared for the urgent housing needs of the wounded. It was important to secure SAPA's public approval of the venture, which was readily forthcoming, in order to show that the veterans themselves were behind the effort.[125]

In November 1943, Lady Kemp purchased for $13,500 the eighteen-room, five-bathroom, Tudor-style house at 78 Admiral Road, standing on a lot 76 by 134 feet. With the help of her daughter, Katherine, who paid for the furnishings, Lady Kemp presented the house as a gift to the CNIB.[126] Of great importance from the perspective of the blind, the building had very simple and uniform floor plans. "The suitability from a sightless man's point of view" was decided by Baker, Turner, and Viets, all of whom knew what would be safe and acceptable for housing blinded veterans.[127]

However, before any of this could come to pass, public wrangling over Toronto's zoning legislation for the Admiral Road property jeopardized the CNIB's plans. A municipal by-law prohibited other than purely residential properties on Admiral Road, and the possibility existed that the CNIB's use of the building would include light rehabilitation training. A number of local property owners, including Judge T. Ernest Codson, stood firmly and vocally opposed to any rezoning, considering it a threat to their quiet lifestyle and possibly to property values in the neighbourhood. Despite government-inspired public rhetoric and the perhaps idealized view of loyal Toronto's commitment to the war effort, gratitude for the wounded's sacrifice did not automatically manifest as a willingness to assist. A meeting of the city's Property Committee was held in early December 1943 to discuss the CNIB's application for a by-law amendment to allow the conversion of the newly purchased building for its intended purposes. Baker opposed the recalcitrant homeowners at a Property Committee hearing, but to no avail. On a strict interpretation of the by-laws, the Property Committee rejected Baker's views and ruled against the proposed amendment.[128] Baker sedately stated that he was "much disturbed" by the whole affair.[129]

The Property Committee's refusal infuriated some city councillors, who felt that Judge Codson had "overawed" the committee members. Alderman John Innes, who chaired the Property Committee and had voted to support the CNIB's petition, was outraged:

> The property rights of owners ... are absolutely nothing compared with the welfare of soldiers who have been blinded in our defence. The whole thing makes me sick. We talk our

> heads off about how much we are going to do for the soldiers when they come back. Yet, when a few do come back now and ask us to permit them to live in a decent location we refuse them because of the selfish opposition of a few property owners. If it weren't for the sacrifices of these men these property owners wouldn't have any property to be so choosy about.

Innes labelled the decision "monstrous" and "hypocritical," and said that if Canada's war wounded were not better treated, then "this country will be in a sorry mess."[130] Another official aghast at the unexpected turn of events was city Control Board member Robert H. Saunders, who publicly vented fury at the members of the Property Committee: "It would be the most unChristian act ever performed at the City Hall if we refused to allow these soldiers to have the best that can be given them."[131] The veterans' community also loudly and publicly supported the CNIB and the war blinded. Frank G.J. McDonagh, president of the Canadian Pensioners' Association of the Great War and a good friend of Baker's, termed the deplorable situation almost "beyond belief." The Canadian Corps Association and the Canadian Legion also voiced outrage.[132]

The imbroglio became a cause célèbre, with numerous emotional newspaper accounts in early December 1943 pillorying the seemingly heartless and unpatriotic homeowners. Seventeen of twenty-five residents in the neighbourhood of 78 Admiral Road informally polled by the Toronto *Daily Star* claimed that they supported the opening of the war-blinded facility, with only four expressing opposition and four remaining "neutral." Undoubtedly typical of the large number of Toronto families with members on active service, or who had already paid a crushing price in the war, Mrs. Aylmer Lyons told the newspaper, "My son, Flight-Sergeant Walter Lyons, was killed last year. I think that everything we can do for returned disabled soldiers should be done." By contrast, however,

Mrs. L. Starkman said of the proposed CNIB site, "I don't want it. There are plenty of quiet places besides here. It would cheapen the neighbourhood."[133] While the uncharitable Mrs. Starkman seemed to represent a minority view among Toronto's residents, this wartime debate implies the need to nuance some commonly held assumptions about the willingness of Canadians to "do their bit" for the war effort or on behalf of men and women in uniform.

City hall was inundated with petitions, letters, and telephone calls in support of opening the residence. One alderman opposed to the amendment claimed that an important civic matter was being decided in the press by "threats, propaganda and hysterics." These were highly charged times during which non-conformity to patriotic views supportive of the fighting forces was socially unacceptable and viewed as morally reprehensible. Outraged citizens even telephoned the reluctant property owners to harshly condemn them. "They even told me I ought to be in Germany," said Mr. Slesinger. Another, Mrs. H.C. Simpson, claimed that she did not want her "heart wrung out day in and day out by the sad sight of blinded soldiers passing by."[134] The war blinded had become a test case for public patriotism and charitable sentiment, and Baker reminded city council that "human values should come before property values." In the end, concerned Torontonians did not let the men down. During heated four-hour deliberations on 13 December, three of the six aldermen members of the Property Committee changed their stance and the by-law amendment passed in city council, overturning the earlier judgment of the Property Committee.

Despite the public furor and the pressures to conform with wartime patriotic views, some property owners appealed to the Ontario Municipal Board to overturn the city council's by-law amendment, notwithstanding the fact that Baker by that time had made it clear that the building would be used as a residence only. The disgruntled homeowners, by now only a few diehards, complained to the board that the CNIB had used the press to pressure the city. In

January 1944, the board avoided taking sides on this contentious issue, which pitted established zoning procedures against a wartime moral imperative. Washing its hands of the matter, the board returned the file to the city for final resolution.

Baker, pleading before a "completely silent council," insisted that the war blinded would cause no disturbances, promised that the CNIB would carefully supervise the premises, and assured the city council that local residents' property values would not suffer. It must have been a sad day for Baker, obliged to convince his city's representatives that sightless veterans were not only deserving but actually non-threatening. "I hope we won't give worry to anyone," remarked Baker upon leaving the hearing. One of Canada's best-known veterans was reduced to making excuses for sightless veterans in need. In response to Baker's parting comment, *Globe and Mail* columnist Frank Tumpane wrote on 25 January, "Don't worry, Colonel. Don't worry too much about that. For there are many in Toronto who recognize the full measure they owe these men. No necessity exists for speaking softly, Colonel. Thunder might be the proper retort." An outraged Tumpane intoned that the "senses of those we choose to call heroes were subjected to the desolation of being named intruders." In describing one young veteran blinded in Sicily and at that time waiting for a place in a residence, Tumpane wrote, "It is certain that when he gripped his head in his hands he had no thought of Admiral Road or some of its squeamish residents ... He could have loved the sight of familiar things as dearly as those who stayed behind him and did not go to Sicily ... Guard the welfare of these men, Colonel ... and don't give anything else a thought."[135]

One member of the Women's Electors' Association, who was present at the council meeting, exclaimed, "I feel ashamed, unclean, that any should try to prevent the best possible treatment being given to blinded heroes." The city upheld the amendment, Mayor Frederick J. Conboy voting in favour.[136] It was a pity that such efforts were needed to obtain the residence and sanctuary for the veterans and that, as *Globe and Mail* columnist Jack Hambleton claimed, "Toronto has been subjected to unfavourable criticism from one end of the continent to the other." The vast majority of Torontonians and Canadians, however, were willing to accommodate the nation's war blinded and assist with their rehabilitation.

Governor General the Earl of Athlone, accompanied by his wife, Princess Alice, formally opened the renovated residence on 23 March 1944, while several hundred people looked on, including a number of war-blinded veterans of the First World War, five from the Second, civic and government leaders, members of the clergy, and Toronto-area military dignitaries representing all three services. "I am proud to be able to present this house as a haven for the new war blinded ... and I wish it to be known as Baker Hall," announced Lady Kemp. Baker was as "astonished" as everyone else to learn of her gesture in naming the building for him.[137] Baker richly deserved the recognition. Lady Kemp handed the key to the building to Alexander Viets, first vice-president of the CNIB and Canada's first war-blinded soldier of the First World War. She formally transferred ownership to the CNIB in July 1946.[138] Within a month of its opening, six recently blinded veterans were in residence in Baker Hall's comfortable surroundings.

In late 1943, the CNIB Women's Auxiliary requested of long-time member Elsinore C. Burns that she take on the chairmanship of the all-volunteer Baker Hall House Committee, "whose responsibility it was," wrote Burns afterwards, "to see that life at Baker Hall should complement and round out the formal training" carried out at Pearson Hall. This meant that the men could be observed in a social setting, as well as have an opportunity to compare notes, feel at ease in familiar surroundings, study, practise their Braille, or simply relax. The new residence was always intended as a site of latent training as well as a place for the men to call home until such time as they were returned to their families or found employment. The federal government assumed the financial burden for operating Baker Hall "as a matter of training responsibility," according to Burns.[139] Certainly, the men had to stay somewhere and their board, like their rehabilitation, was a public charge, not that of the institute.

Up to twenty residents were accommodated at a time for nine months or more, depending on how long they required for their vocational training at Pearson Hall or the nearby CNIB training annex. If there was room at Baker Hall following completion of their training, the men were welcome to stay. About fifteen staff and volunteers – home teachers, social workers, VADs, and others – helped make life enjoyable for the veterans. As Elsinore Burns noted, in the homey atmosphere of Baker Hall, many "special comforts, entertainment, and much hospitality" were provided by "friends" of the war blinded.[140] There were a number of welcome diversions: a music room with a piano and radio, a library with books, magazines, and talking books, and a sun room suitable for card games and other distractions. These were complemented by a small gymnasium on the top floor and the use of two telephones. But there were also rules for the men to follow while billeted at Baker Hall. The House Committee expected that the men would display common etiquette and politeness in their dealings with each other, keep noise to a minimum, with none after 11:00 p.m., and assemble promptly for meals.[141]

A sense of fraternity, identity, and belonging was essential to the men's morale and often, even, success. Bonds were formed at Baker Hall that would last a lifetime. The 1946 CNIB annual report stated that "the community life of the residence enables newcomers to meet others with the same handicap and to discover how they handle the small crises of everyday living. The more advanced trainees are always ready to initiate the new arrivals in the ways of seeing in the dark."[142] "We all agree," wrote Burns, "that the stimulating effect of shared study and shared social activities has helped to make us a family, and Baker Hall a home."[143]

Maurice Campeau was among the first six arrivals in March 1944. "At first I felt uncomfortable – the house was too nice," he wrote nine months later of his first day there. "We went to sleep hoping that everything would be alright ... But now I realize that with the opportunities for different fields of work that the Institute finds for us, we can hope to have the chance sometime to have nice homes ourselves."[144] Lloyd Tomczak arrived at Baker Hall in January 1946, accompanied by his mother. "I first met Jimmy Hunter by going up the stairs on the wrong side and bumping into him," recalled Tomczak. "He told me what he thought of my stupidity, a message that I cannot put into print. But I never forgot the rule after his little sermon." He noted that from time to time, someone would reach for a bottle and soon feel "no pain, a condition not uncommon to all of us at one time or another."[145]

Bill Mayne "right away" felt among friends at Baker Hall. For example, John Simmons, a young veteran of the merchant navy, introduced himself and befriended Mayne even before he had had a chance to unpack his suitcase. To some extent, recalled Mayne, this sort of camaraderie was even more valuable than the vocational training. Being part of so friendly a group and being in the company of others who had been in Japanese captivity was one of the "greatest features" of his time at Baker Hall. His friends inspired him, and he grew confident in their company that his handicap could be beaten.[146] Blindness was physical, but overcoming its effects could depend on psychological and emotional strength.

For his part, First World War veteran Harris Turner sensed the fraternal and caring atmosphere of Baker Hall when he and his wife attended a dance there after the Second World War. They were greeted by Misses Sutherland, Burns, and Elsie Thorne, all in evening dress. "Their warm welcome made us feel immediately at home," and the fact that the women were in evening dress gave Turner, blinded some thirty years previously, "a tremendous lift. In some subtle way it conveyed to me that after being pitied, coddled, extravagantly praised, cautiously handled like delicate children and set apart as a group of beings different from all others, we ... were to be treated from now on as ... people to be relied upon to respond normally to normal customs and average conditions of civilized living."[147] And the women of Baker Hall cared deeply for their charges. Underscoring the family-like atmosphere, Edith Farmer, Baker Hall's superintendent, wrote an open letter to "my dear boys" that appeared in the Baker Hall news-letter in December 1944. "And when I say 'my,' I really mean that you are mine," she wrote. "Surely you all know that each and every one of you have been dear to me in your own special way ... No mother ever had more considerate sons."[148]

Members of the Canadian Red Cross were present to help when Baker Hall opened in March 1944, and they maintained their regular presence and contact with the war blinded until the facility closed in June 1950. These uniformed Red Cross women mainly served as the much-appreciated VADs, but also among them were dieticians, office administrators, and members providing transportation or accom-paniment to the men when they left Baker Hall to shop or for recrea-tion. All were dedicated volunteers specifically assigned to duty with the war blinded. Their commitment helped many men overcome the early rigours of their condition and training.[149] Speaking of the VADs, Lloyd Tomczak recalled thirty years later that "their humour combined with a human touch gave us all that lift we needed at a crucial time in our lives." And he insisted that "no one could touch the quality of welcome put forth by Miss Burns."[150]

The women were well prepared for their roles. A class "A" VAD took 240 hours of preparatory courses approved by the Canadian Nurses' Association and the Canadian Hospital Council. A Class "B" VAD completed 80 hours of training. In 1942 some VADs were re-cruited for service with the Royal Canadian Army Medical Corps for service in Canadian hospitals. The Red Cross and St. John Ambulance provided VAD training and organization. The VADs wore their organ-izations' uniforms and were secondary in authority to fully-fledged military nurses. Their work in Canada was unpaid, but depending on the nature of their assignments, they received room and board, free travel while on duty, and allowances for their uniforms, upkeep, and incidental expenses.

A handful of Toronto-area St. John Ambulance VADs who had previously worked with SAPA members were dispatched overseas in 1943 for service at St. Dunstan's at Church Stretton. Among the qualifications preferred by St. Dunstan's were "the sympathy and tact so essential when helping blind men to regain a feeling of confidence [and] being able to dance, discuss current events, read aloud well, play dominoes, and ride a bicycle." They proved enormously successful and others would soon follow. According to one account, these VADs "were ... called on to display the special brand of courage and ability required for working and living with sightless and horribly maimed men and women undergoing treatment at St. Dunstan's, both at the surgical unit at Stoke Mandeville [separate from Ovingdean] and at the rehabilitation centre in Church Stretton."[151] They displayed the same professionalism at Baker Hall.

One anonymous VAD published a brief account of her tenure at Baker Hall in a Red Cross magazine. "Such a beautiful house and so full of memories! I'm sure that all the VADs who have been on duty there feel, as I do, that it was never really a duty, but rather a pleasure, to spend a few hours there ... We remember the cribbage games, the shopping trips, dancing lessons, the parties, tea in the garden, and most of all the happy weddings in this house. We had quite an interest in the weddings, as several of the boys married Red Cross girls."[152] At least seven such weddings had taken place or were planned by the summer of 1946. For example, in 1945 Marie Ravenscroft, who volunteered at Baker Hall, wed J.J. Doucet, blinded in Italy from a gunshot wound while serving with the Royal Canadian Regiment. The same year the first of several weddings was held at Baker Hall, when Fred Koenig, whose hands were mangled in the same explosion that blinded him, married a woman with whom he had been in correspondence. Reverend Sydney Lambert, SAPA's honorary president, performed the ceremony. In June 1946, Lambert again officiated at Baker Hall for the wedding of Harvey Simmons, blinded while serving in the 19th Field Regiment, Royal Canadian Artillery, and Myrtle Fox.[153] In all, some thirty men were married while resident at Baker Hall and ten weddings and receptions took place there. No less than twenty-one of these men married women they met while at Baker Hall.[154]

Another story of a blinded soldier marrying is useful for the insight it provides from the bride's perspective. David Ferguson, serving with the North Nova Scotia Highlanders, was blinded by a shell burst near Caen, Normandy, in June 1944 while digging a slit trench. His recovery was aided by his remarkable attitude. "When the Doc told me that I was blind for life," he recalled, I was not surprised ... because I knew it as soon as I felt my face after the explosion. I was so grateful to be alive that I didn't give a darn about anything else. Right then, to me life was the sweetest thing a man could ever possess." In April 1946, Ferguson married Red Cross VAD Patricia Weston, a school-teacher. "He's a veteran and I'm proud of him," she said not long thereafter. "It was a little difficult when we first got married but there were so many compensations that difficulties became pleasures ... There are many times when I forget that he is blind and the only reason I married him is that I love him. I don't think it wonderful and marvellous or even self-sacrificing to marry a blind person. I only hope we have a long life together and that he goes on in the world." Ferguson was more to the point: "I think she had a lot of courage. She's brave and wonderful. She's life to me." Their reception was held at Baker Hall. Both enrolled at the University of Toronto where he earned a BA.[155]

In 1946 the Junior League of Toronto began providing daily volunteer readers for the war blinded attending university. It was common for the same girl to read to a student-veteran for the duration of a three-year program. The St. Alban's Girls' Club also provided readers and walking guides from 1946 to 1950. The Arthur Murray

School of Dancing offered weekly lessons, the teachers giving freely
of their time and "helping the lads to learn all the new steps as well
as to regain confidence and poise." The Toronto Musicians' Protective
Association provided volunteer Sunday afternoon concerts and also
played at Baker Hall dances. Various groups and clubs provided useful items, such as radios. Sometimes individual volunteer readers un-
affiliated with any group dropped by. For example, Ted Read arrived
in April 1944, shortly after Baker Hall opened, and stayed involved
until its closure "to give a helping hand and to do anything in any
way, for any of the boys." From 1945 to 1948, a local barber, Pasquale
Leone, established an improvised barber shop at Baker Hall and offered his services without charge on Sundays.[156] Daily teatime was
aided by volunteer tea hostesses who arrived to assist the House
Committee, "lending homelike graciousness to the tea hour." Others
sent fruit, flowers, cakes, cigarettes, and sweets, while various enter-
tainers lent their spare time as well.[157] Despite the small number of
war blinded, Torontonians were well aware of their presence and
responded warmly and generously.

In September 1945, a Sir Arthur Pearson Stag Night Committee
was formed to organize a monthly program of speakers, musicians,
and even quizmasters for the residents of Baker Hall. These evenings
were a major morale boost for the blinded veterans. The speakers
at the final Stag Night were famed composer Sir Ernest MacMillan,
former prime minister Arthur Meighen, and, appropriately, Edwin
Baker.[158] The strong emphasis on social events and pleasantries
helped the men cope and provided them with a semblance of normalcy. The Stag Nights had the goal of cementing intergenerational
ties among the war blinded, as is shown in the wording of the inaugural invitation from the Second Word War blinded to those of the
First World War: "appreciating all the things that you chaps have done
for us" and "to bridge the gap between the last war blind and this ...
we can all have an enjoyable time winning over again not only the

battles of the last war, but also of the present struggle which has just ended."[159]

The formal use of Baker Hall by the war blinded came to an end in 1950. The CNIB sold the building for $35,000 in June 1951, with the proceeds, by prior arrangement with Lady Kemp, set aside for the erection of a blinded women's residence. The institute rightly felt that Lady Kemp had proven "one of the most generous and unflagging supporters the organization has ever had."[160] In her introduction to a souvenir booklet she wrote for the residents of Baker Hall, Elsinore Burns wrote tenderly to the war blinded, "It is not necessary to remind any of you how interested we shall always be in where you are, and what you are doing. We shall continue to watch your careers with the same joy in your progress."[161] She, and the whole of CNIB and SAPA, remained true to this pledge.

In 1947, the late influx of so many new trainees, mainly Hong Kong veterans, had obliged the CNIB to lease a home on Bernard Street to handle the overflow. But only 74 of 145 men "definitely regarded" as war blinded, including veterans of Hong Kong, had completed training to 31 March 1948. In March 1950, Saunders reported that 134 veterans thus far had entered the training cycle, with 18 still in attendance.[162] There were relatively few new arrivals and these henceforward could be handled on an ad hoc basis either in Toronto or through the CNIB facilities in the districts. The Pearson Hall training centre closed in December 1950, with DVA support continuing for several more months to accommodate the two men then undergoing training.[163] Ironically, the closure took place notwithstanding the Korean War, which had been raging since June 1950 and to which Canadian troops had been committed, though in modest numbers. Baker noted in early 1951 that the institute had already made preparations to care for any blinded men resulting from service in Korea.[164]

Between March 1944 and June 1950, when Baker Hall closed, 140 Canadian war-blinded veterans, some three-quarters of the total identified in the immediate postwar period, availed themselves of the CNIB's rehabilitation and training services; 125 of these resided at Baker Hall. Others lived with family members while training in Toronto. Of these 140, 68 were resident in Ontario, 22 came from Quebec, 14 from Manitoba, 10 from British Columbia, 9 from Alberta, 7 from New Brunswick, 2 from Saskatchewan, 2 lived in England, 1 was from Nova Scotia, 4 were deceased by June 1950, and no place of origin was listed for one former resident. By 1950, four had recovered sufficient sight to be deregistered as blinded.[165]

The men's varied occupational histories testify to the many employment possibilities open to the blind as well as to the perseverance of many of the men. The following list summarizes the trainees' occupations at June 1950.[166]

32 concession stand managers
 2 concession stand assistants
 8 industrial workers or machine operators
 7 CNIB staff
 7 studying at the University of Toronto
 6 upholsterers
 6 cafeteria managers
 1 cafeteria assistant
 4 handicraft workers
 3 agricultural workers
 3 small store owners
 3 weavers on their own account
 2 woodworkers on their own account
 2 physiotherapists
 1 working in labour relations
 1 salesman
 1 recreation officer

    1 commercial fisherman
    1 employed in a printing shop
    1 helping run a family hotel
    1 Dictaphone typist
    1 executive director of the Canadian Arthritis and
       Rheumatism Society
    1 in trucking business
    1 employed at the National Research Council
    1 in tourist trade
    1 elevator operator
    1 Veterans' Land Act holding
    1 housewife
    1 continuing medical treatment
    2 occupations not listed
    5 at home; no occupation decided
    5 unemployed
   17 still in training

In early 1951, Fred Woodcock undertook an extensive survey of all the Second World War blinded casualties to firmly establish their number and to determine how many had been trained and whether they had found gainful employment. To 16 January 1951, Woodcock's research yielded 194 war-blinded Canadians of the Second World War, of whom 57 were veterans of Hong Kong and victims of maltreatment in Japanese POW camps, and 137 were blinded elsewhere, mainly in ground combat in the European and Mediterranean theatres of operation. Perhaps surprising was the number of blinded veterans who did not or could not undertake training, or who did not complete training with the CNIB: 58, or 30 percent. Moreover, 40, nearly 21 percent, were unemployed or unemployable, the vast majority of these being also untrained. Most of these men had severe wounds or disabilities extending beyond their blindness. More positively, a similar 1948 survey had shown that fully 75 percent of trained blinded veterans were employed, implying that a much higher percentage of those who *could* work, did so.[167]

Later in 1951, six of the veterans identified by Woodcock had died, while five of them had regained sufficient sight to be struck from the rolls of the nation's war blinded for pension and aftercare purposes. This left 183 veterans eligible for aftercare, added to the 150 surviving blinded from the First World War (of whom 31 lived abroad). These 333 Canadian war blinded constituted, more or less, the high-water mark of SAPA's membership, even though, by one estimate thirty years later, about 460 Canadians were blinded during the Second World War or became blind in the postwar period due to service-related wounds, injuries, illnesses, and physical deterioration.[168]

In 1948 Baker had stated that "despite the loss of sight in early manhood and, in many cases, serious additional disabilities, this group of young men has provided an inspiring demonstration of our claim that, despite blindness, the remaining talents can be usefully applied where there is a determined spirit."[169] In harnessing that spirit, Baker, the CNIB, SAPA, and DVA had restored hope to the nation's war blinded, who were able to walk into the future with dignity.

5 Older and Wiser: Canada's War Blinded in the Aftermath of War, 1945-70

They cannot see, as they march, the impression they make; the still thoughtful faces of spectators are dark to them but they must sense the respect, the gratitude and the admiration they inspire.

– Toronto *Telegram,* 19 June 1957

The Second World War and the years that followed proved a watershed for the Sir Arthur Pearson Association of War Blinded (SAPA) and the war blinded in general. While the war had tragically more than doubled the organization's membership, the postwar years marked the ascendancy of a younger generation of Canadian war blinded. These new members helped reshape SAPA's goals and outlooks, took on a growing leadership role in the group, and increasingly assumed the responsibilities that had been in the capable hands of the First World War generation. These years also saw the passing or retirement of many key players in the early development and successes of the organization.

Canada, too, was experiencing major changes. In the 1950s and 1960s, economic depression and world war yielded to massive economic growth, a vastly increased standard of living for most Canadians, and the uneasy peace of the Cold War. Population growth was phenomenal and, across the country, hundreds of thousands of new dwellings were built, as was the infrastructure to provide for those living in them. Canada also incrementally developed its welfare state, a series of social programs through which the federal government promised to deliver a basic minimum standard of living to all citizens. These emerging policies, such as unemployment insurance, family allowances, improved seniors' pensions, the Canada Pension Plan, universal health care, and welfare payments to the poorest, became available to all Canadians as a matter of right or entitlement, and not only to those society deemed impoverished. These provisions assisted thousands of veterans fallen on hard times.

A precursor of the emerging Canadian welfare state had been the veterans' civil re-establishment programs following the First World War. These were followed after 1945 by a series of complex pieces of legislation aimed at smoothly reintegrating discharged military personnel into civil society. These legislative initiatives, including some dealing specifically with disabled veterans' needs and pensions, were known collectively as the Veterans Charter. The veterans' postwar agitation for increased pension allotments needs to be seen in light of the provisions of the Veterans Charter and also within the context of the country's burgeoning economy and the rapid growth in government social programming.

This chapter will treat the postwar experiences of Canada's war-blinded veterans and deal with some shifts in the business of SAPA, such as the creation of a scholarship fund for young blind Canadians. While there was evolution, there was also continuity, and the period 1945 to 1970 was marked by occasionally vexing membership issues, emotive reunions, the war blinded's continuing integration into a broader veterans' community, ongoing pension struggles, the deepening fraternity linking the military blind with the civilian and an older generation with a younger, and, ultimately, the necessity of carrying on. The post-1945 Canadian war-blinded aftercare program showcased the administrative abilities of the blinded veterans and further demonstrated the capacity of most to endure the new physical limitations imposed upon them.

Pensions and Veterans' Solidarity

Improving federal pensions for Canada's veterans depended on co-operation among the diverse veterans' organizations and the ability of these groups to present Ottawa with a powerful common front. Few veterans worked harder toward this goal than the war blinded. Prominent SAPA members Edwin Baker, Fred Woodcock, Bill Mayne, and Bill Dies devoted enormous time and effort, often under the aegis of the National Council of Veteran Associations in Canada, to arranging for a united front on a range of pension-related questions. SAPA also pursued its own agenda, based on the particular needs of its members and the perception that pension authorities did not fully appreciate the psychological hardships they experienced as a result of their blindness. By the late 1960s, all veterans had achieved considerable success in their struggles with a sometimes recalcitrant government – and SAPA had been in the thick of the fight from the beginning.

SAPA and the National Council of Veteran Associations in Canada

Edwin Baker had long seen the value of veterans' organizations co-operating to petition federal authorities for additional pension and other re-establishment benefits. In the late 1920s, he had been in-volved in creating the Associated Veterans Organizations of Canada, an umbrella group mainly intended to pressure Ottawa on pension issues. In January 1932, the group's five member organizations, including the Canadian Legion, had jointly presented a brief to the federal government, with Baker representing SAPA. By the end of the decade, the coalition had dismantled, partly due to divergent or increasingly specialized interests and also because no outstanding major issues required its continued existence.[1]

The SAPA-Amputations Association "alliance" had borne fruit in the past and, with the outbreak of the Second World War, SAPA and the War Amputations of Canada (so named since 1940) had sought to "foster a united veteran front on the Canadian war effort and on all matters affecting ex-servicemen ... and their dependants."[2] Baker was concerned in 1942 that Ottawa would merely brush aside veterans' general dissatisfaction with government regulations concerning allowances for pensioned veterans' wives and children. What was needed was a robust veterans' unity on the matter. Perhaps a new veterans' grouping, involving the greatest possible number and variety of members, would convince Ottawa that the issues put before the government were important and that ignoring them entailed some political peril. Baker wanted the veteran community, already bolstered in number by thousands of the Second World War cadre, to negotiate from a position of greater strength.

In the autumn of 1942, six veterans' organizations – the Canadian Legion, the Army and Navy Veterans in Canada, the Canadian Pensioners' Association, the Canadian Corps Association, the War Amputations of Canada, and the Sir Arthur Pearson Association of War Blinded – met to reach a consensus on how they might co-operate to further the cause of returned men. But some old rivalries persisted, especially between the Legion and the Canadian Corps Association, and, as Baker noted laconically, "After many weeks it was finally concluded that the Canadian Legion could not be expected to participate."[3] Accordingly, in April 1943, the remaining five groups, most with long-standing friendly ties between them, formed the umbrella organization and lobby group the National Council of Veteran Associations in Canada (NCVA).

Baker was named the organization's first chairman, and SAPA was further represented at NCVA executive meetings by its president, J. Harvey Lynes. The war blinded's already high profile in the veterans' community and with government officials was significantly augmented. The NCVA's operating principles were simple: "no matter may be sponsored in the name of the National Council unless unanimously agreed to by the five member organizations." Moreover, no new veterans' groups would be admitted to membership unless they agreed to this condition and all member groups were in favour of granting membership. On the other hand, nothing prevented individual member groups from making separate representations to the government.[4] In the 1950s, Harry Coyle, a Second World War veteran and SAPA member, opined on the value to SAPA of membership in NCVA: "The importance to the small groups lies in the provision that each member organization has only one vote, and each proposal must be unanimously agreed to before it is acted upon. Thus the war blinded share authority equally with its comparatively giant kindred associations and a brief submitted by them may go to Ottawa supported by thousands of veterans."[5] That had been Baker's point all along.

In response to a 1952 public inquiry, Baker recalled that the NCVA was formed "to promote understanding, co-operation and if possible uniformity in recommendations, proposals, and active efforts for the welfare of ex-servicemen, disabled and otherwise, in Canada." By then the NCVA had grown to six member organizations. Although Baker cited no membership figures for the Canadian Corps Association, the Canadian Paraplegics Association had about 200 members, SAPA 300, the War Amps 3,000, the Canadian Pensioners' Association 50,000, and the Army, Navy and Air Force Veterans in Canada 70,000.[6]

One major goal of the NCVA was to "eliminate controversy" among veterans' groups and promote co-operation and joint action. Previous infighting, especially between the Legion and the Canadian

Corps Association, occasionally had hampered the veterans' community's ability to forcefully negotiate with government authorities. The NCVA was "purposefully" without bylaws or a constitution, to avoid similar internecine conflict. According to Baker in 1952, since the NCVA's inception nine years previously, it had "been able to discourage practically all public controversies between our member organizations and between ... our Council and the Canadian Legion." Since four NCVA members were associations of disabled or pensioned veterans, and their resolutions and petitions were shared unanimously by a variety of groups, their demands, usually quite specific, carried more practical and political weight.[7]

The NCVA's first order of business was to pressure Ottawa to establish a new veterans' hospital and residence in the Toronto area to replace the aging Christie Street Hospital. In this instance joined by other veteran and patriotic groups, including the Legion, the NCVA-led campaign proved successful. The sod-turning ceremony for what would become Sunnybrook Hospital took place, appropriately, on 11 November 1943. SAPA was represented at the event by Harvey Lynes.[8] The NCVA exerted swift and growing influence in government policy-making decisions, though whether it was ever the predominant force in effecting change is difficult to determine. The Legion, too, wielded great political clout by dint of its large membership.

Throughout this period, SAPA remained stubbornly interested in removing the marriage deadline respecting allowances for the wives and children of war pensioners. As things stood, pensioned veterans marrying after 1 January 1930 received no spousal allowance, nor was there any allowance for children born after May 1933. SAPA members felt this unnecessarily disadvantaged men, perhaps especially disabled men, who married and had families later in life. Despite little movement on this issue in the short term, by 1945 SAPA, through the NCVA, had obtained a concession concerning the widows of pensioners rated at least 50 percent disabled. Henceforth women who had married these disabled veterans between 1 January 1930 and 1 April 1944 were eligible for widows' pensions.[9] Though not all pensioners were covered, this was a significant step forward.

Jurisdiction over several key components of veteran-related legislation was divided among several different government departments. The NCVA lobbied Ottawa to completely reorganize the cumbersome Department of Pensions and National Health and carve out a new department of government "exclusively the responsibility of one Minister," which the NCVA proposed should be called the Department of War Veteran Affairs, to deal exclusively with veterans' issues. The Canadian Legion, too, mounted its own very strong campaign in favour of this structural change. Again, Ottawa recognized this pressing need and responded positively to the combined veterans' prodding: the new Department of Veterans Affairs came into existence in October 1944.[10]

Insisting on Their Entitlement

The NCVA burst onto the scene during the war, when patriotic impulses and support for veterans' causes were high and commonly shared across the country, and the group's influence in Ottawa was probably disproportionately strong. But its member organizations refused to let the momentum slow following the war's end. In early 1948, SAPA spearheaded an NCVA brief to the Department of Veterans Affairs on increasing basic pension rates for disabled veterans and their survivors. Copies of the brief were dispatched to the Canadian Legion "with a suggestion that a united front if possible should be presented at this time."[11] Baker, in his capacity as chairman of the NCVA, also sent Milton Gregg, the minister of veterans affairs and a winner of the Victoria Cross during the First World War, a powerful and emotive letter pleading on behalf of greater pension entitlements.

"We, the members of the National Council of Veteran Associations in Canada, have a broad realization of the problems confronting ex-servicemen of this country, and especially the disabled," wrote Baker, who also bombarded the minister with a list of recommendations aimed especially at ameliorating the conditions of veterans with disabilities. Baker hoped to impress upon the minister the sad plight of many disabled veterans whose livelihoods depended on equitable treatment by pension authorities at a time of increasing postwar inflation. In order that war-disabled veterans could obtain pensions sufficient to maintain themselves in dignity, Baker warned the minister that "every precaution must be taken to ensure against confused thinking and ill-conceived economizing ... certain to work hardship on the war disabled."[12]

Since wartime price controls had been eliminated, wages and costs had risen far more quickly than the compensation paid to disabled veterans, whose struggles to find suitable and reasonably paid employment had been well documented since the First World War. Despite a strong economy, times were getting tough for the lowest-income Canadians, often including the war disabled, and not all of Canada's war-blinded veterans could make ends meet. Basic pension amounts had been little changed since 1939, while Baker claimed that the purchasing power of the dollar had been halved in the previous decade. The NCVA insisted on a basic minimum pension rate of one hundred dollars per month for those deemed 100 percent disabled. It had been seventy-five dollars since 1921.[13]

As for disabled veterans' spousal and survivors' pensions, the NCVA sought the elimination of the recently obtained 1 April 1944 marriage deadline intended mainly for First World War veterans, especially given that the latter had by then "substantially dwindled" in number. The group also wanted widows' pensions, which Baker "understood to be a measure of compensation for the loss of a husband whose death was due to his wartime service to the State," to be raised to eighty dollars monthly. This amount did not constitute a living wage. The amount allotted for children being supported by a widow needed to double to thirty dollars monthly, the same rate allocated per child to orphanages or children's shelters. "It is somewhat of a paradox to expect a widow to provide adequate food, shelter, clothing and education for young children at one-half the rate allowed to an orphan," Baker bitterly wrote Gregg.[14]

Then there were the non-pensioned widows. If a man had been pensioned at less than 45 percent disabled or if he was disabled but not pensioned, the NCVA sought an increase to $50 monthly for his widow. As for attendance allowance, sometimes formally referred to as "helplessness" allowance, the NCVA sought an increase to $1,200 per annum. "It should not be necessary to comment on this item," wrote Baker to the minister, "since it must be obvious to all that the very seriously disabled cannot possibly pay for necessary assistance on an allowance of $750." He went on to note that housemaids' annual wages were up to $900 plus board, whereas cooks "insisted" on no less than $600. Orderlies were "unobtainable" at even $1,200 per annum for eight-hour days. "We consider that $1,200 per annum is a minimum requirement for minimum essential assistance," Baker wrote.[15]

Baker hastened to add at the end of his lengthy letter to Gregg that the hardships encountered by Canadian disabled veterans "have arisen largely as a result of the post-war adjustment processes and economic disturbances." Their needs were compounded not only by the rise in the cost of living but also by the "improvement in standards of living since 1918." The veterans had given their all; they wanted just compensation. To refuse would be to "deliberately ... restrict them to sub-normal conditions of living." Baker would not allow them to be so condemned and confidently stated that "we can never believe that this is the desire of the people of Canada." In the end, both sides agreed to a compromise 25 percent increase.[16]

In 1952 the definition of blindness from a pension perspective was a maximum vision of 6/60 metres, with attendance allowance granted in instances of 2/60 or less. As of 1 January 1952, pension compensation for 100 percent disability had risen to $125 monthly with a spousal allowance of $45 monthly. Children's allowance for boys up to and including sixteen and girls to seventeen if they were in school was $20, with another $15 for a second child and $12 for subsequent children. Pensions for widows were set at $100 with $40 for the first child until twenty-one years old if still in school. The attendance allowance was $80 monthly. Veterans deemed unemployable received a war veterans allowance of $50 monthly for a single man, $90 if married. But these recipients could not earn any income exceeding $60 and $100 monthly, respectively. A blind veteran could not simultaneously receive a war pension and a civilian blind pension, which the federal government had awarded since 1937 and which, by 1958, had risen to $75 monthly to all civilian blind aged eighteen and over.[17]

In 1956, SAPA sought and obtained the NCVA's support for the war blinded's principal remaining demands of the federal government. The first was for widows of totally blind veterans to continue getting a full pension for a year following the veteran's death and not see it reduced to $100 the day after his death. Second, SAPA desired an increase in pensions for war-blinded veterans because most earned low incomes and needed more financial assistance than many other disabled, but sighted, veterans. SAPA sought an increase to $200 per month for those 100 percent disabled due to blindness. Third, the war blinded wanted free hospitalization for non-pensionable conditions: "As a major disability group," stated SAPA's resolution, "we *know* there is a direct connection between our pensionable disability and many other conditions that crop up, from time to time, but there is no legal means ... to provide us with free hospitalization and treatment for these conditions. Coming within this category are injuries incurred by falls, etc.; nerve conditions pursuant to the frustration and strain of blindness and its many ramifications contributing to general health breakdown." Universal government-sponsored health care was still more than a decade away, but aging veterans' needs seemed to make the measure more urgent and perhaps more acceptable.

Fourth was the issue of attendance allowance and the lack of consistency in its provision. If a war-blinded veteran was deemed to have useful vision of less than 2/60, he received an allowance of $960 per annum. But oculists' reports varied, and administrators' leeway in assessing remaining useful vision led to some hard feelings on the part of those war blinded not in receipt of the allowance. This even led to some "dissension" among SAPA members. The problems arose among those with very little guiding vision who were assessed at between 2/60 and 4/60. They felt they were closer to those without vision at all than to those in the 5/60 to 6/60 range, some of whom had reasonable guiding vision. Like the totally blinded, they required assistance and services in their daily lives and were obliged to "pay for services rendered." Accordingly, SAPA felt that a new minimum category of attendance allowance, valued at $480, or half the regular amount, was in order for these cases. The resolution further called for the maximum allowance to be increased. Months later, pension authorities had not conceded the principle of a minimum allowance, and Fred Woodcock, the CNIB aftercare officer, requested that SAPA's barely sighted veterans in the 2/60 to 4/60 range contact him with lists of things that their disability rendered very difficult for submission to the Canadian Pension Commission.[18]

At the 1957 SAPA AGM, Mayne noted that most of the work to prepare the NCVA resolution for an increase in veterans' disability pensions had originated from SAPA. Furthermore, SAPA representatives had attended all meetings of the NCVA, and had been part of delegations presenting briefs to parliamentary committees in 1948, 1952, 1954, and 1955 and directly to Minister of Veterans Affairs Hughes Lapointe in 1957. According to the SAPA executive, these efforts had resulted in "many improvements in all phases of veterans' legislation of benefit to the war blinded, to other disabled groups and to all veterans." These included increased pensions and allowances and a new system for computing pensions in the case of multiple disabilities.[19]

Knowing how hard their wives' lives had been as a result of marrying a blind man, the SAPA executive was "whole-heartedly enthusiastic" that SAPA "pursue to the utmost" its initiative to allow pensioners' widows a full year of pension benefits following a veteran's death. Given the small number of spouses eligible, this increase, estimated in 1959 as $85 monthly for one year per widow, meant an insignificant difference to the treasury. A 1959 SAPA brief to the House of Commons Standing Committee on Veterans Affairs recalled "the thousands upon thousands of tasks dependent upon sight which the wife must perform for her blind husband ... These range from the choosing of clothing as to colour ... the countless hours of oral reading from newspapers, magazines and books, the verbal descriptions of countless physical objects ... Picture then, the complete, the total, and absolute dependence of the blind veteran upon the eyes of his wife, the eyes which have become his visual contact with the whole world."[20] SAPA's initiative was only partially successful: the authorities agreed to maintain the pension only until the end of the month in which the veteran died. It wasn't much, but success often began slowly, beginning with small victories and the acknowledgement of the principles involved.[21]

In a 1968 brief to the Standing Committee on Veterans Affairs, SAPA movingly reiterated the value of the blinded veterans' wives:

> Can anyone assess the cost of blindness to the wives and families of the blind? Even we who live under these conditions cannot fully appreciate the full extent to which we depend on the eyes of our loved ones. We do, however, have tangible

> proof of this dependence when the wife of one of our com-
> rades dies ... Our wives ... are on duty every minute of every
> day ... as reader, guide, valet, chauffeur, interrupting their
> normal routine to perform 101 little tasks which require sight
> ... we depend on their eyes to keep us in touch with the every
> day world – its colour, its beauty, its shape, its size, its constant
> activities; in other words, what you, sighted persons, see every
> waking minute of every day.[22]

At the 1959 AGM, the issue of men's surviving widows' pensions
again was raised with a "lively" and emotional tone to the discussions.
In an interesting twist, James W. Doiron, of Penetanguishene, Ontario, and one of SAPA's earliest members, noted that his wife had
died the previous year and that the amount allocated to her as a
spouse of a 100 percent pensioner was no longer paid, imposing on
him some financial strain. Others shared similar experiences. Accordingly, Woodcock felt that there also should be continuance of a war-
blinded widower's spousal allowance, though nothing came of this
proposal. Doiron summed up his life as a war-blinded pensioner: "We
can do much of most things, start a few and finish none." Fellow First
World War pensioner R.S. Morland, from Vancouver, concurred, adding, "Nothing can replace my sight."[23]

SAPA was adamant that Ottawa provide free hospitalization
for total-disability pensioners. Despite the fact that he was a 100
percent pensioner, one prominent SAPA Second World War member,
Chris J. Davino, noted that he had been denied free treatment at a
veterans' hospital because he earned more than $35 weekly! In the
unanimous opinion of SAPA members attending the 1959 AGM, this
contravened section 13 of the Pension Act and constituted a "typical"
misunderstanding on the part of Department of Veterans Affairs
(DVA) and hospital staff. In addition, the war blinded desired a $50
increase to their monthly pensions of $150 to compensate for the

complexities of their "way of life" and the "ramifications of just living normally." Besides, this increase would bring their income into line with a "general labour market scale of wages."[24]

On 16 March 1959, nine SAPA members, plus Judge Frank McDonagh of the War Pensioners, a long-standing friend and honorary life member of SAPA, appeared before the House of Commons Standing Committee on Veterans Affairs. Baker, suffering from exhaustion and "nervous tension" for most of the past year, was unable to attend. Bill Dies stated before the committee that war blindedness had been consistently "underrated" as a pensionable disability, "which was partly due to the blind veterans themselves, in that the abilities and accomplishments of the war blinded had to be overemphasized in order to retain their former sighted positions in a social structure based entirely on the ability to see." In especially pressing the needs and claims of the aging First World War veterans, Dies spoke of his own experiences: "Any help that you can offer me now ... is just about too late ... because I happen to be one of those who, for 42 years, has gone around in the dark amidst frustration after frustration, and it was only because of pre-war and post-war friends and associations and a great deal of intestinal fortitude that I have survived to this date." But his plea was more about the future, not the past; about principle, not compensation. He went on, speaking of Canada's Second World War blinded, "I do not want these young fellows to struggle along the way as some of us have had to struggle ... Be sure also that ... money could not pay me for what I have lost ... there is not enough money in the country."[25] Overall quality of life could not be measured only in dollars and cents.

In support of Doiron's views, expressed at the 1960 AGM, that there existed in Ottawa a "lack of official understanding of the seriousness of the handicap of blindness," an unnamed member outlined his lifelong struggle to obtain a pension entitlement as a result of blindness caused by exposure to mustard gas during the First World War. He had been obliged for years to live on the meagre subsidies provided through the war veterans allowance (the "burn-out" pension) and the "generosity and charity of friends and neigh-bours." Though he eventually won his case for attributable blindness with the Canadian Pension Commission, this veteran still claimed that the government had saved $45,000 at his expense. SAPA wanted all 100 percent disability pensioners on account of blindness to be granted the immediate minimum attendance allowance, and all vet-erans who were completely "black" blind to be automatically given the maximum. Many SAPA members were only 80 percent disabled because of blindness, yet 138 members, more than half, were deemed 100 percent disabled and received no attendance allowance at all. This was the crux of the men's dissatisfaction.[26]

By 1959 the maximum available for attendance allowance had jumped to $1,800 annually, and virtually all members felt that the $1,200 allotted to the totally blind should be raised to the maximum, a position that Woodcock pointed out was also the consensus among other groups of disabled veterans. The allowance for those with some guiding vision could be increased to $1,440. Doiron noted that the blinded had to pay for many basic services, such as snow shovelling and even basic home maintenance, as did the other disabled veter-ans. He believed that the blinded veterans needed the additional at-tendance allowance "in order to live as the people of Canada want us to live."[27]

At SAPA's annual banquet following the 1960 AGM, a strong DVA representation, including the minister, A.J. Brooks, and the deputy minister, Lucien Lalonde, mixed with the mayor of Toronto, Nathan Phillips, and representatives of no less than eight veterans' associations, including arch-rivals the Canadian Legion (renamed the Royal Canadian Legion that year) and the Canadian Corps Association. As often happened, a SAPA event had brought the sometimes div-ided veterans together. In fact, the members of SAPA's Executive Committee "unanimously agreed this was the most successful func-tion with possibly the greatest representation of veterans' groups gathered at one dinner." The minister was said to be very pleased.[28] Less than two months later the Canadian Pension Commission (CPC) increased the attendance allowance for the totally blind to $1,440 per annum from $1,200. Although SAPA had sought $1,800, this was a promising start. Woodcock, not satisfied with Ottawa's decision, busily prepared a list of all SAPA members according to degrees of remaining vision, light perception, and other categories, to assist in determining attendance allowance entitlements for the whole of the war-blinded community. Similarly, SAPA was preparing a list of its members in receipt of war veterans allowance payments to assist with determining attendance allowance needs. Woodcock dispatched to the CPC more than a hundred members' letters describing their needs and demanding increased allowances.[29]

Canada's war-blinded veterans were aging and needing more help. But SAPA's and the NCVA's efforts had begun to pay off and disabled veterans had at least been receiving fair and sympathetic hearings by federal authorities. In fact, that year several SAPA leaders were able to compare Canada's treatment of its war blinded with that provided elsewhere in the Commonwealth – and Canada was not found wanting. Thirteen delegates attended the first Common-wealth War-Blinded Conference, held in London in July 1960. From SAPA, president Bill Mayne, secretary Fred Woodcock, and Bill Dies attended. Information on all the war-blinded organizations was shared, and Woodcock reported that Canada's pension program was the clearest and most generous in the Commonwealth. He was also surprised to learn that, at St. Dunstan's, the chairman in council with his board of directors administered the whole organization, with little input from the British war-blinded veterans themselves. This was not the Canadians' way. Mayne noted that Canadian blinded veterans were easily the "luckiest" in the Commonwealth and added that the South African delegates at the London conference knew virtually nothing of their country's pension legislation. Woodcock thought it was "amazing" how "backward" other countries' veterans legislation appeared when compared to Canada's.[30]

Similarly, in March 1965, J.J. Doucet, SAPA's president, travelled to St. Dunstan's for its fiftieth anniversary celebration. During meetings involving the Commonwealth's war blinded, Doucet felt "indeed proud to be Canadian, for during this discussion I realized how forward-looking and generous our country has been in the treatment and rehabilitation of her disabled veterans" – at least from a comparative perspective.[31] Whether Doucet's views mirrored those of the majority of SAPA members is difficult to say. But despite Dies's honest account before the Standing Committee on Veterans Affairs in 1959 of his own struggles with blindness and with pension authorities, few Canadian war pensioners appeared as well treated as the war blinded in the post-Second World War period.

Nevertheless, the veterans continued to agitate for an increase in attendance allowance. On 4 April 1961, seven SAPA members with several different disabilities presented an emotional brief to the CPC. Directly as a result of this meeting, on 10 May, T.D. Anderson, the chairman of the CPC, wrote SAPA that attendance allowance had been raised to $1,680 from $1,440 for the totally blind. Still short of the desired $1,800, this amount was deemed acceptable and SAPA laid the matter to rest.[32]

The tireless Woodcock continued throughout the 1960s to battle Ottawa over pension allotments and other war-service entitlements for the war blinded, sometimes adopting a testy tone uncharacteristic of SAPA's dealings with federal authorities. He sought a formula whereby the war blinded would be compensated based on the degree of visual loss, commensurate with the disability assessments for members of other groups such as the Canadian Paraplegics Association, the Canadian Pensioners' Association, and the War Amputations. How did blindness compare with a double-leg amputee using prosthetics? In one sense, limbs could be "replaced," though glass eyes could never be made to see. The war blinded, perhaps becoming increasingly militant, or at least envenomed, as they aged, felt they deserved greater compensation, in comparative context, as a result of their particularly onerous disability.

Second World War veteran Robert S. Hunter, who had had difficulties re-establishing himself, wrote Woodcock a letter that was read at SAPA's 1964 annual meeting. "My life prior to my blindness," wrote Hunter, "consisted of driving a truck, farm labour, lumbering, mining and other such unskilled casual labour. Due to my disability I cannot do any of these things now ... I consider myself to be worse off physically than [a double amputee]." He went on, "For one who is totally blind it is out of the question to propel powered machines such as automobiles, boats or even lawn mowers." And while there were still some specific employment possibilities open even to the totally blind, for "95 percent" of jobs generally, "he would find himself cancelled out due to lack of sight. So much for his money-earning capacities."[33]

Quality of life issues mattered as well. Hunter noted that "there are many types of sport, recreation and vacation activities which are of absolutely no benefit to the totally blind. Hunting and fishing have lost their savor and of what use are glorious scenery, theatrical spectacle or the creations of man's art and skill?" He concluded that "my lack of sight has not impaired either my physical or mental abilities ... but it has so fiercely curtailed my power to govern my circumstances throughout every moment of the day and night, and under whatsoever conditions I find myself, that those same abilities, without the God-given power of sight, are impotent." Not all of the war blinded would have agreed with such gloomy sentiments, but many SAPA members felt this growing dejection. In 1968, a SAPA brief to the Standing Committee on Veterans Affairs noted that the war blinded were "rapidly losing touch with modern developments in many fields. The casual daily sighted glances at print, pictures and material objects are denied to our group, who depend mainly on hearing and sense of touch."[34]

Ken Langford of the Paraplegics Association, chairman of the NCVA since Edwin Baker's retirement in 1962, prepared a draft document on the issue of disability assessment. The gist was that the CPC's Table of Disabilities seemed arbitrary and off the mark. The NCVA wanted multiple disabilities to count in the calculation of pension allotments since, as Woodcock phrased it, multiple disabilities "make the problem of carrying on just that much more difficult." If a veteran was deemed 60 percent disabled for a primary disability, and a further 25 percent for a secondary disability, the CPC awarded the veteran 25 percent of the remaining 40 percent, rather than adding the two figures. The difference in this example was a pension of 70 percent versus 85 percent. The veterans wanted severely and multiply disabled veterans, for example a totally blinded man who had also lost an arm, to obtain more than a 100 percent pension. The disabled sought recognition for the totality of their postwar struggles and a redefinition of what being 100 percent disabled really meant. Accordingly, the NCVA felt that a blinded veteran with some guiding vision should receive $333 monthly (185 percent of the amount at the time), a totally blind veteran should receive $657 (365 percent of the current amount), while one totally blind with an arm amputation should receive $801 (445 percent of the current amount). Paraplegics would be on par with the totally blind.[35]

J.J. Doucet, who was elected SAPA's president in February 1964, told that year's AGM, "I am totally blind. When I came back from [active service in] Italy I was operated on the forehead, which paralyzed me completely on the right side. I have a brace on my right foot and wear arch supports. I cannot use my right hand ... yet I am right-handed." Judge Frank McDonagh, an NCVA executive member who served as a co-coordinator and spokesperson for the different NCVA groups on this matter, replied that, if Ottawa adopted

the veterans' proposals, "the CPC would take each one of those individual disabilities and assess it and then they would take the arith-
metical total as being the rate of your pension and they would do
away with this artificial ruling that they have made of a maximum
of 100 per cent." The whole matter hinged on the principle of the
divisibility of disability.

But Woodcock realistically reminded the group that the CPC
thought in terms of dollars and federal budgets and that common
sense had to prevail in the veterans' demands. McDonagh, too, said
that asking for too much could be counterproductive. For example,
a quadriplegic requiring twenty-four-hour care at home would probably need up to $22,000 a year to pay for specialized care and at-
tendance allowance. "We felt that if we went down to the Minister or
anybody else," wrote McDonagh, "and suggested $22,000 they would
say 'your application is absurd – put the man in hospital and leave
him there.'" But the additional costs might not be so exorbitant given
that in February 1964 there were only 607 totally disabled pensioners: 253 war blinded, 174 members of the War Amps, and 180 in the
Paraplegics Association. SAPA presented its brief to the minister on
22 July 1964, the strong delegation consisting of Baker, Dies, Doucet,
and Woodcock.[36] The veterans' proposal was ambitious, however,
and the issue would take years to resolve.

Successive veterans affairs ministers and officials, and most
members of the fourteen-person CPC, remained sympathetic. SAPA
felt that, on most issues at least, more gains could be made through
collaboration and goodwill than by confrontation. SAPA had built up
a supportive constituency within the DVA bureaucracy. In 1965 Gerry
L. Mann, DVA's chief rehabilitation officer and a good friend to SAPA,
noted that the war blinded were "easy to work with and so appreciative of efforts on their behalf." The same year, Minister Roger J. Teillet
appointed a task force with the cumbersome title of the Committee
to Survey the Organization and Work of the Canadian Pension Commission, under the chairmanship of Mr. Justice Mervyn Woods. SAPA

delegates presenting a brief to the committee on 18 January 1966, among them Doucet, Dies, Mayne, and Woodcock, the spokesman, made up a "cross-section of the various types of disabilities," not just blindness. Woodcock stated that "the committee received our presentation with sympathetic understanding and we felt that it was the first time that we have been able to discuss all aspects and problems of the war blinded." The War Amputations also submitted a lengthy brief that further outlined the "difficulties of the totally blind."[37] The timing of the review was critical, since many war-blinded veterans depended on pensions for their survival. In the late 1960s, only about half of the surviving Second World War veterans (most in their late forties and early fifties) were employed, and forty-five of these, nearly half, had found work with the CNIB.[38]

After two and a half years of gathering information, the 1,350-page Woods Report was tabled in the House of Commons in March 1968. On the whole it sustained many of the veterans' arguments, and the report's 148 recommendations for changes to the pension system overwhelmingly favoured the veterans' causes. However, one recommendation angered all veterans: the Woods Committee recommended that disability pensions be subject to income tax if the veteran's total annual income reached a certain limit. That May a furious Woodcock wrote Woods:

> For fifty years we have had to gradually build up ... public confidence in [the war blinded's] ability to perform, and by a gradual process of motivating and encouraging the blind to accept a job, however menial, regardless of their intelligence and abilities ... With a few exceptions, the jobs are of the low-paid variety, monotonous, with no hope of promotions in competition with sighted employees. One of the paramount incentives has been that the ... war blinded could work and earn any amount without it in any way affecting pensions and allowances. If the War Disability Pension is to be subject to

Income Tax ... it will destroy the incentive ... I shudder to think
of all the implications ... I feel certain that many who now, in a
sense, merely augment their pension income, would terminate
their employment, in spite of loss of self-respect. There is,
however, an over-all exercising among our group of courage,
determination and unwillingness to give in to all that their
handicap entails, which ... should be encouraged rather than
discouraged. They have never been complainers – but then,
what else could be expected of men who volunteered to give
their all – and almost did![39]

The income tax proposal was never carried out.

In May 1968, ten veterans' organizations, with the Royal
Canadian Legion in the lead capacity, met in Ottawa to discuss the
Woods Report recommendations, which, in general, the veterans'
community supported wholeheartedly. But rather than proceeding
with an open and immediate evaluation of the report by referring it
to the Standing Committee on Veterans Affairs, the government, believing that implementing the recommendations would prove exces-
sively costly, instead proceeded with a thorough internal study of
veterans' issues with the intention of producing a formal white paper.
This angered the veterans, since DVA minister Roger Teillet and his
successor, Jean-Eudes Dubé, had both promised repeatedly that the
Woods Report would be submitted to the standing committee as
soon as the report was available. Finally, following more than seventy
meetings of a DVA committee specially struck for the purpose, the
government released its White Paper on Veterans Affairs in September 1969. Ottawa planned to offer the veterans less than the Woods
Report recommended. The resulting outrage from the veterans
united them in purpose as never before. Joint action and careful
planning allowed each veteran group to present powerful separate
but coordinated briefs, followed by a formal united one, before
the Standing Committee on Veterans Affairs. The veterans were

able to show persuasively that Ottawa's cost estimates were exaggerated, but they also remained realistic enough to suggest several compromise positions on some of the Woods Committee recommendations.[40]

The very month that the White Paper was released, six SAPA members, accompanied by Cliff Chadderton, the head of the War Amputations who also had been a veterans' member of the Woods Committee, made a strong representation to the standing committee on various elements of the white paper. He especially fought the reduction in pensions to men who had lost one eye on active service and later suffered from sympathetic blindness. Chadderton, a veteran of the Royal Winnipeg Rifles, had lost a leg in combat during operations to clear the Scheldt Estuary in October 1944. He went on to lead the NCVA, a position he held at the time of writing. His early interest and demonstrated strong support for the war blinded earned him an honorary SAPA membership in 1970. In fact, SAPA considered him, as well as Legion officials Don Thompson and M.M. McFarlane, the "work horses" behind the forceful petitioning of the authorities to implement the recommendations of the Woods Report.[41]

The parliamentary committee generally upheld the veterans' views, and its recommendations were tabled in the House of Commons and approved by Parliament in March 1971. The main concessions were the recognition of a veteran's total disability being in excess of 100 percent, and pensionable at a higher rate, and the inauguration of what became known as exceptional incapacity allowance, an additional amount for a severely reduced quality of life.[42] The arduous struggle had demonstrated as never before the value of joint action by all veterans' organizations. The Woods Report led to the greatest legislative change to the pension system since the Second World War.

So close was the veterans' community's solidarity at this time that the Royal Canadian Legion awarded its new Friendship Award to each of the other groups that worked so diligently to pressure

Ottawa to adopt the Woods Report recommendations. SAPA mounted the Legion's award – a medallion and an accompanying scroll – in a very prominent location in the SAPA lounge at the CNIB's Bakerwood headquarters, its Toronto location since 1956. Bill Mayne, the CNIB's aftercare officer since 1970 and SAPA's secretary, believed it had been "the greatest total effort" the veterans had ever mounted together in order to secure the benefits that they felt they deserved.[43] The veterans had won.

The War Blinded outside Canada

All combatant powers of the First World War had experienced war-blinded casualties and, by the outbreak of the Second World War, had had more than two decades of varying experiences in their care and rehabilitation. As such, the post-1945 period offered guiding precedents as well as the opportunity for more advanced medical care, greater understanding of re-establishment needs, and the improved delivery of pensions and other benefits. Not all nations followed Canada's lead and few had the equivalent of the CNIB, with its core of war-blinded leaders, to assist the new generation of sightless casualties. Some comparison with the situation in the United States and the Commonwealth is helpful to place the Canadian pension and aftercare programs in a broader evaluative context.

In 1941 the American Association of Workers for the Blind (AAWB) set up a blinded soldiers' committee to assess the implications of large-scale blinded casualties if the United States entered the war. Among the twelve members was Canada's Edwin Baker. Baker's views were influential, and the AAWB called on the US government to establish a specialized civil re-establishment program for the war blinded distinct from other disabled veterans and to involve the blinded in the rehabilitation process – a clear attempt to emulate Canada's successes.[44]

As a sign of the growing links between the Canadian and American war blinded, during the war two of the latter visited the CNIB in Toronto to learn about Canadian retraining programs. Eventually, one of these Americans was sent to a specialized eye-treatment hospital in San Francisco and the other to the Valley Forge General Hospital in Phoenixville, Pennsylvania, a US Army hospital designated as a treatment centre for eye casualties. Each of these war-blinded veterans served as "first contacts" for all newly blinded American servicemen. Already by the end of 1943 there were approximately 100 American blinded servicemen, a number that approached 1,500 by war's end, with hundreds of additional cases emerging in the postwar years.[45]

St. Dunstan's was very prominent in the international community of the war-blinded, and the Americans also sought Sir Ian Fraser's advice. Seventeen American servicemen attended St. Dunstan's during the war. While visiting the wartime United States, Fraser insisted to the US authorities that it was critical to set up a major administrative facility devoted solely to the needs of the American war blinded. Finally, in June 1944, Old Farms Convalescent Hospital was established in Avon, Connecticut, on a two-thousand-acre tract. Complicating matters, however, and denying the American war blinded the critical opportunity for shared and uniform experiences, the US Navy insisted on operating its own rehabilitation facility at the nearby Philadelphia Naval Yard. Further, the Old Farms training centre was "not in the form that [Fraser] had hoped," and he was "disappointed" during a 1947 visit to the United States to learn that the war blinded there had received only basic adjustment training and perhaps some typing and Braille courses. Although a variety of occupational courses and the chance to engage in social activities were offered, most of the American war blinded were discharged after a mere three or four months of training. It seemed that the "great majority" lived off their pensions without, in Fraser's view, becoming productive citizens or gaining the confidence and self-respect that gainful employment so clearly brought to the war blinded in Britain or Canada.[46]

One problem seems to have been that the Americans remained in military service (and pay and discipline) during their preliminary training. Only upon its completion were they discharged into the care of the Veterans Administration for vocational training. The military ambience did little to improve morale. Moreover, once the Veterans Administration assumed responsibility for the discharged casualty, it normally contracted with state blinded associations for vocational rehabilitation and aftercare services. This decentralized approach, with uneven standards, did not offer the same benefit as a system that brought large numbers of men together to train and share their experiences.[47] Recognizing the limits of this system, in March 1945 some of the American war blinded undergoing rehabilitation training at Old Farms formed the Blinded Veterans Association (BVA), a mutual-help organization not unlike SAPA. But the BVA could only do so much, given that most of its members remained sadly ill-equipped to meet the employment challenges imposed upon them by their disability.[48]

American historian Frances Koestler is dismissive of the US military and government's efforts on behalf of the war blinded and believes that whatever successes the men achieved were due to their own initiatives. The American war blinded concurred with this view. In most cases, according to Koestler, the men were "determined not to succumb to self-pity, and it was their unflagging morale that helped inspirit the rest."[49] Inter-service rivalry, a refusal by the military to fully consult civilian experts, a Veterans Administration seemingly in utter "disarray" in the immediate postwar period, and the fact that the United States had suffered a staggering 650,000 wounded during fewer than four years of war combined to deny the American war blinded the same conditions, practices, and unity of spirit as existed in Canada or Britain.[50] In 1947, one senior Veterans Administration official, resistant to the major funding and organizational stresses that ongoing war-blinded retraining foretold, asked baldly, "Why all this fuss about the blinded veteran? He will be just as blind three years from now." Koestler further reports that as late as the 1970s "ignorance, indifference and internal pressures caused by heavy workloads were resulting in inequities in the [Veterans Administration's] treatment of [the] war-blinded."[51] These were simply not the prevailing attitudes, policies, or experiences in Canada.

In 1952-53, a postwar statistical census of the by-then nearly two thousand American blinded from both world wars showed some interesting parallels to and also divergences from the Canadian experience. The US survey indicated a very clear correlation between those who maintained positive outlooks and socialized with other blinded people and successful social readjustment and rehabilitation. This finding reinforces the critical importance of a fraternal organization like SAPA in helping to lay the groundwork for the men's future success and happiness. The Canadians seemed to have been doing most things right. Only 616 of the surveyed Americans, or 31.6 percent, reported themselves as associating with other blinded people, and barely half the men were employed. Married blinded veterans were nearly twice as likely to be employed as those unmarried and much more likely to display "positive attitudes towards life."[52] As Baker proudly reported to the January 1947 SAPA AGM, Lloyd Greenwood, an American air force veteran and the founder and executive director of the Blinded Veterans Association, stated that his organization was seeking to "develop along lines similar" to SAPA.[53] By 1947 the US Veterans Administration recognized the BVA as a veterans' advocacy group and the following year the BVA established its headquarters in Washington to better exercise that function. Not all US war-blinded joined: in 1960 there were 900 dues-paying members, a number which would rise to 1,200 by 1971.[54]

One important distinction from the Canadian experience was that, while supportive, the American Foundation for the Blind was not the parent organization to the BVA in the same sense that the

CNIB sponsored and fostered SAPA. In 1962, Woodcock reminded SAPA members to "realize CNIB's uniqueness, in that veteran and civilian blind work together for the good of all blind in Canada. To [my] knowledge there is no other organization in the world that can boast of similar coordinated cooperation."[55] In 1955, having taken a cue from the Canadian experience, the BVA appointed two of its members to serve as aftercare officers, but this position was not formally financed by the Veterans Administration. The timing was no accident: Fred Woodcock, the Canadian aftercare officer, had attended the BVA's conference that year and strongly urged such a move. John Mattingly, president of the BVA, attended the 1957 SAPA AGM and reunion, as did Kathern F. Gruber, an experienced teacher of the blind who had worked with war-blinded veterans at the American Foundation for the Blind.

Incredibly, only at the end of 1972 were "exploratory talks" held between the Veterans Administration and the BVA aimed at providing a contract to the BVA to offer returned veterans a "field service program" akin to the CNIB's aftercare services, something that the Canadian organization had been providing since its inception in 1918. Even taking into account differences in scale, the US experience made the Canadian situation appear highly functional.[56]

Close contact was maintained between SAPA and the BVA, often through the personal links established by Woodcock, who was held in such high esteem by the American group that it made him an honorary life member in 1960. Woodcock also received the American Legion Annual Amity Award for his services to blind veterans around the world. At the BVA's Hartford convention in 1967, Woodcock received a standing ovation from the American war blinded for his informed presentation to the BVA on the issue of blinded veterans' widows' pensions. Heeding his advice, and learning from SAPA's long experience in the matter, enabled the BVA to present a successful brief to lawmakers in Washington.[57]

In a postwar review of the situation of the war blinded in the Commonwealth, Ian Fraser reserved his highest praise for the CNIB, SAPA, and Edwin Baker. In his estimation, Canadian facilities and programs were second only to St. Dunstan's itself.[58] Accordingly, during the Second World War, Canadians needed less assistance from St. Dunstan's than did troops from the other dominions. For example, Australia had nothing comparable to Pearson Hall or even to New Zealand's Blinded Servicemen's Trust Board, which Fraser described as a "little St. Dunstan's." No centralized training facility was established in Australia, evidently due to that dominion's sparse population and the exceedingly long distances between major population centres. War-blinded Australians instead organized groups in each individual state that were linked through a national umbrella group, though these organizations remained unsupported by a national association like the CNIB. Relatively few South Africans were blinded and these benefitted from a small organization replicating St. Dunstan's as far as possible. One of the South African war blinded, trained as a physiotherapist, re-entered the army in that capacity – according to Fraser the world's only blinded soldier on active service during the Second World War.[59]

St. Dunstan's itself trained more than 1,000 blinded veterans during the Second World War, about 300 of whom later regained at least some useful sight. As of 1946, St. Dunstan's still had 1,673 veterans from the First World War on aftercare, with an average age of fifty-six, plus 666 men and 20 women from the Second. Hundreds more would be admitted in subsequent decades as a result of delayed service-incurred blindness.[60] By 1961, there were 2,600 St. Dunstaners, including 1,350 from the Second World War or subsequent conflicts. Some were from Allied nations such as Belgium, the Netherlands, France, and especially Poland, including those who had fought the Germans as members of an underground resistance movement. British civilian members of auxiliary services, such as

air-raid wardens, fire and rescue workers, and coast observers blinded on active service, or whose blindness was attributable thereto,
also counted as St. Dunstaners. Three hundred other British war
blinded did not pass through St. Dunstan's, preferring the Scottish
National Institute for the Blind at Newington House, Edinburgh. This
was a choice St. Dunstan's respected, though the Scottish facility
could not rival St. Dunstan's.[61]

Aftercare in the Postwar Era: Some Case Studies

According to the CNIB's 1940 annual report, the institute had a register of 11,992 blind Canadians. Although the war blinded constituted
less than 2 percent of the total, they continued to exercise an influence out of proportion to their numbers. For example, Edwin Baker
had been the CNIB's managing director since 1931, and before then
its general secretary. Alexander Viets was the institute's first vice-
president, and Bill Dies, Viets, and T.E. Perrett, OBE, were on its council. Harris Turner, a journalist before and after his war blinding, was
the institute's director of publications.[62] Several of the war blinded of
the Second World War also became prominent members of the CNIB.
Many others worked in various managerial and other positions in its
field operations and local branches. For example, Ross C. Purse and
Bill Mayne, both Manitoba veterans of the battle for Hong Kong, held
influential positions, Purse becoming managing director in 1973.
These men ensured a close continuing bond between the CNIB and
SAPA and made the war blinded's aftercare needs a priority.

    The CNIB's mandate to deliver aftercare services to war-blinded
veterans on behalf of the federal government continued in the postwar decades. The formal and informal delivery of aftercare should
be understood alongside other factors, including the extensive
CNIB-structured retraining and job-placement programs described
in the previous chapter, other DVA-initiated services and funding for
disabled veterans, and veterans' access to federal service-related

pensions and the many other provisions of the Veterans Charter. The CNIB aftercare officer facilitated and co-ordinated the delivery of government-sponsored services and also, wherever possible, tried to ease the financial, social, familial, and psychological hardships that veterans might face. Employment satisfaction and job prospects were important areas of investigation for the aftercare officer, as were family finances and general quality of life. Often, knowledge of these situations could only be obtained through a personal visit to ascertain conditions in the home and to interview the veteran. Blindness imposed an especially harsh handicap on these young men and, although many managed a remarkably positive social re-establishment, not all were able to reintegrate easily, or even successfully.

Pursuing a policy initiated by Baker, aftercare officer Fred Woodcock criss-crossed Canada in the decades following the war, visiting the war blinded in their homes and communities and filing extensive reports of his findings with recommendations for action. In 1952 Woodcock wrote that the aftercare officer "listens, advises and endeavours to solve their problems – works solely in the interests of the veteran."[63] For example, in the early 1950s Woodcock visited Quebec, including outlying districts such as the Gaspé Peninsula, home to some war-blinded veterans of the Royal Rifles of Canada captured at Hong Kong. He noted that "quite a number of this group did not take advantage of our War Blinded Training Centre [Pearson Hall] and now that they have settled down and appreciate the stagnant position of a non-employment situation, expressed their regrets at not having come in for training." Despite this, "this group is vastly improved" from a visit he had made several years previously, when grimness pervaded their outlooks. In 1959 he journeyed nearly 4,200 miles over a three-week period to visit all the war-blinded veterans in the Maritime provinces. The local CNIB offices greatly assisted him and, according to Woodcock, the SAPA members were highly appreciative of the many services offered by the CNIB and SAPA.[64]

By 1952, Ottawa was paying $130 yearly per war-blinded vet-
eran to the CNIB for aftercare services, a figure raised to $175 in
1964.[65] The hard-working Woodcock co-operated closely with officials
from DVA, the Canadian Pension Commission, and other veterans'
associations. He screened the files of all non-war-blinded veterans
who had lost their sight and were registered with the CNIB to ascertain whether he could assist them to pursue a pension claim and
whether they were admissible as members of SAPA.[66] In addition,
Woodcock prepared a small booklet entitled "War Blinded Veterans
Aftercare Benefits and some Concessions for the Registered Blind"
and sent a copy to every veteran on aftercare.[67] DVA assumed financial responsibility for the CNIB aftercare officer, his staff, and his office expenses as part of its aftercare service. The budget included
allowances for entertainment and travel, as well as postage, printing,
stationery, and 4 percent of all CNIB head office costs, including util-
ities and administrative staff.[68]

There was, naturally, a close correlation between the employment profile of the war blinded, their ages and health, and the degree of aftercare services they needed. Of the First World War veterans,
73 percent of those resident in Canada had retired by 1952. These
veterans spanned fifty-five to eighty-seven years of age, the average
age being sixty-five. Six were still practising massotherapists, and
eight remained self-employed. Of the nearly 200 Second World War
veterans that year, 71.5 percent were employed, with nearly one-
third operating concession stands or CNIB-run cafeterias. Of the 54
unemployed veterans, 28 were unable to work for health reasons
while another 6 were too "unstable" to find employment. By 1964, 40
SAPA members were employed by the CNIB and 97 were employed
elsewhere. Of the 78 First World War veterans, 65 were unemployed
or retired while 13 still worked. Of the Second World War veterans,
125 were employed and 53 were unemployed or retired.[69]

With these statistics serving as context, below are some case
files begun by Woodcock following his aftercare investigations and

supplemented by subsequent aftercare officers, especially Bill Mayne. As Chapter 4 dealt with a number of cases of war-blinded veterans undergoing retraining and rehabilitation, here the less familiar but equally representative and routine aftercare work will be explored. Many veterans developed blindness incrementally or suffered worsening vision as a result of the wartime aggravation of an existing condition. Notwithstanding the origin of their blindness, all were in need of care and encouragement. The cases have been selected for their different life-course histories and each represents many others like it.

One unusual case was that of Dr. William R. Feasby, a well-known scholar physician, who, at the end of his career, cut short by his death in 1970 at the age of fifty-eight, was a medical director at Toronto's Queen Elizabeth Hospital and a director of the CNIB. A lieutenant-colonel in the Royal Canadian Army Medical Corps during the war, he served in military hospitals overseas, especially studying respiratory diseases. But he was also a patient, suffering from corneal dystrophy, a pre-enlistment condition 100 percent pensionable, since it was determined in the postwar period that wartime service had aggravated it greatly. As early as 1942, Feasby's deteriorating eyesight had been examined by St. Dunstan's ophthalmologists. He was found to have sufficient vision to carry on in his duties without being admitted to St. Dunstan's, though the expectation was that his condition would continue to worsen.[70]

Yet few knew during the war that Feasby was visually impaired to this degree and, in the immediate postwar period, that he was categorized as legally blind. What is curious about his case, though not unique, is that Feasby was not interested in obtaining CNIB or DVA services, evidently because he did not want his wife and children to be made aware of the degree of his vision loss. Even without aftercare services, for which Feasby became eligible in 1951, Woodcock admitted that "Dr. Feasby apparently is publishing medical literature and doing very well." Woodcock added a marginal notation to his report that seemed part instruction and part warning: "Do not contact this man." A 1955 eye clinic report stated that Feasby "wears special glasses which are fairly satisfactory in bright light."[71] Incredibly, Feasby also served as an official historian under contract to the Department of National Defence. While aided in his efforts by researchers toiling through the archives in Ottawa, his accomplishment in publishing, in 1956, the two-volume *Official History of the Canadian Medical Services, 1939-1945*, is impressive given his increasingly failing sight.[72]

The case of Harold B. Hines was more typical. A Nova Scotia truck driver in November 1943, at the age of nineteen, Hines enlisted in the Royal Highland Regiment of Canada (the Black Watch). Suffering multiple shrapnel wounds and a gunshot wound in the thigh during combat in Normandy and the Netherlands, Hines remained in service, perhaps in part due to the grave shortage of trained infantry in the Canadian Army at the time. Finally, on 17 December 1944, he was completely blinded by shrapnel wounds in the Netherlands. Hines was pensioned at 100 percent disabled and received a 100 percent attendance allowance. He trained at St. Dunstan's and Baker Hall in 1945 and very successfully managed a concession stand in Nova Scotia. Woodcock stayed in close contact with him, sending him warm letters full of news of the other men with whom Hines had trained at Pearson Hall. Hines married, helped raise two children, and was able to manage on his own for many years. In a report of 4 September 1975, aftercare officer Bill Mayne, who had visited Hines, noted that although he was unemployed, he remained in good health in his early fifties and seemed "quite happy and content" since returning to live on the family farm in Central Argyle. Hines stayed involved in his community and was an active member of the Royal Canadian Legion. Like many other war-blinded veterans, Hines appreciated the CNIB's aftercare services, the provision of specialized equipment, and the visits from the aftercare officer.[73]

Merrill B. Latham, also from Nova Scotia, enlisted in 1943 at the age of seventeen and served as a private in the West Nova Scotia

Regiment, serving in Italy from December 1943 to December 1944. That month he suffered a gunshot wound in the head, the loss of his right eye, and disfigurement in the left frontal area of his head. Incrementally over the decades, his remaining vision eroded. In 1960 he moved to Calgary and found employment with the Corps of Commissionaires until 1973, at which time his vision no longer allowed him to carry on. In 1974, married with two adopted children aged twelve and ten, he was more or less confined to his home and rather discouraged. In 1975 he became a 100 percent war-blinded pensioner, obtained CNIB aftercare services, and became a member of SAPA, even contributing three hundred dollars toward the 1992 Ottawa reunion he and his wife attended.[74] At a critical juncture, SAPA's support, activities, and mere existence seemed a lifeline to Latham, as to other war-blinded veterans whose careers came to an early end.

Cecil E. Capson, from Moncton, served as a private in the Royal Canadian Regiment and was severely wounded in Italy. His left eye had been enucleated and he had only light perception in his right. He was a 100 percent pensioner also in receipt of attendance allowance. By 1948 he was married with one son, though not working. It is not clear how his family made ends meet, but in 1964 he wrote Woodcock asking for a loan. By 1977 Capson was divorced and living with his son's family. Apparently needing the camaraderie of the similarly afflicted, he regularly attended SAPA reunions.[75] His story of financial strain and marital discord represents the experiences of other war-blinded veterans.

Earl A. Friedman's numerous vision problems did not prevent him from serving in the Royal Canadian Air Force (RCAF) from 1941 to 1946. The Torontonian suffered from pre-enlistment retinitis pigmentosa, glaucoma, and cataracts, all of which were aggravated while on active service. Married with two daughters, Friedman, who worked as a postal clerk, went from being a 50 percent vision-impaired pensioner in 1953 to 100 percent in 1959. According to a 1976 CNIB report on his case, Friedman had been "experiencing visual problems for years but he is as yet unable to face his condition or to accept assistance." He turned to the CNIB only in the 1970s when marital and possible employment problems caused him "extreme anxiety." But his refusal to face the possibility of complete blindness head on led him to sever his links to the institute after only a few months.[76] Friedman's state of denial was not unique.

Jack Ashworth, from Ontario, joined the army in 1939 at the age of nineteen and served two and a half years before being discharged in 1942 due to his failed vision. He started working for the Meekin Brush Company in Hamilton in 1943, making wooden handles. He was married and in receipt of a 95 percent disability pension. In 1960 he was earning $70 a week and doing very well for himself, but he lost his job the next year when the company switched to plastic handles. In 1962, deteriorating eyesight due to hemorrhages attributable to his military service made it impossible for him to work for some time. His disability pension was $240 a month. Ashworth qualified for aftercare services and CNIB training and worked in the institute's occupational and "Blindcraft" shops. Later he worked as a part-time janitor at a CNIB facility where, by 1973, he was earning $2 an hour and was much appreciated as a worker.[77] Ashworth's experience was typical of the CNIB's provision of sheltered work for a number of war-blinded veterans in need.

Leonard Blemkie, also from Ontario, born in 1922, served in the army overseas and, while not totally blind, suffered from tunnel vision and loss of night vision as a result of retinitis pigmentosa. In 1948 Blemkie found a job at a lumber company in Toronto but worried that if his employer learned how little he could actually see, he might lose his job. As we have seen, other veterans sought to mask their disability. At first he was rated at 50 percent disability and received only a 20 percent pension (a mere $28 a month) on the grounds that four-fifths of his disability predated his military service. In 1955 he and his wife separated and Blemkie, left with three children, needed an emergency loan of $500 and a further longer-term loan of $1,200.

CNIB's aftercare officer arranged for the money since Blemkie was re-mortgaging his home and seemed a safe risk. He still worked at the lumber firm, earning the good wage of $60 a week.[78]

In June 1962, Woodcock wrote the Canadian Pension Commission seeking an increase in Blemkie's pension. He portrayed Blemkie as a hard-working man obliged to care for his children after his wife "deserted" him, leaving him with an eight-year-old, a three-year-old, and a baby, and thereby immediately creating some financial difficulties. Woodcock felt that Blemkie had had a "tough row to hoe since the last war" and that to "maintain a home for the children and himself" had been quite a struggle for a man whose eyesight continued to deteriorate. The small lumber business which he had started in the countryside in 1960 was not doing very well, and his pension had been cut when it was ascertained that his vision allowed him to drive from time to time (though he should not have done so). But more recent official assessments of his condition had gone in his favour: Blemkie was labelled 80 percent disabled, for which the government would assume a 40 percent responsibility. Accordingly, he was paid a pension at 32 percent of the applicable rate for a 100 percent disabled veteran for whom the government assumed complete responsibility. Woodcock's intervention had had some effect but there was no more that he could do.[79] The administrative and social complexities of Blemkie's experiences were not unknown to other blinded veterans.

Robert S. Howard, another Nova Scotian, joined the RCAF in 1943 at the age of seventeen and served overseas. He suffered from macular degeneration incurred while on active service, though his refraction problems were a pre-enlistment condition not aggravated during the war. Following his discharge, Howard's vision had not failed to the extent that he required CNIB re-establishment training. He was not considered war blinded and he was not pensioned as such. However, a creeping loss of useful vision obliged him, in 1959, to seek the help of the CNIB and federal pension authorities. In June of that year, Woodcock visited Howard in Stellarton, Nova Scotia, for a meeting that lasted late into the night. Howard, then thirty-three, was fighting the reality of his blindness, had become depressed, and, according to Woodcock's report, had not yet "learned to be blind." Howard displayed a "bitter attitude" made worse by enforced idleness. Woodcock tried to convince him to go to Toronto for CNIB training, though it does not appear that he ever did so. The CNIB aftercare officer did not mince words with Howard: "I would not listen to any of Bob's excuses," he wrote. But at least this war-blinded veteran lived in a multiple-dwelling structure which he owned. He was married with one child, although three more were born following his 1959 pensioning.[80]

By the 1970s, Howard's vision was severely restricted. While he was not completely helpless, he wore dark glasses permanently, even in the home. Bill Mayne visited him in September 1975 and found him to be "very unhappy and frustrated ... trapped by his disability." Howard rejected offers of in-home disability training and dog-guide training, a decision, Mayne believed, stemming from a lack of the very self-confidence that CNIB training instilled. But Howard bounced back, finding strength in both the CNIB and SAPA. By 1979 he was much more active outside the home and became involved with the Pictou County CNIB advisory group. As a further display of aging members' continuing interest in and even reliance on the camaraderie SAPA provided, in 1992 he, too, donated one hundred dollars for that year's reunion. A decade later, his morale had improved so much that he was involving himself heavily in the affairs of SAPA. "Bob and Bertha have been the backbone of the SAPA Maritime Branch and active at the national level of the Association for decades," wrote Krysia Pazdzior, SAPA's associate executive director, to William Marsipont, a Royal Canadian Legion service officer in Stellarton in November 2002. She also referred to Howard as a "dedicated long-term" member of SAPA. By this time living in New Glasgow, he and his wife celebrated their fifty-fifth wedding anniversary in 2001.[81]

G.A. Sheppard, from North Gower, Ontario, in the Ottawa Valley, joined the RCAF in September 1941 at the age of twenty-two. He served with Eastern Air Command in Canada and Labrador. Prior to his enlistment he had obtained his senior matriculation and been employed with the Canadian Legion. He was discharged in October 1945 and was accidentally blinded in August 1946 while completing a rehabilitation course at the Ontario Training and Re-establishment Institute (OTRI), a training centre for military personnel in Toronto. A refrigeration coil charged with sulphur dioxide exploded, burning both his eyes and leaving him with only guiding vision. Sheppard may have been the only war-blinded case to lose his sight in a post-discharge incident. Worsening matters was the fact that his wife was pregnant at the time. He was a patient at the Christie Street Hospital from August 1946 to January 1947 and, upon his discharge, survived on welfare, being unable to secure employment. At first there was no pension compensation for disabled OTRI trainees, although this was eventually implemented and made retroactive.[82]

"Mr. Sheppard suffers from strong light and as a consequence keeps his head down away from the glare, and there is a constant need for him to dab his eyes with a handkerchief to absorb the con-stant flow of liquid from the tear ducts," wrote Fred Woodcock. He added that Sheppard and his family lived a "meager existence." More-over, DVA had inexplicably failed to notify the CNIB of his case until November 1947. Woodcock immediately met with him and arranged for CNIB retraining and a DVA-funded allowance for him and his family of $104 monthly, as opposed to the City of Toronto welfare amount of $41 plus $25 for rent. Woodcock also arranged a CNIB loan of $100 for Sheppard until his pension was paid. He trained as a concession stand operator and moved to Ottawa to operate one in the Confed-eration Building on Parliament Hill. By 1950, he owed the CNIB $500 despite having received $2,800 in retroactive compensation from DVA. Woodcock became frustrated; the CNIB could help, but it was not a cash cow.[83] Part of the aftercare process was to teach responsibility to the veterans and instill a sense of purpose into their lives. This was often no easy task.

Frank Arno, a blinded Hong Kong prisoner of war, suffered from tuberculosis and mental disorders and was never able to readjust to civilian life. Extremely neglectful of his health, and in and out of Sunnybrook Hospital, his postwar history was a long downward spiral. There was little the aftercare officer could do in this case and several others like it. DVA administered Arno's pension on his behalf but, following one clerical miscue, he received a lump-sum payment of $1,359, which he promptly spent entirely in binging. He died in 1971.[84] Arno's case was particularly desperate, but there had always been a small percentage of war blinded who could not cope. However, the surviving records show that most tried, which alone is some measure of success. Buttressed by DVA's financial support, the CNIB and SAPA helped willingly and most veterans gladly accepted their efforts. Sometimes it was not enough.

SAPA Membership

In a laconic 1942 entry in the SAPA minutes it was simply recorded that the group had changed its name from the Sir Arthur Pearson Club of Blinded Soldiers and Sailors to the shorter but more all-encompassing Sir Arthur Pearson Association of War Blinded.[85] But the extension of SAPA membership to the blinded casualties of the Second World War portended far greater changes than merely that of the group's name.

Many SAPA members believed at the onset of the Second World War that modern warfare would result in massive casualties, including a large number of war blinded. They therefore expected the organization would quickly grow in size. Despite these fears, the ratio of blinded to overall casualties was, in fact, similar in both world wars, taking into account the higher incidence of delayed blindness following the First World War. Nevertheless, in 1945 SAPA president Harris Turner noted the sad truth that the war had, in fact, revitalized SAPA through dramatically increased membership.[86] This new conflict obliged SAPA to reaffirm and, to some extent, revise its membership criteria. Since its inception, the group had sought to define itself and protect its identity as an organization made up of veterans having lost their vision during, or as a clear result of, military service in wartime. The debate over membership lasted for decades, and a difference emerged between SAPA's own stricter criteria and an increasingly inclusive DVA view concerning a blind veteran's (but not necessarily a war-blinded one's) eligibility for CNIB-delivered, federally funded aftercare services.

If Ottawa wished to pay for additional veterans' aftercare, the CNIB was pleased to co-operate. But SAPA did not need to accept as members those whom it considered blinded through causes mainly unrelated to war service. The First World War veterans, especially, wished to maintain compliance with SAPA's original membership guidelines. Hence grew the distinction between, on the one hand, the strictly defined war blinded and, on the other, the smaller number of blinded veterans deemed ineligible for SAPA membership but who nevertheless received similar services. The CNIB aftercare officers, Fred Woodcock and then Bill Mayne, were responsible for the delivery of aftercare services to hundreds, even thousands, of Canadian veterans who had become CNIB clients and for whom Ottawa assumed some responsibility. In 1966 Woodcock explained that "when the Canadian Pension Commission, on behalf of the Federal Government, accepts some responsibility for a veteran's loss of sight and he receives a pension – in any amount – and is registered with the CNIB as a blind person, he is entitled to Aftercare services under a mutual agreement between DVA and CNIB." In that year, for example, there were 320 veterans on aftercare, 83 from the First World War and

237 from the Second. These men and women were officially considered "war blinded," but not all were SAPA members according to the association's own stricter membership criteria.[87]

In 1943 SAPA's Committee on the Constitution and By-Laws affirmed that members "must be one hundred percent disabled in respect to vision, *some portion* of which is due to war service and pensionable" (emphasis added). One hundred percent disabled meant vision not exceeding 6/60 or 20/200 in the better eye following the use of corrective lenses. But how was "some portion" defined? For SAPA, it had come to mean at least 80 percent due to war service. The next year the association began offering membership to blinded servicemen immediately following their discharge from the armed forces.[88] In the years to come, the group slightly eased membership requirements, partly in recognition of the nebulous origins of vision loss and sometimes with a view toward the precipitous mortality rates in its ranks.

Less than a decade following the end of the Second World War, the SAPA executive had to grapple with the recurring, pressing, and thorny problem of membership eligibility. Older members, and some newer ones, were passing away with distressing regularity; should the criteria be slackened somewhat to allow for the organization's survival? SAPA's Membership Committee minutes admit to some "controversy" over the matter. Evidently, some war-blinded veterans felt that relaxed government rules for service attributability and aftercare treatment could lead to a growing SAPA membership of *blind* veterans, though not fully *war blinded* ones. The difference mattered; the former group was increasing in number more quickly than the latter. Decisions had to be made respecting their membership in what amounted to a rather exclusive veterans' association. In November 1952, the committee, chaired by long-time SAPA executive member Bill Dies, who was in a good position to judge eligibility requirements, recommended that seven First World War veterans and six from the Second (including four veterans of Hong Kong) be admitted as SAPA members. Seven applicants, including one Korean War veteran, were rejected for the time being, although three of them were later admitted.[89]

As in the 1920s and 1930s, SAPA's mortality rates remained high. In the decade following the 1947 reunion, 90 blinded veterans, 66 from the First World War and 24 from the Second, had died, averaging nine a year. In 1957, there were 335 Canadian war-blinded veterans on aftercare of whom 278 were members of SAPA. There were also 650 blind veterans with no aftercare entitlements, and Woodcock was often able to help them benefit from veterans' legislation. That year twenty new SAPA members were approved, including five from the First World War. Six of the Second World War cases suffered from multiple sclerosis, a condition sometimes leading to loss of sight and, in these cases, deemed at least in part attributable to war-related service.[90] In 1961 a British pensioner living in British Columbia was granted membership – his recent blindness being attributed to gassing at Ypres in 1917, nearly forty-five years earlier. Another veteran of the same increasingly distant war was added to the rolls in 1963.[91] Others would follow. Several British St. Dunstaners moved to Canada and were eligible for aftercare privileges, taking advantage of the reciprocal arrangements between St. Dunstan's and the CNIB. One, Alice Gimbrere, a war-blinded veteran of the Women's Royal Naval Service, had trained as a physiotherapist and became SAPA's third female member.[92]

In 1959, sixteen new members joined the organization, eight from each war, including three multiple sclerosis cases from the Second World War. These more than offset the twelve deaths recorded in the previous year. Though a somewhat greater willingness to take in new members kept membership fairly stable, eighteen more First World War members died in the year ending February 1962. At that time, only four new membership candidates were being considered. Thirteen more First World War veterans died in the following year, and six more in the year ending February 1964. Several Second

World War veterans died annually as well. By September 1964, there remained only 78 First World War members from a total of 256.[93] SAPA was shrinking.

In March 1957, the Membership Committee recommended to the executive that SAPA's membership rules be slightly amended to allow blind veterans admittance to the organization "providing any portion of disability in excess of 2/5ths aggravation is due to war service and pensionable." As a result, nineteen aftercare recipients, sixteen from the Second World War, would have qualified.[94] This would have been "lowering the bar" in requiring that a minimum of only 40 percent of a blind condition be attributable to the aggravation of an existing vision disorder while on active service. Not all existing members were in favour. In June of that year, Bill Mayne, in his president's report to the AGM, made clear the organization's views: "qualifications for membership are *extensive* or total loss of eyesight through causes attributable to war service" (emphasis added).[95] The proposal was not enacted.

The issue dragged on for years. By 1959 most of the recent candidates for membership, while certainly legally blind, had only 40 percent of their service disability pensions allotted on account of their registered blindness. There was a difference between aggravated on service and incurred in service, with the former rarely meeting the 80 percent membership qualifying level, despite the fact that Ottawa granted them aftercare privileges. In some cases, blindness was not even the men's primary disability. Some of SAPA's First World War veterans, especially, felt that membership should be limited to veterans with no less than 50 percent of their blindness attributable to war service and pensioned therefor.[96] Even this would have been a major concession: being "war blinded" had always been the organization's litmus test for membership. Dies, influential, and with as long a "corporate memory" as any member, felt that only those who were in receipt of at least an 80 percent disability pension for blindness be admitted. The registration level of the CNIB was 6/60, legally blind, and the pension authorities pegged this level as 80 percent disabled. This eligibility minimum was approved by the executive. Woodcock noted in 1963 that there was a "strong feeling" among SAPA members on the issue and that the membership had of late "been much more strict in [its] interpretation."[97]

At the 1965 AGM, the matter came to a head. The general consensus was that the term "war blinded" meant something and that it was important to protect this distinction. Harris Turner wondered if SAPA should even desire new members. He asked, "Wouldn't it be better to carry on until the last two shake hands and say: 'Which one?'" On hearing this, the members present broke out in "hearty applause." Harvey Lynes, SAPA's first president in 1922, noted that to modify entrance requirements would tarnish the memory of departed war-blinded comrades who were proud members of SAPA because of its distinctiveness. A motion to maintain the selectivity of the group was unanimously carried "with enthusiasm." Eighty percent disabled on account of blindness it would be.[98] SAPA treated the matter very seriously. Samuel Clark, who had been wounded early in the Second World War, had since then benefitted from improved vision to such an extent that in 1965 he was no longer deemed eligible for aftercare services. Accordingly, and with sincere "regret," SAPA removed him from the organization's active membership. Two other members that year also had their memberships revoked for a similar positive reason.[99] Their opinions on losing membership in SAPA do not appear to have been recorded.

Frequently, veterans were unaware that they were being considered for membership in SAPA. When DVA registered with the CNIB a veteran who was entitled to aftercare privileges, SAPA automatically reviewed the man's case and, if deemed acceptable, prepared a membership form for approval at the next AGM. Being a member of SAPA entailed no fees, though members could purchase a SAPA lapel pin and SAPA beret on a voluntary basis. In addition to routine association correspondence, all new members received a brief history of SAPA, a copy of the SAPA constitution, and a membership card.[100]

In the year ending May 1967, six war blinded on aftercare were admitted as SAPA members while twelve First World War veterans and four from the Second died. No fewer than 1,437 blind veterans were registered with the CNIB at this time, of whom 75 from the earlier and 240 from the later conflict received aftercare. Fifty-six First World War and 171 Second World War veterans were SAPA members, leaving 88 veterans on aftercare outside of SAPA membership.[101] For the next several years, SAPA's numbers remained reasonably stable and the organization viable, notwithstanding an aging membership.

Bonding Two Generations of War Blinded

Edwin Baker understood that the hundreds of thousands of returning Second World War veterans would bolster the strength of the veterans' movement. But the growing veterans' community needed to show the unity it sometimes had lacked in the past. In a 1943 address to the Canadian Corps Association, Baker remarked that "there is a tendency among some organized groups of the first Great War Veterans to live in the past and to overlook the needs of these new men coming along. Unless veterans of the present war are made welcome, they will inevitably develop new associations of their own."[102]

Some in SAPA believed that the advent of a Second World War generation of war-blinded veterans held the potential for disharmony and cliquishness among members. At first, some First World War SAPA members saw a looming "problem" in uniting the generations and in forging a consensus for the benefit of all. Could or would the Second World War veterans be "made welcome"? Harris Turner certainly felt so. In 1945 he wrote that most of the discharged war-blinded veterans of the Second World War were "keen young men who, while realizing what they have lost, have developed a spirit of optimism and independence and can be counted on to live up to and surpass any of the achievements credited to the men who lost their sight a quarter of a century ago."[103] This generous view was a prescient observation.

In fact, in 1946 the SAPA president, Bill Dies, wrote that the needs of the blinded from the Second World War had injected older SAPA members with a "fresh interest and a new incentive in contributing to the successful readjustment of war casualties." He also felt that SAPA's social functions were infused with "renewed vigour by reason of the influx of younger members." The older generation's experience, coupled with the newer generation's dynamism, revitalized the organization and reaffirmed its raison d'être.[104] By 1947 the prevailing view in SAPA was that the bonding of the two groups had been "substantially successful."[105] According to one Second World War SAPA member, the younger generation of war blinded "soon realized the value of the Association" as it fought doggedly for better pension entitlements and other veterans' benefits.[106]

The 1947 reunion went a long way toward solidifying these inter-generational relationships. The old hands had "extended a sincere and hearty welcome" to the younger members, some of whom nearly immediately acceded to the SAPA executive. For example, David Dorward, a future SAPA president, joined the executive for the first time early in 1944, and Fred Woodcock, capable and industrious, soon after the war became SAPA's vice-president and later its long-serving secretary – in addition to his onerous duties as CNIB aftercare officer. At the January 1945 AGM, eleven memberships of Second World War veterans were approved, with seven of the men in attendance and interested in the affairs of the association. The passing of the torch had begun. In 1949, Woodcock became SAPA's first Second World War-veteran president.[107] The members of the Second World War group proved able and worthy successors to those remarkable men who had blazed the trail on which the younger group would travel. Many among the newer generation also developed lasting ties with each other, shared a devotion to the ideals of SAPA and the CNIB, and showed sincere loyalty to both organizations and their founders and leaders. In 1957 Mayne wrote that "Our bonds are those of a common disability, and of service. Ten years ago, when I became a member, I had little conception of [SAPA's] greatness."[108] This sense of empowerment and unity bestowed through membership in SAPA was something that the First World War veterans had known for several decades.

Sir Ian Fraser also recognized the critical necessity for both generations of war blinded to merge their interests, perhaps even their identities. "I felt it extremely important that the new generation should become a part of the old, that the unity of St. Dunstan's should not be impaired by the entry of young men in our ranks, but rather that it should be strengthened." He need not have feared; as with the Canadian experience, the bonds between the two generations of British war-blinded veterans grew strong.[109]

Two decades later, Woodcock complimented the First World War veterans whose ranks in SAPA were by then "rapidly diminishing." Referring to them as "this particular breed of old war horses," he reminded those in attendance at SAPA's 1964 annual meeting that "it is to them we owe the basic framework of veterans' legislation" and that it was due to their efforts that SAPA was held in such "high regard and prestige within the Government and other Veterans' Associations." Similarly, at the November 1968 AGM, SAPA president Chris J. Davino, a Second World War veteran, paid a very warm tribute to the thinning ranks of First World War veterans. Referring to the latter as "senior veterans," Davino remarked that "sometimes we engage in friendly debate as to which of 'our' wars was the toughest. We will all agree, I think, that there is no such thing as an easy war. Our presence here will surely attest to that ... We have enjoyed and do enjoy your association with us." He added that "we envy your glories of Passchendaele, Vimy, and Cambrai which were written in true blood as were ours of Ortona, Dieppe, and Hong Kong." He especially wished to thank SAPA's "Old Reliables," who certainly had shown little sign of institutional "apathy," for "shaping our veteran destiny and [for] your guidance over the rough trails ... We who have come of middle age, salute you." The handful of First World War veterans present for Davino's oration rose in acknowledgement to "sustained applause."[110]

Perhaps unexpectedly, Canada found itself at war again a mere five years following the end of the Second World War. The pleasant afterglow of victory soon yielded to the harsh realities of a dangerous international rivalry pitting the US-led western democracies against the Communist bloc under the direction of the Soviet Union. When Communist North Korea invaded its southern neighbour in June 1950, the democracies responded vigorously to the aggression and, not long afterwards, Canadians were again fighting overseas. Before the conflict ended in stalemate in July 1953, about 25,000 Canadians had served, 516 were killed or died while on active service, and more than 1,200 were wounded. Korea produced a new crop of veterans just a few years after the last ones had returned home from the earlier conflict. Some of them suffered at least partial vision loss, though not many appear to have been blinded outright, and SAPA's membership did not grow as a result of the conflict.

Decentralizing SAPA

Despite the sense that the two generations of war blinded had bonded as individuals, a small minority of SAPA members undertook the vast majority of the association's work. The "heart and soul" of the organization seemed to remain strongest with the First World War veterans, many in their sixties and seventies. In 1964 Woodcock contrasted the First World War veterans' continued interest in SAPA with the lackadaisical approach of too many Second World War veterans who, according to Woodcock, seemed beset with the "attitude of 'sit back and let George do it,' which does not speak well for the future of our organization."[111] Of course, the First World War veterans were retired, whereas most from the Second World War still worked. During his 1956 president's report before thirty-five members at the SAPA AGM, Bill Mayne lamented the lack of spirit, even the "apathy," infecting the SAPA membership in general. "My impression," he wrote, "is that there is a great lack of interest on the part of many members" and that "in Toronto this lack of interest is most apparent." He attempted to cajole those present: "The qualifications for membership in this Association are extensive or total loss of sight. We have a common bond of disability and of service. I feel that we would do well to spend more time together." He returned to the charge at the 1957 AGM, at which 124 members were present due to that year's reunion: "During this Reunion, and for some time after, the interest by our members in this Association will be high and keen. As time goes by, however, that interest will slacken and wane. Any such lessening of interest is disastrous to any organization, but more so to our Association, with its membership so small in numbers and so scattered across Canada."[112]

Extraordinarily proud of SAPA, Mayne went on, "It is true that we received tremendous assistance from DVA and the CNIB, for which we readily give our most sincere thanks, but let us not be too modest. Let us be frank and say that our successes result partly from our desire to succeed."[113] The men's successful re-establishment and their ability to move forward had stemmed from their own strength of character, not merely from the provisions of the Veterans Charter. At the 1960 SAPA AGM Bill Dies, who had replaced Mayne as president, also warned against members' complacency, and encouraged the younger members to become more interested in SAPA and to continue working on behalf of all blinded veterans.[114]

Perhaps a SAPA restructuring, even decentralization of sorts, would make the association more immediate to members and rekindle interest in its affairs and goals. The vastness of Canada's geography worked against the war blinded. As early as 1949, aftercare officer Fred Woodcock wrote of a "problem" maintaining SAPA unity and expressed a strong desire to foster "closer contact" among members. While Toronto remained SAPA's centre of gravity, several other large Canadian centres had well over fifteen members. As SAPA's Toronto members had from time to time held local reunions, it seemed sensible to encourage and formalize such an arrangement elsewhere in the country. Because general SAPA reunions were infrequent, and Canada's war-blinded veterans felt especially at ease in each other's company, the SAPA executive authorized the establishment of local SAPA organizations to help keep members in touch and to promote recreational and social activities. Central or "national" authority and control over all operating policies and practices was to be maintained, but SAPA needed to enhance the organization's visibility and relevance among its far-flung members.[115]

The SAPA executive directed that each local SAPA "social club" required a minimum of ten members and was to elect an executive to liaise regularly with its national counterpart. Since relatively few SAPA members from outside Toronto attended the annual general meetings, each local club was obliged to hold at least one social event a year at which members would have the opportunity for raising concerns or asking questions. A local representative could then forward any "individual or collective problem" to the SAPA Executive Committee for study. The whole scheme of decentralizing SAPA was a means of putting more members in touch with more local organizers who could assist them. Recognizing through experience the critical importance of a regional presence, the CNIB, through its aftercare fund, initially allotted to the local groups five dollars per registered local member per annum to fund their activities. This amount rose periodically in the years that followed. Regular reporting from the clubs about their activities, and the SAPA national executive's strict approval process for these activities, limited any tendencies toward organizational fragmentation. Moreover, the executive forbade the social clubs from forwarding resolutions or other SAPA-related information to any other veterans' groups or the press without prior national executive approval.[116]

In November 1948, fourteen of twenty-three war-blinded veterans living in Winnipeg and environs attended the founding meeting of that city's SAPA social club. Within five years their numbers rose to thirty-two, as more veterans from the Winnipeg Grenadiers who had been captured at Hong Kong passed through the rehabilitation process. In January 1949, the SAPA executive formally authorized the Winnipeg social club, its first satellite organization. The similar number of war-blinded Montrealers followed with their own club in 1953. Three years later the Montreal group had thirty-two active members and Winnipeg's twenty-eight. In 1957, clubs were established in Vancouver and Victoria.[117] In Toronto, the national executive served as its own unofficial local club, and its members easily could meet with local SAPA members at large. In 1966 the social clubs were formally termed "branches" of SAPA.[118] In the 1970s a branch was established in Saint John to serve the Atlantic provinces.[119] This reorganization helped to rejuvenate SAPA, heightened its national profile, and allowed members greater input into the organization's affairs. Most importantly, as Mayne had urged in the 1950s, the men could "spend more time together" – a recipe for better morale and the longer-term health of this small veterans' group.

Patriotic Activities

SAPA's minutes attest to the Canadian war-blinded's keen sense of patriotic duty and monarchical fealty. The veterans were certainly not neglected on the occasion of official regal events or visits. Woodcock attended the queen's 1953 coronation, which for him proved "an emotional and inspirational experience." Along with Padre Lambert of the War Amputations, Woodcock represented the NCVA, showing SAPA's stature in the veterans' community.[120] In 1957 Edwin

Baker and Bill Mayne, the SAPA president, were introduced to the royal couple when the queen and the Duke of Edinburgh laid a wreath at the cenotaph in Ottawa. On 30 June 1959, while on a Canadian tour, Queen Elizabeth II visited Bakerwood, the CNIB head-quarters in Toronto. Baker and Dies were presented to Her Majesty on this occasion, which all the Toronto-area SAPA members were in-vited to attend wearing their medals and berets and carrying white canes, so that they might form an informal guard of honour during the queen's visit.[121] In October 1964, the queen was again in Ottawa, and J.J. Doucet, SAPA's president, was presented to her after she again laid a wreath at the National War Memorial. Similarly, in March 1965, Doucet and SAPA member Charles Hornsby, blinded during the First World War, travelled to St. Dunstan's for its fiftieth anniver-sary celebration. The queen entertained three hundred St. Dun-staners and their escorts at St. James Palace, and Doucet was again presented to her, to his great delight.[122]

The matter of evolving Canadian national and monarchical symbols and traditions also evoked debate among the war-blinded veterans, as among Canadian veterans generally. The debate over changing the Canadian flag, specifically, elicited much interest and in 1959 SAPA adopted the position that the design of any new Can-adian national flag should incorporate the Maple Leaf, the Union Jack, and the Fleur-de-Lys. In February 1965, Doucet represented the organization at the formal unveiling of the new Canadian flag in Ottawa. While he described the event as a "very moving ceremony," Doucet also admitted that it was with "a great deal of nostalgia that we saw the Red Ensign, under which we had served in two World Wars, lowered for the last time."[123] With this, he echoed the views of most other veterans.

Similarly, SAPA members expressed varying opinions on the adoption of an official Canadian anthem and the resulting possible downgrading of "God Save the Queen." At the AGM held in November 1966, one of the thirty-three members attending, K. Albrecht, stated,

"We have now adopted the Canadian flag, why don't we also make use of our National Anthem, 'O Canada?'" Surprised that the anthem had been absent from the 1965 reunion, Albrecht insisted that "I think we should put 'O Canada' right beside our Canadian flag. We are Canadians; we receive our pensions from the Canadian Government; don't we owe our country that much that we sing 'O Canada?'" Bill Dies felt Albrecht's timing in raising this potentially divisive topic was "most inopportune" and wished the matter to be put in abeyance. Still, Albrecht insisted that, since it was "dear to [his] heart to recognize our own country first," the SAPA Executive Committee agreed to revisit the matter and report at a later date.[124] There is no evidence that it did so. Most blinded veterans were deeply attached to Canada's British roots, symbols, and traditions. It was decided, especially taking into account older veterans' feelings, that future formal SAPA functions should begin with the singing of "O Canada" but close with "God Save the Queen."

Early in 1967, Veterans' Affairs minister Roger J. Teillet, whom Woodcock often described as "a man of his word," invited the NCVA to appoint an official delegate to the fiftieth anniversary commemoration to be held at Vimy Ridge in April 1967. The minister also invited Edwin Baker to attend those ceremonies to be held in Ottawa. Woodcock inquired of DVA if, in the event a SAPA member or another disabled veteran was nominated by the NCVA, Ottawa would be prepared to fund a trip for an escort for that veteran. Not only was the response negative, but it was made clear to Woodcock that no DVA staff in attendance at Vimy would have time to devote to the needs of a blinded or disabled veteran. Woodcock was highly "indignant," since this ruled out many members of the NCVA, including several of its executive members. Judge Frank McDonagh, a Vimy veteran himself, agreed to represent the NCVA, of which he was an honorary vice-president. Ottawa's policy resulted in the NCVA dispatching a stiff letter and resolution to DVA complaining bitterly about the department's ill-conceived parsimony. SAPA members were "highly incensed," since, as Woodcock pointed out to the 1967 AGM, "to our knowledge, we, the war blinded, have never been a burden, or a responsibility, to any delegation attending a formal function put on by the Government of Canada." Moreover, Woodcock had hoped to send as a delegate long-time SAPA member and CNIB official M.C. Robinson, "who had actually lost his sight while clearing a dug-out in the Battle of Vimy Ridge."[125] Although one of the very few occasions on which DVA let down disabled veterans, this apparent discrimination left a wound.

More happily, and perhaps the result of the furor DVA's uncharitable policies had caused earlier in the year, Woodcock represented the NCVA at the twenty-fifth anniversary ceremonies held at Dieppe in August 1967. He wrote an extensive report of his participation, noting that just before the Canadian delegation's departure for Dieppe, Teillet symbolically lit two miner's lamps from the centennial flame in Ottawa and handed them to Woodcock and to Bob Kohaly, the first vice-president of the Royal Canadian Legion. Woodcock's escort for the trip was John Garshaw, the DVA's casualty welfare officer for the Hamilton area who, like Woodcock, had served with the Royal Hamilton Light Infantry at Dieppe. Designated a member of the Dieppe Survival Group, Woodcock recalled his participation as "a terrific, emotional experience, created by the stupendous crowd reaction from the French people ... The [Dieppe] Chief of Police later informed us that there were 65,000 to 70,000 people jamming the Esplanade." Despite the terrible injuries he had suffered at Dieppe, Woodcock noted that "it made one feel proud to have taken part in the raid."[126] The blinded veterans knew the importance of their service, had suffered decades of living with its effects, and felt the need, as they inevitably aged, to commemorate and be remembered.

The men also needed each other. As had been the case in the interwar period, the years following the end of the Second World

War witnessed a surge in the number of social activities aimed at lifting the men's morale. No events mattered more than the SAPA reunions.

Reunions

Even before the Second World War ended, SAPA began planning for a postwar reunion of Canadian war-blinded veterans. There had not been a reunion of blinded veterans from the First World War since 1931 and this eagerly awaited reunion, held in 1947, would prove an opportunity for the blinded of both world wars to become acquainted with each other and for the younger veterans to become fully involved in the affairs of SAPA, the CNIB, and the Canadian blind in general. In this regard, the association was entirely successful. A decade later, the 1957 reunion offered the war blinded an opportunity to sensitize the entire country to their existence and, more importantly, to their remarkable rehabilitation successes. The 1957 reunion, blending very strong contingents from both world wars, might have been SAPA's public zenith as a veterans' organization representing a body of Canadians who had suffered, in the nation's defence, the privations of a near-lifetime of blindness. The 1965 reunion followed in this vein.

The 1947 Reunion

Planning a major national reunion while the Second World War warblinded retraining, rehabilitation, and residence programs remained in full operation was an enormous and taxing undertaking for both SAPA and the CNIB. Organizing the transportation, assembly, and itinerary of more than one hundred war-blinded veterans plus their escorts for the 1947 general reunion in Toronto, SAPA's fourth, required thousands of volunteer hours. The dedicated CNIB and SAPA communities saw to even the minutest details, often linked to the special and sometimes complicated requirements unique to the blind. The minutes of the SAPA Executive Committee speak of little but reunion planning for three months before the event.

Equal to the task, the energetic and industrious CNIB and SAPA officials and volunteers organized an ambitious program of activities. Bill Dies, SAPA's president, emphasized the usual outstanding support of the Voluntary Aid Detachment workers (VADs), especially Clara Sutherland and Elsie Gorman, "our constant friends," in allowing all these detailed plans to come together so successfully. These women volunteers were simply invaluable to Canada's war blinded and, by extension, to the Department of Veterans Affairs as well. SAPA showed its appreciation during the 1947 reunion by admitting as honorary members nineteen VADs who had been working with the war blinded since the First World War; Sutherland was made an honorary vice-president of SAPA. This mass honorary inclusion is unique in SAPA's history.[127]

The June 23-28 reunion, held at the King Edward Hotel, was expensive, but DVA and the CNIB proved willing and generous benefactors. Between them, they shared the complete costs for any SAPA member and escort to travel to the conference. Lodgings and meals were paid for one week. The costs of bringing the men to Toronto was more than $11,000, with much of the funding coming from DVA's aftercare budget.[128] But SAPA's leaders felt it important that the two war-blinded generations mingle in large numbers as quickly as possible, with the older veterans assisting the younger to understand life's considerable potential despite blindness. Dies noted that "for a week the war blinded of both conflicts played and worked and talked together, getting to know each other better, sharing, experiencing, discussing problems." After it was over, he also felt that the 1947 reunion had helped blur the distinction between SAPA's "old" and "new" boys.[129] Officially, the reunions were held to "renew the ties of friendship, common experience and common purpose which unite" all SAPA members. The first reunion in 1926 had drawn 75 delegates and the second in 1933 attracted 81, but the 1947 reunion, reflecting the fact that SAPA had been renewed by a second generation of war blinded, drew more than 130 members.[130]

The war blinded's reunion attracted the attention and support of top-ranking DVA officials, including the minister, and was aided by a broad spectrum of civic, community, and veterans' organizations. This high-profile involvement with the blinded veterans symbolized the public's postwar gratitude for the men's war service, sympathy for the poignancy of their wounds, and a tacit understanding of the challenges that lay ahead of them. Mayor Robert H. Saunders accompanied Bill Dies in laying a wreath at the cenotaph on Tuesday 24 June, with Padre Sydney Lambert officiating at the service. The RCAF band from Trenton, Ontario, provided the music. The men and their escorts were then treated to a civic luncheon and that evening the CNIB hosted them at Pearson Hall for a relaxed evening of catching up and exchanging information. The next day the Riverdale Kiwanis Club arranged an excursion across Lake Ontario to Niagara Falls. The souvenir booklet published for the reunion noted that "from start to finish the Kiwanians ensured that there would be no lack of high spirits and entertainment." The Niagara Falls branch of the Canadian Corps Association hosted the war blinded at lunch. Many enjoyed a complimentary excursion on the famous *Maid of the Mist* prior to a dinner laid on by the Parks Commission of Niagara Falls.[131] Local and institutional authorities co-operated every step of the way; with the memory of the Second World War still fresh, and the economy sound, nothing was too good for these disabled veterans.

On Thursday 26 June, some of the men played golf, with Second World War SAPA member Ronald Hewlett sinking a twenty-two-foot putt. The government of Ontario hosted a luncheon, with Premier George Drew formally welcoming the blinded veterans. Later that day the men attended a garden party organized by Lady Kemp at her elegant Toronto residence, Castle Frank. The Honourable Ray Lawson, Ontario's lieutenant governor, attended. Lady Kemp used the occasion to state that, of her many philanthropic interests and activities over the decades, the Baker Hall residence for the war blinded "was the happiest investment" she had ever made.

On Friday, 27 June, the national council of the CNIB hosted a lunch at the Royal Canadian Yacht Club, and no fewer than five hundred people attended that evening's banquet and dance at the King Edward Hotel. Minister of Veterans Affairs Ian Mackenzie was the guest speaker. So solid was the relationship between the institute and the federal government, and so successful had proven the on-going retraining of war-blinded veterans, that Mackenzie felt moved to state, with well-meaning exaggeration, that "the CNIB is practically part of DVA." Walter Woods, the well-known and highly respected DVA deputy minister who was especially proud of the DVA-CNIB partnership, was also present. The National Council of Veteran Associations and the Canadian Legion were also represented at this highly publicized event, illustrating SAPA's and Baker's ability to unite these sometime rivals in the Canadian veterans' community.[132] The success of the 1947 reunion would be difficult to match. But the men's strong desire to meet as a body from time to time, coupled with ongoing public and institutional support, meant that the next full-scale gathering was no less successful.

The 1957 Reunion

A decade later, when most of the Second World War veterans had been established but the First World War veterans were aging, SAPA felt it was time for another reunion, likely to be its biggest ever. Baker estimated that the travel costs for the 1957 reunion would be about fifteen thousand dollars. SAPA, of course, had no money of its own. DVA had only five thousand dollars left in the fiscal year ending 31 March 1956 to devote to such an event and seemingly no room at all for SAPA reunion expenditures in the 1956-57 fiscal year. Departmental budgets had been cut almost everywhere, and it seemed a foregone conclusion that additional requests made of the Treasury Board "would not be welcomed." Always accommodating, DVA instead increased the individual aftercare rates it would allot the CNIB for the next three years so that additional money would be available to make up, in good part, the estimated ten-thousand-dollar shortfall.[133] In 1957 Baker, who was part of SAPA's 1957 reunion committee, announced happily to his fellow committee members that DVA, through CNIB, had authorized a twenty dollar allowance per person for SAPA members and escorts from out of town.[134] Although not as much as desired, this meant that with the careful husbanding of resources, the support of the CNIB, and the co-operation of civic authorities, community groups, and businesses, the reunion could go on. The federal government was not in the habit of funding advocacy groups' social gatherings, but it consistently made exceptions for SAPA.

The 1957 reunion, held 16-21 June, reprised some of the highlights of 1947, including a cruise on Lake Ontario to Niagara Falls, a complimentary excursion aboard the *Maid of the Mist*, a tour of the Welland Canal, and visits to the "fruit district." Over the next few days, the T. Eaton Co. and Imperial Oil hosted lunches in honour of the war blinded.[135] Lady Virginia Kemp had succeeded Lewis Wood as CNIB president in 1954, but declining health obliged her to relinquish her post in 1957, at which time she was made the honorary president of the institute. She offered the SAPA delegates another garden party at Castle Frank, despite being critically ill. This was the last social event she held there, as she died on 26 June, five days after the conclusion of the reunion. For several decades she had been a "generous and devoted" friend and sustaining benefactor to the war blinded.[136]

By far the highlight of the reunion, one of the most memorable events in SAPA's history, and one of the proudest occasions for any Canadian veterans' group, took place in downtown Toronto on 18 June. It lasted less than half an hour. Some 150 Canadian war-blinded

veterans of both world wars, wielding white canes, marched in a stirring procession. This remarkable moment, filled with emotion, displayed for all to see that the terrible effects of war wounds on the
human spirit could be overcome and that physical disability need
not rob a veteran of dignity.

S.G. Nicks, the president of the Toronto branch of the War
Amputations of Canada, acted as parade marshal. The war blinded,
including two women, marched from the King Edward Hotel via Bay
Street to the cenotaph in front of City Hall, arriving for an 11:15 ceremony officiated by Padre Lambert. The Salvation Army band led the
way, followed by a SAPA colour party, the SAPA executive, and a pla-
toon of twenty members from each of the navy, army, and air force:
each serviceman guided two blinded veterans, one on each arm.
The city's best Boy Scouts, those having earned the coveted grade
of Queen's Scout, served a similar function. Several cars carried those
SAPA members unable to make the ten-minute walk to the cenotaph.
Mrs. A.R. Mallory, the widow of a popular and recently deceased
SAPA member, laid the wreath with Bill Mayne. The city controller, Mrs.
Jean Newman, extended the city's official welcome in the absence of
Mayor Nathan Phillips and subsequently hosted the veterans at a
civic luncheon.[137]

Of the war-blinded veterans' progression to the cenotaph, the
Toronto *Telegram* stated, "They cannot see, as they march, the impression they make; the still thoughtful faces of spectators are dark
to them but they must sense the respect, the gratitude and the admiration they inspire." Hundreds, probably thousands, had turned
out to watch. According to one press report, not only was this the
first time the blinded veterans of both world wars marched together
"as a unit," but it was the first occasion on which the SAPA colours
were paraded or displayed publicly. The men proudly wore their
SAPA berets and held their white canes "as proudly as any swagger
stick." It was an "impressive sight," wrote the *Telegram*. Another press
report exclaimed, "With their decorations and medals, white canes

held steady, they marched in column-of-route in perfect step behind the band. The column was in threes – two blind and a guide in the centre ... all of them, the old and the comparatively young, heads up, marched proudly." Another account gushed that SAPA was "the most distinguished group of servicemen and women in the realms of the Commonwealth."[138]

Fred Woodcock, the reunion chairman and SAPA secretary, recalled that the parade was the outstanding event of the reunion activities. Although Woodcock had experienced some "nervous apprehension on the part of the Executive regarding parade attendance," he was "overwhelmed at fall-in time, by the mass participation, in spite of the heat. I think most of us now realize the terrific impression made on the citizens of Toronto who witnessed the event, and feel sure that most of us sensed it during the parade."[139]

The 1957 reunion established a record for attendance: of 313 SAPA members (130 from the first war and 183 from the second), including several dozen who were not resident in Canada, 151 were on hand, accompanied by 146 escorts plus 10 invited guests for a total of 307 participants. There were also at least 20 volunteers present.[140] The reunion received prominent press, radio, and television coverage, and, according to Harry Coyle, a war-blinded Second World War veteran, SAPA was "spotlighted before the people of Canada." SAPA members Fred Woodcock, Harris Turner, and Bernard Castonguay were interviewed on the CBC television show *Tabloid,* and film of the veterans' parade and their trip to Niagara Falls was shown in newsreels in all of Canada's large theatres.[141] The heavy and highly favourable publicity for the event was obtained and co-ordinated by the CNIB's public-relations department. Like no event at any other reunion, this parade offered SAPA the opportunity of public display and the recognition that accompanied it. SAPA president Bill Mayne referred to the superbly organized and emotive 1957 reunion as "glorious" and full of "happy and sometimes poignant memories." He felt that the members had offered a "tremendous response."[142] The intense feeling of camaraderie, the exceptionally large number of delegates, the widespread civic, community, and corporate support, and the public and media attention combined to make the 1957 reunion perhaps the most successful in SAPA's history.

The 1965 Reunion

The war-blinded veterans did not have to wait as long for their next reunion, which was held in the Georgia Hotel in Vancouver from 3-9 July 1965. Woodcock noted that the decision to hold the reunion in 1965 instead of waiting ten years was determined by the rapidly increasing mortality rate among SAPA's First World War members. This was the first reunion held outside of Toronto, and co-ordinating it proved a challenge.[143]

In December 1964, Woodcock visited Vancouver for four days to look into the reunion planning and, initially, he "had not been too encouraged" by what he discovered. Long-distance planning was proving difficult for SAPA's Toronto-based executive, and DVA officials in Ottawa and Vancouver became heavily involved in assisting with the program. In fact, according to Woodcock, who served as the conference organizer, Gerry L. Mann, who headed DVA's Special Services Division, served as his "right hand" during the whole of the reunion.[144] One problem was that a Canadian Pacific Railway special train to carry SAPA delegates and their escorts from central Canada to the west coast would cost a whopping eighty-two thousand dollars. The Canadian National Railway then agreed to a cheaper option, accommodating the war blinded by adding two more cars to each of two trains travelling west from Toronto. If members wished to fly, SAPA-CNIB, using funds from the aftercare budget, would reimburse the men up to the cost of rail travel. The 1965 reunion was expected to cost upwards of sixty thousand dollars, and some of the desperately needed money was found in a dormant bequest to the CNIB intended for just such a purpose.[145]

There were 135 SAPA members present in 1965, in addition to wives, escorts, and sixty-eight members' children. This was an excellent turnout given the logistical problems and expenses. Lord and Lady Fraser of Lonsdale (Sir Ian having been elevated to the peerage in 1958 as Britain's first life peer) were also in attendance, adding a special touch to the event. Lord Lonsdale was the guest speaker at the banquet, which was also attended by DVA minister Roger J. Teillet, Judge Frank McDonagh, and A.N. Magill, the CNIB's managing director. For a time Lord Lonsdale even joined the heavily attended SAPA annual general meeting, held during the reunion, and was met with a "hearty round of applause" following some brief remarks. Perhaps more importantly, he came bearing the gift of five thousand dollars to help defray the hefty reunion costs.[146]

The program was ambitious and exhilarating. The British Columbia division of the CNIB sponsored a boat trip for the veterans to the CNIB Holiday Centre on Bowen Island. The men also participated in a deep-sea fishing trip. Some events were held in Victoria, where the men attended a wreath-laying ceremony at the cenotaph, later lunching at the Empress Hotel. One important aspect of all reunions was the opportunity for SAPA members to seek information, advice, and to simply complain if need be.[147] This was part of aftercare officer Fred Woodcock's job, and he was kept busy.

The reunions were well worth the cost and trouble. They helped cement relations between members, encouraged solidarity, rallied morale, and allowed the men to show, for themselves and the public at large, that they formed part of a wider, honoured community. They were also demonstrably capable of independence, and they fed on the pride that came with this.

Some Postwar Matters

With everything else that was taking place, SAPA was also on the move in the 1950s. The erection of a new and much-needed CNIB headquarters was of enormous interest to the SAPA members, who were also, naturally, CNIB clients. But more importantly, they would gain their own meeting space, a lounge much improved over their limited space in Pearson Hall, which was slated to be sold. To June 1954, 93 SAPA members (including 50 from the First World War) donated more than a thousand dollars in total toward the building fund. A SAPA committee was struck to inventory the contents of the club room at Pearson Hall and decide what was required in the new lounge. Baker was a member of the committee and his presence ensured that the war blinded, so intertwined with the activities and history of the CNIB, obtained all that they needed. SAPA's effects included the 1934 St. Dunstan's flag and many photographs, as well as the memorial plaque outside of Pearson Hall, which was to be placed in the new SAPA lounge. Perhaps not surprisingly, given the loss of Baker's son, David, and the patriotic pride animating the association, the war blinded also wanted their lounge to include an honour roll of members' sons killed in the Second World War and a memorial book of deceased members. Some members felt that the old lounge in Pearson Hall had been subject to "abuse" and it seemed that since the end of the war it had "been used for everything but its original intent." Baker agreed that the use of the new SAPA lounge would be "strictly controlled" by a new committee.[148]

The new CNIB headquarters, named Bakerwood in honour of Lieutenant-Colonel Edwin Albert Baker, OBE, MC, Croix de Guerre, BSc, LLD, managing director of the CNIB, and Lewis M. Wood, CBE, president of the institute from 1918 to 1954, opened 16 April 1956. It consisted of five and a half acres of floor space located on fourteen acres of grounds on Bayview Avenue in Toronto. As well as the national headquarters of the CNIB, Bakerwood housed the offices of the Ontario division, a library, workshops, vocational training space, classrooms, and recreation and hobby rooms. An attached residence, specially designed for the blind, was able to accommodate 140. Bakerwood was also home to the "very attractive" Sir Arthur Pearson

Association of War Blinded Lounge. "Dedicated in perpetuity" to SAPA members, the lounge was dignified and comfortable, and symbolized the bonds between Canada's military and civilian blinded, between the organization's origins and its continuing operations.[149] The men attending the 1957 reunion in Toronto found the new CNIB headquarters an "amazing revelation."[150] The CNIB had become a highly recognized Canadian institution, and the war blinded formed an essential part of its history.

SAPA Scholarships

SAPA members had always shared the strong desire to assist the civilian blind in some way, such as participating in various CNIB fundraising campaigns. But in 1958, SAPA struck a committee to investigate how the Canadian war blinded could formally help their civilian counterparts and, in so doing, perhaps create a lasting legacy. By this time, the First World War veterans were in their sixties and seventies, and some among them wished their experiences and the existence of their cherished organization to be perpetually before the public. Accordingly, in February 1959, SAPA adopted the following aim: "to encourage blind and visually impaired students to further their education so that they may live full and contributing lives." To help make this happen, SAPA, with few funds of its own, created the SAPA Scholarship Fund.[151]

The idea of funding scholarships had wide appeal among the war blinded. The number of scholarships, their amounts, and eligibility requirements were debated in SAPA's Executive Committee and in a Scholarship Committee, the latter chaired for years by the busy Bill Mayne. A University of Toronto graduate, Mayne took an immediate interest in facilitating higher education for Canada's most promising young blind students. SAPA's leadership agreed from the beginning that the fundraising would be limited to the war blinded themselves, so that the awards would truly represent their stated desire of helping the civilian blind. Annual appeals from the national headquarters and frequent reminders during branch meetings would encourage members to donate. The early tally of donations showed the fund was popular from its inception. Within a few months, 83 members had contributed $667; by October 1959, 114 members had given $848. From November 1960, the donations became tax deductible.[152] The scholarship fund was the only substantial amount of money held by SAPA, its other expenses being met by the DVA-funded aftercare account or directly by the CNIB.

SAPA contacted the five Canadian schools for the blind – the Ontario School for the Blind in Brantford, the Halifax School for the Blind, l'Institut Nazareth and l'Institut Louis-Braille, both in Montreal, and the Jericho Hill School for the Blind in Vancouver – to forward names of suitable candidates with strong academic potential at the university level. By not undertaking its own evaluation or establishing academic criteria, SAPA relied on the discretion and judgment of the individual schools' superintendents in recommending students for the scholarships, each worth fifty dollars.[153] Though not every school forwarded the names of candidates in the fund's earliest years, the awards were immediately gratifying to grantors and recipients. The three winning candidates in 1960 all "expressed their thanks verbally and in writing ... impressed by the kindness of the members of this Association."[154] In helping fulfill one of SAPA's basic goals, the awards helped solidify ties between the war-blinded and Canada's blind youth. The program was off to a good start – a harbinger of things to come.

In 1961 Fred Woodcock announced at a World Veterans Federation meeting in Paris that SAPA intended to provide a student scholarship to a developing nation and requested applications from member countries. Sierra Leone, Nigeria, and Ceylon (now Sri Lanka) expressed interest, and eventually SAPA sent $50 awards to one Nigerian and one Ceylonese student. The latter applied the money toward the purchase of a typewriter.[155] This proved to be the beginning of a long association between SAPA and the blind students of Ceylon. In 1962 two awards were made to Ceylonese students and one to a Nigerian, while another Ceylonese student received a scholarship in 1963. The recipients from Ceylon attended the Mount Lavinia School for the Blind in Colombo, and SAPA's award was normally presented by the Canadian high commissioner. The money was intended for educational expenses or the purchase of equipment once the recipient was established in a vocation.[156]

Annual appeals to members were made in co-operation with the SAPA social clubs (i.e., branches) and, in February 1963, the Scholarship Committee sent out an appeal letter to the SAPA membership noting that since the fund's inception four years earlier, 139 members had donated more than $2,300. In seeking more, the Scholarship Committee pleaded with members to "remember that we are assisting boys and girls who, like ourselves, are blind. There are no others who need help more than young blind students and there are no others who should be more willing to assist them than we, the war blinded."[157] The veterans knew well the importance of encouragement, education, and funding in helping to build a satisfying future for the sightless.

Most contributors to the fund were among the dwindling number of First World War veterans. Those from the Second would soon have to pick up the pace or else, Mayne believed, the fund-raising effort might collapse. However, in the year ending in April 1968, 104 members gave just short of $2,000 – a healthy participation rate. That year SAPA decided to extend its scholarship program to younger students by granting a twenty-five-dollar scholarship to those from each school for the blind who were entering high school and were deemed by their teachers and principals to have "shown the greatest leadership and morale-building qualities during the year" – qualities which had underpinned SAPA's activities since its inception. The first such awards were made in 1970. After nine years at the helm of the Scholarship Committee, Bill Mayne relinquished his duties in

1968. He had built up the fund from scratch, administered its expenses, and left it in excellent shape, with total assets in excess of $6,700.[158]

The scholarships rapidly became an important raison d'être of SAPA. For example, J.J. Doucet, in his 1965 SAPA president's report, noted that one of his "happiest presidential duties" was to award a SAPA scholarship to Shepsel Schell, from the Ontario School for the Blind in Brantford, so that he could continue his studies at the University of Manitoba. In fact, increasing the scholarship fund and expanding the number and destinations of bursaries became SAPA's Canadian Centennial project for 1967. Interestingly, that year SAPA's secretary, Fred Woodcock, announced that Ceylon's Mount Lavinia School for the Blind would be a prime recipient of the Canadian war blinded's aid, since "they seem to be the most responsive and effective in putting our scholarships to good use." SAPA provided the Ceylon school with a Sony broadcasting unit made possible through a special fundraising effort among members, which yielded $286. There were some outstanding Canadian recipients, too. A 1962 winner was Jim Sanders, who would, four decades later, become the CNIB's CEO. One 1967 winner was Robert Mercer, who would go on to high-ranking positions with both the CNIB and DVA.[159] The scholarship program enabled the veterans to assist young disabled Canadians, imbue their organization with a powerful sense of purpose, and even honour their own successes; they had become donors, not just recipients.

The Changing of the Guard

The quarter-century following the end of the Second World War saw a number of important passages for SAPA. Not the least of these was the loss of some key and respected members. In April 1949, Alexander Viets, one of the CNIB's and SAPA's founders, and a veteran of both the South African and First World Wars, died suddenly at home following a heart attack, aged seventy. A large contingent of Canadian war blinded attended the funeral.[160]

Two dear friends of the war blinded died in 1959. Lewis Wood, a founder of the CNIB and its president for thirty-six years, died in March, and former VAD Clara Sutherland passed away in May. Of Sutherland, the SAPA minutes recorded, "No one individual ever devoted more time to Canada's war blinded than did the 'sweetheart of SAPA.'" Of Wood: "The full extent of his efforts on behalf of the blind and many other disability groups will never be known or realized." Both funerals, like Lady Kemp's two years previously, were well attended by SAPA members.[161]

In 1954 Baker relinquished his post as SAPA's secretary after three decades and was replaced by the equally able Woodcock, who was also the CNIB's aftercare officer. Baker accepted the position of honorary vice-president of SAPA although his involvement with SAPA was beginning to wane. He was by this time sixty-three, and almost the whole of the SAPA executive were now Second World War veterans. In addition to Woodcock, Bill Mayne was increasingly active in the association's affairs and had become one of a handful of Second World War veterans to inherit the mantle of the First World War organizers. In January 1956, Baker missed a SAPA AGM for the first time.[162]

Baker's partial withdrawal from the affairs of SAPA was due to the complexities of his role with the CNIB, especially as the institute was preparing to inaugurate its impressive new headquarters in Toronto. He was also exhausted. But other members' lack of interest in their organization did contribute to a general slackening of SAPA activities. For example, there were none of the usual SAPA social functions in 1955 and the services of the Pearson Hall House Committee were not required for the first time. By 1949 such social functions had become the principal function of the House Committee. Money was no concern since the CNIB made available $850 per annum to cover SAPA's incidentals and entertaining.[163] Following their retraining, however, many Second World War veterans were simply getting on with their lives.

Baker, whom Woodcock described as "our great leader of the blind," retired from the CNIB on 30 June 1962. Lord and Lady Lonsdale attended the CNIB annual meeting in Toronto that year and paid Baker high tribute. No fewer than eighty-eight SAPA members joined Lord Lonsdale to fittingly fête Baker, the man who had done so much to restore their hope. He had become Canada's Arthur Pearson. Upon his retirement, the CNIB announced the E.A. Baker Foundation for Prevention of Blindness, and ninety-six SAPA members donated more than $1,100 of the $60,000 raised.[164] Giving and donating had become one of SAPA's main roles.

As evidence of his prestige and his ability to group disparate veterans' views and agendas, Baker was not only an active executive member of SAPA, but also the honorary president of the War Pensioners of Canada, a life member of both the Royal Canadian Legion and its rival organization, the Army, Navy, and Air Force Veterans in Canada, and, for more than thirty years, a member of the executive of the War Amputations of Canada.[165] He served as chairman and then honorary chairman of the NCVA from the group's formation in 1943 until his death. He symbolized the bridging nature of SAPA's presence in the veterans' community and was responsible for the war blinded's high profile among Canadians.

Baker was among the first group to be honoured with the Order of Canada, an award inaugurated to coincide with the centenary of Confederation in 1967. His official biographer, Marjorie Campbell, sent her best wishes and congratulations: "I am pleased and proud to see your name where it belongs among the original Companions of the Order of Canada." Baker replied, "I am honoured to accept, realizing it pays tribute to a large company of fellow Canadians. I am particularly honoured to be in the first group selected and accept it with deep humility."[166]

Edwin Albert Baker, among Canada's best-known veterans, and almost certainly its most famous blind citizen, died suddenly from an aortic aneurism at his home in Collins Bay, Ontario, on 7 April 1968 at the age of seventy-five. He was survived by his wife and three of his four children. He was buried in Cataraqui Cemetery, near Kingston. The eulogy for Baker, given by the Reverend John Neal, was reread to the thirty SAPA members attending the 27 April AGM. They responded with a "deep, sorrowful silence." Baker's loss was keenly felt by the entire SAPA family. He had been the association's secretary for twenty-seven years, from 1927 to 1954, the CNIB's general secretary from 1920 to 1931, and its managing director from 1931 to 1962. Neal's eulogy demonstrated the degree to which Baker had touched many thousands of blind and disabled people across the world and how he was revered in these communities. Baker had shown people how to "turn stumbling blocks into stepping stones," applying the lessons taught by Sir Arthur Pearson half a century earlier. "He has left in his wake," stated Neal, "a living memorial in his work for the blind and for the prevention of blindness. Many have been blessed because he has lived. A great man has passed among us and we shall not forget him."[167]

In July 1969, SAPA received yet another boost from Baker, though he had been deceased more than a year. Baker had bequeathed £1,000 to St. Dunstan's but the British organization had returned the money, equivalent to more than $2,500, to Baker's family. John Baker thereupon transferred the money to SAPA to "be spent for any purpose decided by the Club, not excluding outright cash gifts to any veteran who may be in need, particularly those from the First World War." With this, SAPA's E.A. Baker Benefit Fund came into being.[168]

Not long after Baker passed away, another of SAPA's well-known First World War veterans, Bill Dies, died on 11 December 1968 at the age of eighty-one. Woodcock recalled that Dies's affectionate nickname was "the old war horse" and that he had been a life-long activist on behalf of the war blinded and for veterans' rights generally. An arm amputee in addition to being totally blind, Dies had joined the CNIB in 1941 as its sales manager, retiring in 1955. He also had been a member of the Army, Navy, and Air Force Veterans in Canada and the War Amputations of Canada. Dies was among the founders of SAPA and had remained active in its affairs throughout his life.[169]

Fred Woodcock retired from the CNIB in March 1970. Bill Mayne, whom Woodcock strongly endorsed, succeeded him as CNIB aftercare officer and also as SAPA secretary, since the two posts had traditionally and wisely been associated. In a farewell speech to the January 1970 AGM, Woodcock spoke "feelingly" of his service to SAPA and the CNIB, and noted "satisfactions, heartaches, and sincere friendships" that he would long remember. Seventy-two people attended a dinner in his honour at the King Edward hotel in March 1970.[170] The guard had changed.

The postwar decades had been vibrant, fertile ones for SAPA and the war blinded. The members had attracted public attention to their achievements, fought successfully for improved pensions and a better standard of living, and, generally, carried on with their lives in sometimes arduous circumstances. The last decades of the twentieth century would witness the passing of the last war-blinded veterans of the First World War and the aging of those from the Second. In the absence of Canadian participation in any large-scale conflicts and the consequent lack of blinded casualties, SAPA's numbers declined rapidly. Increasingly, the surviving veterans concentrated on seeing one another more frequently and in creating a viable legacy project that would enshrine in perpetuity their memory and that of their association. In doing so, Canada's war blinded remained consistent with their founding ideals: to help themselves so that they might help others.

6 Twilight, 1971-2002

Him that overcometh, shall inherit all things.

– Rev. 21:7

The last several decades of the twentieth century brought enormous changes for the Sir Arthur Pearson Association of War Blinded and for all Canadian war-blinded veterans. While SAPA's guiding principles continued unchanged, its declining and aging membership presaged the absorption of Canadian National Institute for the Blind (CNIB) aftercare services by Veterans Affairs Canada (VAC) and some major restructuring as the next millennium loomed.[1] Given changing government policy and budgetary priorities, and the association's own considerable self-examination, SAPA's organization and operations evolved enormously in the period 1971-2002.

This chapter will treat these momentous changes, which included the introduction of exceptional incapacity allowance, a marked breakthrough in veterans' pension benefits; the granting of active SAPA membership to blind veterans on aftercare whose disabilities resulted only in part from active service; sweeping modifications to the aftercare program that caused an institutional split between

SAPA and the CNIB and created a confused CNIB-SAPA-VAC relationship; the final SAPA reunions; and the creation of a self-perpetuating
SAPA scholarship foundation, one of SAPA's final but most important
achievements. As the veterans entered the autumn of their lives with
dignity, the government generally responded to their needs with
understanding, and the CNIB remained the war blinded's pillar of
support.

The Last Forty Years of Pension Regulations

Exceptional Incapacity Allowance

On 2 December 1970, with representatives from the various veterans'
organizations present in the House of Commons visitors' gallery,
Minister of Veterans Affairs Jean-Eudes Dubé introduced Bill C-203, a
major amendment to the Pension Act. The main elements of the bill
were a 10 percent increase in veterans' pensions and allowances, the
granting of exceptional incapacity allowance (EIA) ranging from $800
to $2,400 per annum for especially suffering veterans already pen-
sioned as 100 percent disabled, and a 50 percent pension to all Hong
Kong veterans held as prisoners of war by the Japanese. At the same
time, attendance allowance, so critical to the war blinded, was raised
to a yearly maximum of $3,000. These provisions stemmed from the
recommendations made in the 1967 Woods Report, introduced in
the House of Commons in March 1968, and by various subsequent
parliamentary committees and sub-committees. The new legislation
received royal assent 30 March 1971. The Royal Canadian Legion was
pleased, noting in a press release that Bill C-203 "constitutes a major
step forward in veterans' pension legislation ... it will, we believe,
remedy many inequities."[2] Bill Mayne, the CNIB's war-blinded aftercare officer and the SAPA executive secretary, noted that the "close
co-operation" between the National Council of Veteran Associations

and the Legion to pressure Ottawa had likely been responsible for the establishment of EIA, a program he termed "one of the most significant benefits ever established."[3]

Bill C-203 amended section 57 of the Pension Act, which had previously allowed veterans a maximum total disability pension of 100 percent, notwithstanding the fact that the combined disabilities of some exceeded 100 percent as calculated in the table of disabilities. These veterans could get additional treatment, but no more money than was payable for a 100 percent pension. Exceptional incapacity allowance changed all of this, recognizing the hardships of pensioners more than 100 percent disabled whose quality of life was especially severely hampered by their disabilities, and compensating them with additional funding.[4] Section 57 of the Pension Act defined the conditions under which EIA could be awarded: "In determining whether the incapacity suffered by a member of the Forces is exceptional, account shall be taken of the extent to which the disability for which he is receiving a pension has left the member in a helpless condition or in continuing pain and discomfort, has resulted in loss of enjoyment of life, or has shortened his life expectancy."[5]

After the introduction of EIA, totally blinded veterans (without even light perception) who had a second disability obtained the maximum annual award of $2,400 (grade 1). This was the same as quadriplegics and triple or quadruple amputees. If veterans suffered from total blindness, with or without light perception, but without other disabilities, they received $2,000 (grade 2); with light perception but no light projection, $1,600 (grade 3); with light projection permitting orientation in familiar surroundings indoors, $1,200 (grade 4); and with the ability to count fingers and to move around in protected areas outdoors, $800 (grade 5).[6] For the war blinded, EIA was a significant and long-sought-after entitlement. Their condition, especially as they aged, led to obvious "exceptional" circumstances rendering life difficult and expensive, and this had now been recognized by the federal government.

EIA was strictly linked to definable ills resultant from a pensioned condition. To obtain attendance allowance, the disability imposing the need for assistance did not need to be pensionable; the critical element was that the disabled veteran be pensioned to some degree. To obtain EIA, however, it had to be established that the veteran's deteriorated condition was a direct consequence of a specifically pensioned disability and met the definition in section 57 of the act.[7] This was not always an easy task for Canada's war-blinded veterans. Almost immediately, Bill Mayne determined to undertake the major project of canvassing all SAPA members to review their level of disability and current pension and allowance entitlements, and to encourage them to obtain up-to-date medical assessments of their disabilities. He hoped to ensure that all war-blinded veterans received the maximum allowable EIA for their particular circumstances, and he was prepared to argue the merits and specifics of each and every case with federal authorities.[8]

Mayne hoped to find an ally in his endeavour in the Pension Review Board (PRB), a new body independent of the Canadian Pension Commission whose mandate was to review veterans' appeals of claims for pension or benefit adjustments rejected by the CPC. The PRB served as the final appeals authority in the administration of the Pension Act. Early on, the PRB showed itself willing to adopt a generous approach in its application of the "Benefit of the Doubt" clause, section 70 of the act. In addition, the new legislative amendments established the Bureau of Pensions Advocates, which was intended to help veterans prepare their appeals to the CPC and the PRB.[9]

But Mayne wished to push further. In 1973 he orchestrated, with the War Amputations' Cliff Chadderton's assistance, an appeal test case. Chris Davino, a war-blinded veteran with a secondary disability, who had some light perception of little real use, appealed his EIA award and sought an increase to $2,400 from $2,000 per annum. SAPA's view was that light perception alone equated to total blindness. Not all ophthalmologists agreed, and the two associations

wished to raise sufficient doubt to warrant a ruling in favour of
Davino.[10] However, SAPA's consulting ophthalmologist was unable to
agree that having only light perception equated to total blindness,
since the ability to perceive light has a social and psychological
value. For example, a blind person with light perception normally
can tell day from night and whether lights are on in a room. But the
doctor did agree that this minimal difference was of no occupational
use and therefore not relevant for measuring a person's disability for
pension purposes. This contention formed the basis of Davino's appeal. The stumbling block was that the award of EIA also took into
account overall quality of life issues, which would include any sense
of psychological well-being advanced by light perception.[11] The case
was in the hands of the PRB before the end of the year.

In addition, SAPA appealed four cases of veterans with some
guiding vision who did not receive EIA despite additional disabilities including deafness. The cagey Bill Mayne was himself among
the four cases, and his idea here was to test the appeal process to
learn what the pension officials needed in terms of supporting evidence and to discover what questions were asked of the veterans.
In this way, SAPA could hone its skills in anticipation of further
appeals.[12]

Even high-profile SAPA cases wound their way slowly through
the system. Fred Woodcock, for instance, listed all his physical disabilities resulting from his war service and blindness. He described
frequent pain behind his artificial right eye and nausea when at-
tempting to "see through a small blurred vision area in the lower
temporal field of the left eye with [the] aid of a magnifying glass." He
was deaf in one ear with diminished hearing in the remaining ear.
His shoulders had been badly injured and he had suffered recurring
pain in them ever since. Moreover, injuries to his back and right leg
had worsened over the years, weakening him and occasionally ham-
pering his mobility. By 1974 he was unable to undertake any physical

work, and his aging wife, according to Woodcock, had been obliged to take on "many more personal tasks for me." He also suffered from shrapnel infection, loss of equilibrium, and hives. Accordingly, that year he sought an increase to the maximum allowable EIA, given that the sum of his disabilities easily exceeded the 100 percent benchmark. Mayne, Woodcock's successor as national aftercare officer, took the latter's case in hand, but to no immediate avail.[13]

In the meantime, in August 1974, Mayne, uncharacteristically testy, submitted a lengthy and impassioned appeal to the CPC to review the awarding of EIA to the war blinded. Specifically, he sought to have the commission award grade 5 EIA to all war-blinded veterans deemed 100 percent disabled and he wanted the totally blind without additional disabilities to obtain grade 1 EIA rather than grade 2 as was called for in the act. In reviewing the merits of the war blinded's collective case, the CPC felt obliged to compare the lot of the blinded veterans with that of other veterans with different very severe disabilities in receipt of grade 1 EIA, against the EIA award stipulations defined in the act. The commissioners felt that the totally blind were not as helpless as others in the grade 1 category, that their pain and discomfort was not the equal of these grade 1 pensioners, that the blinded had no less ability to enjoy life than these other veterans, and that there was no hard evidence that blindness shortened their life span. "It is not considered," wrote the commissioners in their ruling, that the war blinded's "tensions and frustrations (pain and discomfort) are comparable to that of a coughing breathless asthmatic, a cardiac cripple with angina decubitus, or of a bedridden multiple sclerotic, all of whom are conscious of and under the tension and anxiety of approaching death."[14]

Similarly, with respect to grade 5 EIA for all 100 percent pensioned, though not totally blind veterans, the CPC rejected Mayne's claims. The commissioners again were forced to compare the war blinded's lives to those of existing grade 5 recipients, in this instance bilateral below-knee amputees. The commissioners adamantly believed that the double amputees were more helpless, in greater pain, less able to enjoy life, and certainly not likely to have life expectancies greater than those with at least some vision, no matter how restricted.[15]

Mayne was furious with the ruling, and especially annoyed that the decisions had been based on comparison with other classes of disabled veterans, a standard of measurement Mayne felt was "unfair" and ignored the psychological impact of blindness, especially when combined with the aging process. Ironically, Woodcock had purposefully sought such a comparison in the 1960s, believing it would serve the war blinded's cause; the shoe was now on the other foot. In January 1975, Mayne dispatched a seven-page letter to Dr. C.N. Brebner, the CPC's chief medical advisor, reiterating his views and insisting that the "helplessness of the totally blind pensioner is grossly underestimated."[16] One can sympathize with both sides here, since Mayne's forcefully expressed and passionate convictions lacked the kind of empirical evidence the CPC needed to justify reinterpreting section 57 of the act. Comparison to other disabilities seemed the only means of assessment. Mayne's repeated pleas went unheeded. A further ten-page letter to Brebner less than a month later (Mayne did not seem disposed toward writing to the CPC chairman, A.O. Solomon) got him nowhere. Responding to yet another of Mayne's complaints over the CPC's assessment procedures, Solomon wrote Mayne in July that a comparative analysis was the best means to proceed and that "the Commission[ers] felt that they could not consider the war blinded as a group separate and distinct from other disabled veterans."[17]

Finally, and hardly surprisingly given their earlier rulings, in 1975 the CPC and the PRB rejected the SAPA test cases noted above. Happily, however, the CPC did agree to award EIA at a higher level (from grade 3 to grade 2) to blinded veterans with some light perception but no light projection.[18]

Stymied on the principle of automatically awarding totally blinded veterans grade 1 EIA, in June 1977 Mayne, in company with Cliff Chadderton and Andrew C. Clarke of the Canadian Paraplegic Association, met with Minister of Veterans Affairs Daniel MacDonald to request a rate increase for EIA. MacDonald, an enormously popular minister with SAPA members, was himself a disabled Second World War veteran, having lost his left arm and leg in combat in Italy in 1944. Not hearing back from MacDonald, Mayne wrote to the minister in November to remind him that, in 1970, a parliamentary committee had recommended that grade 1 EIA be set at $3,600 annually, not the $2,400 eventually enacted. According to Mayne, the veterans in question were unduly "economically disadvantaged," unable to gain access to the highest-paying jobs while at the same time suffering additional living costs as a result of their conditions. SAPA sought the additional $1,200 annually for grade 1, and proportional increases for the other grades, plus the mandated annual consumer price index increases, which would set the new maximum EIA rate at approximately $4,900, reckoned Mayne, as opposed to its current $3,950. There were 267 war-blinded veterans on aftercare resident in Canada (not all were SAPA members), of whom 187 were pensioned at 100 percent. Eighty-two did not qualify for EIA and 105 did, of whom 22 received it at grade 1, 35 at grade 2, 8 at grade 3, 22 at grade 4, and 18 at grade 5. Fifteen additional aftercare recipients lived abroad, of whom eight obtained grade 2 EIA and one grade 5. The aggregate cost to the Crown of their EIA benefits was $282,200 per year. Increasing the rates by nearly 25 percent on average for these veterans would add about $65,000 in annual costs.[19] It did not seem like much, but MacDonald, obliged "to look at more than just the emotional factor," also had to take into account additional costs that would accrue for payments to the 930 non-war blinded veterans in receipt of EIA, a program whose annual costs of approximately $2.2 million would rise by nearly 50 percent if the Department of Veterans Affairs (DVA) accepted the SAPA proposals. MacDonald concluded that, given the generous federal payments made to EIA-obtaining veterans, the idea of their being "financially disadvantaged" was a "hard sell."[20] Matters stood where they were.

In 1982, the CPC requested that Mayne's successor as aftercare officer, SAPA executive secretary David Dorward, serve on a special committee to make recommendations to improve the EIA guidelines and the fixed table of disabilities. The War Amputations of Canada, the Royal Canadian Legion, and the Bureau of Pensions Advocates were also solicited to participate.[21] This challenge interested the pugnacious Dorward, who, although mainly insisting on the changes for which Mayne had lobbied unsuccessfully for years, fought hard in the next few years to relax pension policy to include as many disabled, suffering veterans as possible.

Using the pages of the *SAPA Chronicle*, the association's newsletter, and other means, Dorward consistently reminded SAPA members of their possible EIA eligibility if they were, according to the wording of the legislation, in a helpless condition, in continuing pain and discomfort, unable to enjoy life, or likely to have a shortened life expectancy. To Dorward, the EIA eligibility of the war blinded, under these points, seemed obvious. For example, he pointed out, "When blindness and aging are combined ... the need of sighted help increases, rapidly and extensively." He also felt that the emotional anguish and psychological pain of blindness needed to be taken into account when assessing whether a veteran's disability was "exceptional." Blind people could not enjoy life to its fullest potential. They were also beset, Dorward believed, by the "regrets for opportunities missed [and the] acceptance that things will never improve." These burdens "cast a pall" over their ability to make the most out of their lives. Despite a lack of specific medical or scientific evidence suggesting that the war blinded had shorter life expectancies than other veterans, "blind persons draw pensions for a shorter time than their sighted counterparts" and life insurance for them was more expensive to obtain.[22]

He built a strong case. In a 1984 letter to L.M. Hanway, chief pensions advocate with the Bureau of Pensions Advocates, Dorward decided to "stress the psychological" issues facing aging, war-blinded veterans. In a rare admission that some among Canada's war blinded had difficulty adjusting to life without sight, Dorward wrote, "Too many of the war blinded could not adjust to blindness; in consequence they tended to become bitter and withdrawn with age. They had difficulty making friends with sighted people and now live alone with their wives brooding on their glorious youth and suffering from 'if only's.'" It is difficult to know if Dorward was exaggerating the case to make his point with Hanway, or if the war blinded had become, with age, increasingly wearied and discouraged. Dorward believed such suffering constituted a clear-cut example of the "loss of enjoyment of life."[23] Mayne continued to believe that the war blinded's "successes in various vocations have served to diminish the seriousness of our disability in the eyes of the CPC." "Do not be embarrassed to lay it all out," he counselled members, lest the authorities gain a skewed impression of the degree of the veterans' disabilities.[24] Had the war blinded become victims of their own civil re-establishment successes?

In 1992, following an in-depth pension review, the CPC granted twenty-nine of forty-four SAPA members upgrades in either or both EIA and attendance allowance.[25] The years of cajoling Ottawa might have paid off for some, but the results also came years too late for many suffering war-blinded veterans who had gone to their reward since the introduction of EIA. Still, Dorward – by this time SAPA president – employing a softened tone and approach, indicated his sincere pleasure with the "prompt, professional and efficient" response by VAC on inquiries made on behalf of SAPA members. Any denied requests, he hastened to point out, were the result of "legal or technical rather than humanitarian reasons." The war blinded and government officials maintained a harmonious and productive working relationship. As Dorward wrote to Marcel Chartier, chairman of the

CPC, "I am particularly struck by the sincerity of everyone involved ... We are a shrinking number of very proud individuals who wish to maintain our dignity and independence for as long as possible."[26]

On 17 August 1994, Bill Mayne and SAPA executive director Jim Sanders presented a brief to the Senate Sub-Committee on Veterans Affairs. Sanders stated plainly that "blindness alone does not create an insurmountable barrier. With the right opportunities, the right training, and the right attitude, blindness can be reduced to a daily nuisance, at times a difficulty, but never a barrier." They stressed that the veterans' "true barrier" resulted from long-term blindness prematurely aging them and inordinately stressing and complicating their lives in their declining years. Blindness, they insisted, amplified the standard problems of aging and made the war blinded different from any other veterans' group. Sanders and Mayne emphasized the point that SAPA members' spouses, by far their main sources of support, were also aging and experiencing undue strain in assisting their husbands. Sanders and Mayne requested that the sub-committee recommend to the CPC that a 100 percent disability pension for blindness should automatically entail Grade 1 EIA. At that time, SAPA had 134 members with an average age of seventy-five. There were two First World War members left and two from the Korean War. It was important to move quickly. Most of the members receiving EIA did so at grades 4 or 5 and would stay in that category. Accordingly, the change would entail little additional government expenditure and, given the unique set of circumstances posed by blindness, the CPC's decision would not set a precedent for other disabled veterans. The sub-committee, chaired by SAPA-sympathetic Senator Jack Marshall, agreed to recommend to the CPC that EIA claims assessments take into account the psychological and physical burdens imposed on veterans by the joint effects of aging and blindness. Marshall promised that he would make a "strong pitch" on behalf of SAPA: "We hope to be able to do something for you that you deserve and that is justifiable."[27] But the wording of the legislation seemed unassailable, and the matter was laid to rest.

Pensions

Notwithstanding the differences of opinion between the veterans and the government, SAPA's relationship with Veterans Affairs Canada remained amicable, respectful, and, in many ways unique among veterans' groups. SAPA continued to robustly but reasonably represent its members' interests while, for its part, the department showed goodwill and meted out measured increases in pension benefits and entitlements. The personal relationships between SAPA-CNIB and departmental officials, often including the minister, appeared genuinely warm and friendly.

In the 1970s, the gentlemanly Bill Mayne, whether acting in the capacity of CNIB aftercare officer or SAPA executive member, adopted a conciliatory yet forthright approach with the department, softer than Fred Woodcock's had been and decidedly more congenial than David Dorward during his tenure as aftercare officer. Yet even Dorward, while SAPA's president, came to realize the benefits of taking a collaborative tone with an already sympathetic ministry. Frequently, informal contacts with VAC or CPC officials solved problems before they became cause for public grievance. SAPA's membership was shrinking and time was drawing shorter; even minor progress in tough budgetary times would be a success. In 1974 Mayne wrote that "wherever and whenever approached, DVA officials and staff are always helpful, co-operative and sympathetic. They are prepared to do all within their power to assist the war blinded."[28] This seemed contrary to the perhaps more publicized conflictual relationships DVA occasionally maintained with other veterans' organizations. Despite its small size, SAPA's important role as a member of the National Council of Veteran Associations (NCVA) placed it in the forefront of veterans' advocacy, if not publicly then certainly with DVA. Some important and hard-won pension legislation gains resulted from SAPA initiatives or, at least, long-standing SAPA and NCVA pressure. Mayne became chairman of the NCVA in March 1975, while Woodcock was the honorary chairman.[29]

Canadian Pension Commission officials certainly claimed to see their primary role as helping veterans, rather than stubbornly guarding the public purse. Speaking at the October 1978 SAPA AGM, Howard J. Clarke, deputy chairman of the CPC, noted that "the Commission attempts to find sufficient evidence to grant an award. Our purpose in life is to grant pension entitlement and all we require is sufficient credible evidence to permit us to do so." The system was generous: the CPC paid all travel costs, including any lost wages, for an applicant to appear before the entitlement board. An advocate was provided at Crown expense. At that time there were 850 applications a month for various upward entitlement adjustments. The federal government was paying pensions to 109,000 disabled veterans and 26,000 surviving dependants. Moreover, living disabled veterans combined for more than 123,000 spouses and children for whom additional benefits were disbursed. A 100 percent disability pensioner received $8,151 a year, and the overall pension cost to the treasury was approximately $450 million annually.[30] In this context, SAPA's requests seemed minor and affordable, or at least the war-blinded veterans thought so.

A brief piece on veterans' legislation included in the CNIB's 1973 annual report, probably written by Mayne, remarked that "1973 is truly a milestone in the history of veterans' legislation. It established the formula for the basic rate of pension for handicapped veterans, a goal that has been sought since 1919." The self-congratulatory piece noted that SAPA, working with and through the NCVA, and with the Legion, DVA, and the CPC, had been instrumental in achieving this long-desired goal. "Under the new agreement," stated the annual report, "the basic rate was equated with the composite grouping of five unskilled classifications of the Federal Civil Service." Veterans had sought this particular formula for decades. In 1973 the basic annual rate for a single 100 percent disability pensioner was $4,704, being the average salary paid to the composite group. The spousal allowance was 25 percent of the basic rate, with 13 percent accorded the first child, 22 percent if there were two children, and 7.5 percent for each additional child. Widows received 75 percent of the basic rate.[31]

But what could not be foreseen was the immediate onset of hyperinflation brought on by the economic and energy crises that followed the 1973 Arab-Israeli War. By October 1975, Canada's consumer price index (CPI) had risen 11.4 percent in the previous year, and it was far from clear whether pensions would rise to meet these growing costs.[32] The Pension Act allowed for a rise in pension allotments every 1 January in accordance with the rise in the cost of living, as measured by the CPI. In 1972 veterans' pensions rose 3.6 percent, in 1973 4.5 percent, in 1974 6.7 percent, in 1975 10.1 percent, in 1976 11.3 percent, and in 1977 8.6 percent. The problem was that the pensions formerly had been based on the annual wage average of the composite group and these wages had risen faster than the cost of living. Veterans felt entitled to the percentage increase of the composite group's wages and not that of the CPI. By 1977, the veterans estimated that the composite group earned some $540 per annum more than the basic rate plus CPI increases. Further, if the CPI were to fall, veterans sought assurance from Ottawa that their pensions would remain unaffected.[33]

On 26 October 1977, notwithstanding strong public appeals by the NCVA and the Legion, Minister of Veterans Affairs Daniel Mac-Donald stated in the House of Commons that the government would maintain the current system. "I know this is a disappointment to veterans' organizations," he said, "but good Canadian citizens that they are, I am sure they will realize that this is a year of restraint and we will not be able to introduce improvements until our fiscal position improves."[34]

Nearly a year later a compromise was reached: effective 1 July 1978, the basic rate was to rise by $310, bringing it more or less to par with the average annual wage of the composite group. There also would be subsequent periodic increases. Mayne referred to this as the culmination of a "lengthy and intensive campaign" to which SAPA was heavily devoted.[35] Finally, in 1985, a year Mayne called "rewarding," federal authorities agreed that the annual upward pension adjustments would be made in accordance with whichever was greater: the rise in the CPI or the basic salary increases of the composite group.[36] In the grand scheme of things, this decade-long negotiation went the veterans' way rather quickly. Though counting only 185 members by February 1977, Mayne described SAPA as a "forceful, active, viable organization" that "plays a leading role in veterans' affairs through the instrument" of the NCVA. SAPA proudly, and justifiably, considered itself "one of Canada's leading veterans' organizations."[37]

In 1980 DVA launched the Aging Veterans' Program, renamed the Veterans' Independence Program in 1986, to help veterans and their families live happily and safely in their homes for as long as possible. The provisions called for assisting veterans with household tasks and outdoor maintenance that might have become onerous. There was no means test, and the program immediately proved a boon to SAPA members who needed help with snow removal, lawn cutting, homemaking, and home repairs.[38] In 1984 the *SAPA Chronicle* published an "open letter" to all members from the eighty-eight-year-old J. Harvey Lynes. "We owe it to our wives and ourselves to take advantage of this program," he wrote, "but, if you don't, you are endangering the program for your fellow veterans and for those wonderful girls who have grown older along with you." Echoing a concern of Dorward's, Lynes reminded SAPA members that if the program were not taken advantage of, it would "die on the vine" because VAC officials for the most part were "so much younger than we that they were not even born at the time of the Second World War."[39] Many

SAPA members naturally availed themselves of the Veterans' Independence Program.

SAPA Membership and Attrition

Debating Eligibility

In June 1971, Bill Mayne, who chaired SAPA's Membership Committee, reintroduced a hot topic of debate that would exercise SAPA for the next several years, as it had in the past. In reviewing DVA files of blind veterans, which the CNIB shared with SAPA to ascertain whether any cases should be reclassified as war blinded, Mayne's committee noted to the association's executive that there were sixteen to eighteen possible candidates for admission.[40] This would necessitate close inspection of each case to determine who, exactly, could be defined as war blinded – a matter which had bedevilled SAPA intermittently for years.

Finally, in March 1972, the Membership Committee recommended for admission to SAPA only three of the membership candidates who, while not conclusively war blinded by SAPA's definition, were in receipt of DVA-funded, CNIB-delivered aftercare services. This led to a "serious discussion" of the whole matter by the Executive Committee. If these men were admitted as members, they would also be eligible to attend the SAPA reunion that spring and be compensated for their travel from the already-stretched aftercare fund set aside for this purpose. While federal authorities considered each of them at least 80 percent disabled attributable to blindness (SAPA's strict disability minimum for admission), it was not always clear what portion of this blindness could be properly linked to wartime service. SAPA's eligibility requirements called for a veteran's vision disability to be not just at least 80 percent but be *all* war-related. According to SAPA, the government was proving increasingly "compassionate" in dealing with attributability, and the question before SAPA's leadership was whether the association should be more lenient as well. Further, since DVA was paying for the reunions, the department might favour having all blinded veterans, even non-SAPA members, be eligible to attend them and thus eligible for SAPA membership in all but name. The time might even come when all those receiving aftercare benefits would, perhaps should, automatically become SAPA members.[41] What if DVA insisted? What would a firm SAPA refusal portend for the association's aftercare and reunion funding in the future?

In 1972 about ninety aftercare-obtaining, non-SAPA members were registered with the CNIB, and Mayne felt that DVA might "quite properly" insist that they be allowed to attend SAPA reunions, though no Veterans Affairs officials raised the issue that year. He thought that SAPA might offer these veterans some lesser form of member- ship status, such as the long-discarded associate member category. The national executive's mood appeared to be softening in the matter, perhaps due to accelerating members' attrition. After much discussion at that June's AGM, the three aforementioned members were admitted by a strong majority vote of the ninety-one members present. Overall membership recently had fallen to 196, and the number of non-members on aftercare had risen to ninety-six. The pendulum was beginning to swing; a firm decision could not be delayed indefinitely.[42]

Harvey Lynes, SAPA's original president, was adamantly opposed to any lessening of SAPA's membership criteria, suggesting that the aftercare veterans be welcomed at social events only and not be admitted as active members of the association. Fred Woodcock, in a rare show of concurrence with Lynes, agreed wholeheartedly. The association's heavyweights having forcefully weighed in, SAPA's decision that June was to "resist any pressure from DVA to include non-member aftercare veterans in SAPA activities including reunions." Lynes's motion to this effect was overwhelmingly carried. In com- parison, St. Dunstan's policy was far more receptive. Blind veterans who had as little as 40 percent of their vision loss attributable to wartime service could benefit from St. Dunstan's services. Moreover, St. Dunstan's subsidized certain classes of veterans whose pension entitlements were not at the rate of 100 percent.[43] SAPA seemed a bit doctrinaire on the matter, but the war-blinded veterans sought to avoid "diluting" their association with blind veterans whose afflictions often had little to do with wartime service.

More than a year later, the gate-keeping Membership Committee recommended to the executive that seven aftercare veterans be admitted to SAPA. All were 80 percent or more disabled "with respect to loss of vision." Leonard J. Little, an elderly Windsor veteran, had had his blindness attributed to his exposure to mustard gas on the western front some fifty-six years previously. All were welcomed into the association.[44] In October 1974, SAPA admitted thirteen members based on the DVA files that the CNIB submitted to SAPA. Four of these seemed obvious, including one veteran who had lost an eye to a gunshot wound, eventually leading to optic atrophy in the other, and another First World War veteran who had suffered corneal scarring due to mustard gas.[45] In this way, SAPA's membership numbers remained reasonably stable, and even rose somewhat – an important consideration since the DVA-financed aftercare budget was based on the association's total membership. In other words, financial considerations might overcome the philosophical and constitutional hurdles to admitting blind veterans. Rejecting indefinitely the CNIB's aftercare cases whose disabilities were not fully war related could prove costly to SAPA. And admitting new members who would probably not have met SAPA's requirements decades earlier was a means of maintaining the association's membership at a level at which DVA aftercare funding would suffice to subsidize major social activities like reunions.

Mayne admitted that "the screening of blind veterans granted entitlement to aftercare services for eligibility to membership in SAPA is not an easy task."[46] For example, many aging veterans developed diabetes leading to blindness, and one major problem confronting SAPA's Membership Committee was whether diabetic retinopathy was an eligible cause for membership. Ross Purse, the managing director of the CNIB, a veteran of Hong Kong, and a war-blinded SAPA member, felt that the condition was often "likely the result of war service," since accidents or "traumatic conditions" could contribute to the onset of diabetes. But it was a hard sell with SAPA stalwarts. On the instigation of Lynes, citing the SAPA constitution's eligibility requirements for membership, the 1974 annual meeting delayed approving additional members suffering from diabetes. The whole matter needed more study. It was the same for the numerous veterans suffering from retinitis pigmentosa, a hereditary condition that could nevertheless be seriously aggravated by the arduous circumstances encountered while on military service.[47] For the time being, SAPA members would not admit these cases, either. SAPA remained first and foremost a proud *war-blinded* veterans' organization.

In October 1974, SAPA's membership stood at 197 members in Canada, of whom 35 were from the First World War and 162 from the Second. An additional 6 members resided in Britain and 3 in the United States, for a total of 206. Of those in Canada, Ontario accounted for 71, British Columbia 38, Quebec 34, Manitoba 20, the Atlantic provinces 18, Alberta 11, and Saskatchewan 5. Six of those living in Canada were British veterans.[48] In 1977 five new members were admitted, including one, Eugene Dickson, who had served overseas in the 28th Battalion during the First World War – fully six decades earlier. On the other hand, five First World War SAPA members, and three from the Second, died in the six months ending March 1978. By September of that year, membership had fallen to 177.[49] The writing was on the wall. If SAPA wished to remain vibrant, or even just viable, it would have to be more flexible and accommodating in accepting newcomers.

On 14 October 1978, "a new era" began when the AGM voted to reinstate the category of associate membership and extend it to seventy-five "officially" war-blinded veterans on aftercare whose cases did not warrant active membership in the association. Associate members had no voting privileges and could not hold office. Nevertheless, "for the first time in its history," stated an article in the association's newsletter, SAPA "represents all War Blinded Veterans whose loss of sight, in part or in whole, is the result of war service."[50] Within a year, Mayne's Membership Committee was recommending that all associate members receiving aftercare be upgraded to the status of active members. This was no time to stand on ceremony. In addition, a "stigma" had arisen over the associate member category because some members, especially First World War veterans, continued to view them as illegitimately labelled war blinded. Mayne, however, felt that without the new influx, SAPA would have difficulty remaining "strong and active." SAPA members ratified the appropriate constitutional change at the June 1980 AGM; henceforward, any veteran 80 percent or more visually disabled, eligible for aftercare, and whose disability was due in *some portion* (as opposed to wholly) to war service, could accede to active membership in SAPA.[51]

It was a decision whose time had come: between 1980 and 1983, nine First World War members and fourteen from the Second passed away. The twelve new active members in the period 1980-86 could only partially compensate for this growing rate of attrition.[52] By 1994, three or four members died about every quarter. The rate of members' deaths had accelerated dramatically: thirty-three passed on from 1991 to 1994.[53] At the same time the pool of blind veterans from which to draw new members was also in decline. By 2001, membership was down to sixty-six with an average age of eighty-two: twenty-two belonged to the Ontario branch, seven were in each of the Quebec, Alberta-Saskatchewan, BC Mainland, and Vancouver Island branches, six resided in the Maritimes, two in Manitoba, and eight lived outside of Canada.[54]

In November 1998, SAPA welcomed in membership the Honourable Barney Danson, former minister of national defence in the

1970s, who had lost an eye in Normandy in 1944. Danson was suffering from acute macular degeneration in his remaining eye. Deeply committed to veterans' causes, Danson at that time was heavily engaged in political and fundraising efforts to erect a new Canadian War Museum in Ottawa. SAPA henceforth counted one of Canada's highest-profile and influential veterans among its ranks; but SAPA had always counted among its own, either as active or honorary members, some of Canada's best-known veterans.[55]

Passing the Torch

Up to July 1997, 763 veterans had been active members of SAPA since 1922; a handful of others would join subsequently.[56] Those left were aging very rapidly and some First and Second World War veterans reminisced poignantly about a near-lifetime of blindness and the nature of their catastrophic injuries. As attested by their testimonials at reunions, participation in overseas VAC-sponsored battlefield pilgrimages, and heightened visibility at commemorative events, Canada's war-blinded veterans became nostalgic late in life.

The years were catching up to the veterans; it was a time for reflection on what had happened to them and on what they had endured. Harvey Lynes delivered a Remembrance Day speech at the University of British Columbia in 1976 in which he recalled visiting, with his wife, the bed-ridden and disabled veterans at Vancouver's Shaughnessy Hospital. One such Second World War veteran was Clarence Jimmy Bowes, described by Lynes thus: "He is a blinded soldier; in addition he is paralyzed from the neck down. He spends his days in a battery-powered wheel-chair and until recently spent many hours in the craft shop of the hospital weaving place mats; at that time he had the use of the little finger and thumb on one hand. His demonstration of patience and courage plus tremendous fortitude placed him in a category by himself. His work was so excellent that it won for him recognition in the Canadian National Exhibition in Toronto [and] the Pacific National Exhibition."[57] Lynes was heavily involved in SAPA's affairs until the very end. Just before his death he submitted a lengthy personal note for inclusion in the *SAPA Chronicle,* "from Your Founding President." "As our numbers grow smaller," wrote Lynes, "it is imperative that we draw closer together, never for a moment forgetting our common bond – that of soldiers who suffered total or partial loss of vision in the service of our country." He went on, "We are a unique group who have met life head-on and I am proud of us. We have looked beyond our own disability to help the children and, in so doing, our Scholarship Program was born and has flourished. We have come a long way since the very lean days following W.W.I. Canada now has one of the finest war pensions in the world."[58] Lynes passed away in Arizona on 31 July 1985 at the age of eighty-nine.

Similarly, Lloyd Tomczak delivered a moving address following the June 1977 SAPA reunion banquet. He stated, "On April 14, 1945, I was shot between the eyes by an enemy sniper. Through the grace of God and the skill of a Canadian Army neurosurgeon, I survived that wound." His brother had already been killed while serving with the RCAF. Tomczak went on:

> No one denies that we have all had our moments of anguish, both physical and mental. But are we not so much better off than those whom we left behind? Would they not cheerfully and gladly put up with a disability just to be here with us and have the right to live in this wonderful country? We all know that this is so ... Every day of our lives let us show our appreciation by living each day to the best of our ability in unselfish service to our country, our community, and our fellow man. If we can pass this on to our children, and in turn to their children, we can help to ensure that the memory of their sacrifice will be held sacred for all time to come.[59]

Kay Christie, a highly celebrated nursing sister with the Royal Canadian Army Medical Corps during the Second World War, was one of Canada's most cherished veterans. By 1986 she was the past president of the NCVA, a leading member of the Nursing Sisters' Association, and a SAPA honorary member. She was enormously respected by the war blinded, having been captured at Hong Kong with so many of them. She had valiantly ministered to the men during that seventeen-day campaign and in captivity thereafter, and the SAPA Hong Kong veterans in particular treated her as one of their own, although she was fully sighted. Christie attended the 1986 SAPA reunion and wrote Dorward in May of that year, "It was great to see the SAPA members and their wives again but, as always, time is too short ... It is always fun to join in these little post-dinner gatherings but it was interesting to watch one after another of us begin to wilt, in spite of our heroic attempts to carry on. As the years pass, this has become so evident within every group."[60] The veterans' communities were heading into their collective twilight, and SAPA was no different.

In 1982 Fred Woodcock recalled forty years later that at the time of his wounding at Dieppe "my only communication with the world was one tap on the forehead for no, two taps for yes." "When I was lying alone in the [POW] camp, I wondered how I was going to make a living. I thought a lot about what I could do in blindness, and it worried me." But the willing hands he found among the war blinded, to which he joined his own in assisting others, helped him recover his morale and pursue an outstanding career with the CNIB. Looking back on it all, Woodcock, who received the Order of Canada in 1985, recalled of the war blinded, "We are a select group, a unique family, and we have enjoyed a long friendship."[61] Woodcock died on 31 July 1998. Bill Mayne described him as "kind, generous, persuasive and tough when necessary." To the war-blinded veterans he was "advocate, counsellor, father confessor, comforter, disciplinarian and, always, a friend."[62] The heart and soul of the organization was vanishing.

Other war-blinded veterans were retiring after decades of employment with the CNIB, heralding, to some extent, an altered relationship between the two groups. The disproportionately strong
presence of war-blinded veterans, normally also members of SAPA's
executive, among the CNIB management team had always ensured a
sympathetic disposition within the institute toward the problems of
the war blinded. No better example existed than that of Edwin Baker.
But in the late 1970s that overlap began to diminish. Mervyn Carlton,
who had served with the Winnipeg Grenadiers at Hong Kong, retired
from the CNIB in 1977 after twenty-two years of service, though he
stayed on as SAPA's president. Chris Davino, a former SAPA president,
retired in November 1977 after thirty-two years with the CNIB as a
cafeteria manager. He had been blinded in December 1943 at Ortona,
Italy, while serving with the Royal Canadian Regiment.[63]

Bill Mayne, the energetic CNIB aftercare officer and SAPA fixture
for three decades, retired from the CNIB effective 1 January 1979.
Ross Purse, the institute's managing director, himself a war-blinded
veteran, noted that Mayne had "served us with distinction whenever
and wherever possible." This was an understatement. Mayne ranked
with Baker and Woodcock as among the most influential and respected of war-blinded veterans, not only within the SAPA-CNIB
family but also among DVA officials, the NCVA, the Legion, and the
host of other community and service groups to which he belonged
or with which he dealt. In 1977, on the advice of St. Dunstan's, he
had received the Queen's Jubilee Medal for his advocacy on behalf of
blinded veterans.[64] Ending his employment with the CNIB only meant
that he would devote more time to his beloved SAPA – which he did
with devotion for three decades more. Fernand Huneault, president
of SAPA's Quebec branch, warmly noted that "at one time or another
[Mayne] has helped every one of us with grace and efficiency and
without hesitation ... he may be assured of our lasting gratitude."[65]
Mayne was inducted into the Order of Canada in 1982. SAPA president
Anne Michielin wrote of him in 1995, "Over the years one member of

our Association has given so much in every possible way that it would be impossible to thank him fully. His contribution to the spirit and strength of our Association has been monumental."[66]

Aftercare Changes and Challenges

In 1974 the CNIB launched a full-scale review of its operations and services for blind Canadians. Chaired by Cyril Greenland, the "Unmet Needs of Blind Canadians" inquiry was published in 1976 under the title *Vision Canada*. Anne Michielin, a Second World War veteran and active SAPA member from Alberta, was on the study's steering committee. While she was not specifically representing war-blinded veterans, her participation was a nod to their importance as a specific, organized category of blind Canadians. Bill Mayne organized the presentation of a SAPA brief to Greenland and strongly encouraged individual members and the branches to submit comments on their needs and expectations from the government and the CNIB, especially insofar as aftercare services were concerned.[67]

The results of Mayne's internal polling provide a useful snapshot of the successes, disappointments, and lifestyles of Canada's war-blinded veterans. The comments received painted a generally satisfactory picture, although quite a number of veterans felt that the CNIB aftercare officer and district CNIB officials should be in closer contact with the war blinded and more frequently convey pension and entitlement information, about which the CNIB officials appeared uncertain. The study also showed that numbers of civilian blind found that the more basic services the CNIB provided them compared poorly to the generous government pensions and other funding for the war-blinded veterans. Saskatchewan war-blinded veteran Gordon Buchanan's daughter wrote Mayne on her father's behalf that "we have found that the general reaction is that we are War Blinded and are already being well looked after. Also it is often apparent that as War Blinded do get compensation to enable them to have a better standard of living, there is a great deal of jealousy and sometimes the War Blinded are the recipients of rather nasty remarks."[68] The sad irony of this situation was that a founding principle of SAPA was to promote social policies in aid of Canada's civilian blind, and the organization had successfully collaborated with the wider efforts of the CNIB, for which many leading SAPA members worked diligently for years.

But many respondents, especially if they resided in Ontario, close to SAPA and CNIB national headquarters in Toronto, were highly favourable to the system as it existed. "We, a blind husband and sighted wife, feel all our needs have been well taken care of by CNIB and [DVA]," wrote the Bakers from Ontario. They went on:

> At the outset, we received help and encouragement – we had felt that loss of remaining sight was "the end," but soon found this wasn't so at all. We were helped to carry on with our ordinary way of life as far as possible, and to develop new interests as well. Our morale was boosted tremendously and helps were provided such as a white cane and how to walk with it; Braille watch and clock and kitchen timer (to find one can still brew the tea for the exact number of minutes is in itself a real lift to the morale.)
>
> The most painstaking instruction given in carpentry, and special tools for use by feel instead of sight opened up a new world of interest and enjoyment in a skill which was undiscovered until blindness came. This new hobby has given endless pleasure in its feeling of achievement and in providing some unique and handsome furniture for our home. (I feel very proud of my husband when people comment on our furniture and I can tell them he made it.)[69]

Although the CNIB's delivery of services and information occasionally might have been found wanting, it was far from clear whether DVA or any other authority could dispense aftercare more effectively.

Nevertheless, major changes to the structure of the aftercare program were in the offing.

CNIB aftercare services, for which the federal government paid, became available to a veteran immediately following the Canadian Pension Commission's acceptance of his or her eligibility. Aftercare included adjustment-to-blindness training such as Braille, typing, mobility, crafts, social adjustment counselling, vocational training, and the provision, on a permanent loan basis, of personal equipment including a Braille watch, a Braille writer and supplies, a portable typewriter and supplies, a talking clock, a talking-book tape player, maintenance on all the foregoing, Braille or large-print playing cards and cribbage boards, and a white cane. In 1987 VAC agreed to re-imburse war-blinded veterans up to one hundred dollars for pre-scription sunglasses. By 1990 VAC's "Approved List of Equipment" for blinded pensioners also included contact lenses, dog guides, read/write machines, and other benefits. The following year VAC authorized, in some cases, the Xerox/Kurzweil personal reader, a device employing a synthetic voice system capable of reading aloud typeset or typewritten material placed on its scanner.[70]

As of 1 April 1974, the DVA aftercare rate paid to the CNIB was $416 per annum per blinded veteran. Since the services rendered by the CNIB came from local budgets, the CNIB assigned $188 of this amount to the veteran's CNIB district office for the provision of after-care services, $23 went directly to the accumulating reunion fund, and the balance of $205 reverted to the CNIB's Aftercare Department to pay for a variety of other expenses. These included all of SAPA's expenses, including branch, executive, and annual general meetings, and $25 per veteran sent to the SAPA branches.[71] The money went fast. DVA's funding was conditional on CNIB district social or case workers visiting each war-blinded member annually. DVA reimbursed the institute separately for the retraining needs of newly identified cases.[72]

DVA aftercare monies were specifically earmarked to fund SAPA's social activities, especially the reunions. By 1978, $32 from the annual amount per veteran was deposited into the reunion fund, an increase of 40 percent in under five years. In that same year, Mayne's aftercare office wound up with a surplus of $7,410, which he used to bolster the reunion fund. In the past, up to $11,000 in a single year had been transferred this way. But Mayne realized that, with SAPA's dwindling numbers, DVA's funding formula would "have to be re-negotiated and based on actual Aftercare Services Department costs, as opposed to an average services cost formula multiplied by the number of war blinded veterans."[73] Such a renegotiation was not long in coming, and it did not necessarily advantage the veterans.

Although the aftercare services were dispensed through the CNIB district offices, Bill Mayne, protective of the program on behalf of the war-blinded, noted that "the jurisdiction over and the responsibility for the co-ordination of the total program lies with the [CNIB's] National Aftercare Officer," who liaised with DVA, the CPC, and other veterans' associations.[74] Mayne retired at the end of 1978 after eight years as the CNIB aftercare officer and SAPA executive secretary. In his report to the 1978 AGM, he wrote, "It is not absolutely essential, but it is advantageous that the incumbent War Blinded Aftercare Officer be the Executive Secretary of SAPA. The Aftercare Officer provides the time, the secretarial staff, and the information and records necessary to facilitate the work of the Executive Secretary. The work of the Aftercare Officer with respect to entitlement, pensions and allowances complements and supports the work of the Executive Secretary in the same areas."[75] To maintain the long tradition of this dual role, pioneered by Edwin Baker decades earlier, the CNIB would have to find a successor in SAPA's ranks.

In 1979 David Dorward replaced Mayne in both capacities. Mayne described Dorward as "a determined man, not easily swayed from his judgment."[76] This was an understatement although, as events transpired, both organizations would need a man of Dorward's strength of character to negotiate with DVA. Dorward also took over the editorship of the association's nascent newsletter, the *SAPA Chronicle*, with a concomitant change in tone from Mayne's friendly and fraternal voice to one much more businesslike.

The days of the CNIB Aftercare Office, and the decades-long agreement between DVA and CNIB for its funding, were numbered. In 1981 DVA began preparing to end funding for the CNIB Aftercare Office with DVA counsellors slated to assume the direct responsibility for delivering those aftercare services formerly provided by CNIB staff in the districts. These DVA counsellors would henceforth arrange for the provision of aids and appliances for war-blinded veterans and do the administrative work associated with the war blinded's travel. This change meant, in effect, that war-blinded and blind veterans would no longer have a direct service-related link to the CNIB, whose more than six decades of specialized experience Ottawa was willing to forego. The institutional ties that bound the CNIB to DVA, and which saw a high-ranking SAPA member embedded as an important member of the CNIB management team in a tight, triangular relationship, were loosening. This in turn weakened the ties between SAPA and the CNIB. A new contract between DVA and CNIB for very heavily scaled-back services was slated to come into effect 1 April 1983.

David Dorward was skeptical that DVA could deliver an ambitious aftercare program, and he was extremely angry over the imposed changes. SAPA insisted that, as a minimum, DVA counsellors should advise, visit, and assist the war-blinded, as had the CNIB aftercare officers and local staff. The association also sought the full continuation of DVA treatment benefits: the ongoing provision and repair of aids and appliances, the provision of Braille and typing supplies, travel benefits, training, and up-to-date information concerning pensions and allowances.[77] The department had its own reasons for implementing the new relationship structure. For example, the Aging Veterans Program, which offered household assistance and other benefits to older veterans and was increasingly important to SAPA members, was handled through DVA's regional offices, without expensive intermediaries. It seemed sensible, therefore, for DVA officials to deal in the same manner with the relatively small number of war-blinded and blind veterans as well.[78] But had the department bitten off more than it could chew in the interests of cost rationalization? Canada was undergoing a severe economic downturn at the time, openly referred to as a recession. All government departments had suffered spending cuts and, according to a pessimistic Dorward, DVA's ongoing support for the war blinded might shortly "dry up." Times were tough, SAPA membership was in decline, and adjustments would have to be made.[79] But the restructuring of aftercare service responsibility and delivery proved to be an error of judgment.

Beginning in April 1983, SAPA members' requests for equipment, repairs, or other aftercare needs had to be submitted directly to DVA, a process loudly decried by Dorward at the June 1983 SAPA AGM in Saint John, New Brunswick. As he put it to the members, "Remember, the squeaky wheel gets the grease, ask for what you need and do not take 'no' for an answer." According to the SAPA minute book, "David stated that it was only by persistence that DVA would realize that the war-blinded group was militant and not to be toyed with." Dorward, ostensibly the CNIB aftercare officer, sounded frustrated and desperate, perhaps like a man who had been stripped of a primary responsibility.[80] In his report to the 1983 AGM, he noted that "during the three years since the last reunion, much of my time has been spent negotiating with DVA concerning the changes they wished to make in their program." Although the department had 235 counsellors on staff, Dorward dismissively opined that "many of the counsellors are young, they do not understand disabled veterans, and they go by the 'book' as they know it. More important, they do not believe [that] there is a need for the aftercare office anymore." He had travelled to DVA offices across Canada "endeavouring to educate them in the needs and demands of the war blinded" and hoped they would be "ready to learn."[81] Dorward's fiery tone no doubt made his visits memorable for DVA staff. To what extent this advanced SAPA members' causes remained to be seen.

DVA authorities had informed Dorward, he told SAPA members, that "their staffs of counsellors and experts could serve the war blinded without assistance" from the CNIB following Dorward's planned retirement in October 1984 (he eventually stayed on several years longer). The theory was nice, mused Dorward at the 1983 AGM, but without a war-blinded advocate, SAPA members would henceforth be at the "mercy and whim of the counsellors and [DVA] district directors, who are made up of good, bad, and indifferent people."[82] Dorward also noted that the costs of the 1983 reunion had exhausted SAPA's reunion fund. DVA money to support SAPA's veterans' advocacy (counselling and information dissemination) had dropped precipitously to only $90 per member per annum. (This amount later rose to $100 in 1989 and $150 in 1997, with the understanding that such monies could be used for reunions, though no additional funding would be available for that purpose.)[83] But the war-blinded veterans assembled in St. John were upset at the prospect and "after considerable heated discussion ... the meeting resolved that a demand be made on DVA for funds for another reunion in 1986."[84] It would be a very hard sell.

In 1984, in response to an outcry from SAPA and the CNIB, DVA (since 1984 referred to for non-statutory purposes as Veterans Affairs Canada, or VAC) agreed to maintain some limited funding to the institute to maintain beyond that October the position of director of war blinded and blind veterans services (the new title for the aftercare officer) to serve an advocacy role, only, on behalf of the war blinded. This minor concession was insufficient for Dorward. In March of that year, he wrote to G.J. Parker, VAC's director of benefits, that the department had always sought the advice of the aftercare officer on all matters pertaining to the war blinded, including related spending of government funds. Dorward felt that VAC's restrictions on the role of the director of war blinded and blind veterans services constituted an "unfeeling limitation" and a "dereliction of duty" and that the department's proposed sum of $30,000 annually fell far short of his minimum desire of $75,000 to maintain the director's office and salary. He also wanted $25,000 to fund aftercare library services and $19,500 per year for other SAPA activities, all of which he eventually received, though the office costs were pegged at $73,500. Subsequently, VAC allotted the sum of $61,400, payable directly to SAPA, for office expenses and per capita grants to branches, barely sufficient for the purpose.[85] VAC had shown caution and understanding, despite the department's obvious desire to eventually end such funding. In the same letter to Parker, Dorward vehemently rejected apparent DVA insinuations that his robust stance reflected a personal interest in the continuation of a fully funded office and that he hoped to hang on in that capacity beyond October. Dorward, turning sixty-five, admitted that he had, indeed, requested a two-year employment extension from the CNIB pending a satisfactory outcome of the financial negotiations.[86] But who could champion the war-blinded and blind veterans' causes as effectively as the pugnacious incumbent office holder?

Dorward was almost certainly the most consistently combative of SAPA's executive secretaries; subtle he was not. In August 1984, he visited the DVA offices in Charlottetown and met with "a large delegation" of officials. He succeeded in buying some time: government funding for the office and limited functions of the CNIB director of war blinded and blind veterans services would continue until 30 September 1985, an extension of one year. Thereafter, the department would administer all aspects of the aftercare program directly. In anticipation of this change, Dorward, as Fred Woodcock had done in the 1960s, wrote for the use of SAPA members and VAC staff the comprehensive "SAPA Guide to Veterans Affairs Canada Benefits and Services." In addition, VAC also promised to investigate means of supporting the proposed 1986 SAPA reunion in Montreal. The new funding arrangement would come into force 1 January 1986 directly between SAPA and VAC, without the CNIB as intermediary, enabling SAPA's office functions and branch activities to be maintained at a minimal level.[87]

While the relationship between SAPA and the institute remained close, they were divided for the first time. By the same token, for the first time since it was founded in 1918, the CNIB was no longer an official purveyor of services to the war blinded on behalf of the federal government. One immediate effect of this change was that SAPA took on a greater role in the lives of its members and assumed the direct responsibility of informing them about changes to pensions and entitlements. The *SAPA Chronicle* was a good tool. The role of SAPA branch managers became more immediate, since they now served as points of contact with VAC on behalf of their members' needs.[88] SAPA was decentralizing, to some extent, and in recognition of this, all branch managers were made members of the SAPA executive. In 1985, Bill Mayne, then SAPA's president, thought that cohesive branch organizations would strengthen SAPA's hand in its dealings with VAC regional offices. He also believed that it was the national executive's duty to "ensure that VAC is ever conscious of the SAPA presence." This issue had occupied the association since its founding, but, Mayne wrote, matters were "now a bit more serious."[89]

Another significant change occurred in 1986 when the independent-minded Dorward relocated the SAPA office to his home in Napanee, east of Toronto. SAPA had split from the CNIB not just administratively but physically. The move stirred controversy among SAPA members, especially the Toronto-based executive. Fred Woodcock registered severe disappointment, believing it was silly for Dorward to distance himself from the infrastructure and the case files of the blind veterans and also to be less in touch with issues affecting the civilian blind. How, he asked, could SAPA fulfill its primary constitutional mandate "to further the interests of the blind in Canada, the war blinded in particular?"[90] Mayne recalled in later years that Dorward, for all his outstanding qualities as a champion of the war blinded, sometimes appeared to "resent" the institute's nearly inevitable "controlling" influence over SAPA. In any event, Mayne noted that the "bulk of the work" of the association was undertaken by the executive director (prior to 1986 known as the executive secretary), as had generally always been the case, since the incumbent had for decades doubled as the CNIB aftercare officer.[91] It might have mattered less where he was located.

According to Mayne, Dorward "never relaxed the pressure and never backed away" and "by means of lengthy and frustrating negotiations concluded [the 1986] agreement with VAC with respect to financial support for SAPA operations." The level of financial support was "much-reduced," but at least the principle and precedent of direct government subsidy for SAPA's reunions and administration had been established. Moreover, VAC formally recognized SAPA as an advocate for Canada's war-blinded veterans. Although Dorward felt that the operating grant covering the year beginning 1 April 1986 was below SAPA's anticipated needs, he was pleased with VAC's "generous" donation for the 1986 reunion.[92]

At the AGM held during the Montreal reunion, Mayne outlined SAPA's stark financial environment as well as its unchanged obligations to its membership. In addition to carrying out the routine operations of the association, Mayne noted SAPA's mandate to "provide opportunities for the members to meet and fraternize; to provide an advocacy service; to represent the interests of the Association within NCVA and with other veterans' associations; and, in general, to promote the well-being of the members and the Association."[93] This tall order was accomplished with the continuing support of CNIB and VAC. For example, in 1986 the CNIB assumed the financial burden of printing and distributing the *SAPA Chronicle*, a fraternal gesture that Dorward described as a welcome "boon" to SAPA's meagre finances.[94]

Beginning 1 July 1986, however, and following numerous evidently justifiable SAPA complaints that VAC regional offices were not
effectively delivering aftercare services or informing the war-blinded
of their pension entitlements, the department once again contracted
with CNIB, on a yearly fee-for-service basis, to manage the war blinded and blind veterans' aftercare needs. The extra burden on staff,
complaints from veterans, and the difficulty of the task for non-
blinded administrators contributed to VAC's change of heart. Dorward,
ever persistent, continued to push for SAPA to have a consultative
role in the manner in which CNIB delivered VAC's aftercare. At this
time VAC also allocated a rather paltry $25,000 in sustaining funds
for SAPA's veterans' advocacy role on a year-to-year contractual basis,
but with no provisions for SAPA "socialization or reunions." As a result,
the SAPA national office could send virtually nothing to the branches
for their activities. These were among SAPA's leanest times – a "financial crisis" in Mayne's words.[95] But as Mayne himself recalled some
years later, SAPA was the only veterans' group that obtained public
funding for its social activities.[96]

The SAPA-CNIB Bond Renewed

David Dorward and Bill Mayne both realized that SAPA's future could
best be assured by the appointment of a younger, dynamic executive director who could reintegrate SAPA into the CNIB fold and yet
maintain the war-blinded's interests as paramount. They sought
nothing less than the fully funded re-establishment of the traditional
dual position of CNIB aftercare officer and SAPA executive director. In
1987 they broached the topic with Euclid Herie, the managing director of the CNIB. After some lengthy and at times frustrating negotiations between SAPA, the CNIB, and VAC, mainly about budgets,
staffing, and the status of aftercare provisions within the CNIB organization, this restructuring took place in 1989. The minister, George

Hees, had been personally involved in these discussions.[97] In June 1989, a clearly relieved and thankful Mayne wrote Herie, "Well Euclid, our plans regarding the renewal of the former close relationship of our two organizations are now becoming a reality. It has been a long and tedious effort, but the benefits to be gained are worth the efforts expended ... We are back where we belong."

This transition reflected the simple reality that the war-blinded veterans were fewer in number, aging, and in real need of their friends at the CNIB. The institute would provide services while SAPA would concentrate on veterans' advocacy and its members' social needs. Effective 1 July 1989, the new SAPA executive director was CNIB aftercare director Jim Sanders, forty-two, totally blind but not a war-blinded veteran. Sanders was born with severe vision impairment and had been a registered CNIB client since he was two months old. He had held a number of prominent executive positions with the CNIB and proven himself to be capable, independent minded, and utterly devoted to improving conditions for Canada's blind population. At the time of his appointment, he also took on the challenging Ottawa-based role of managing the CNIB's national and international programs.[98] This frequently involved dealing with government officials, something his SAPA duties would also oblige him to do. Even though he was not a veteran, his appointment became key to a renewal of close and formal ties between the CNIB and SAPA.

The institutional break had been neither total nor lengthy, but the organizations' tight bonds would never again be loosened. "CNIB has agreed that Jim, with our consent, may assume the duties of Executive Director of our Association at no cost to the Association. This is a benefit of no small degree," wrote Mayne in the *SAPA Chronicle*. "Our former close relationship with CNIB is now restored." The CNIB became SAPA's sponsor, assuming the costs of the association's administrative needs, which totalled some $55,000 in 1990 and a whopping $76,000 the following year. To offset this, VAC funded the

CNIB approximately $60,000. This did not affect VAC funding SAPA directly approximately $15,000-17,000 per annum for its advocacy role on behalf of the war blinded.[99]

Sanders, a "damned good man," according to Mayne,[100] established an office on McLeod Street in Ottawa funded by the CNIB and, in a smooth transition in June 1989, the SAPA headquarters moved there from Dorward's residence in Napanee. Sanders also became the editor of the *SAPA Chronicle*, and Krysia Pazdzior its associate editor. She eventually became associate executive director of SAPA and Sanders's key administrative support.[101] Mayne stepped down after six eventful years as president (Dorward referred to him as SAPA's "pillar of strength") and Dorward became the president with Anne Michielin as vice-president. Dorward felt that 1989 was a "watershed" year in the history of SAPA and admitted upon assuming the association's presidency that henceforward Jim Sanders "is the man who will be doing most of the work for the Association." The non-veteran Sanders's appointment had necessitated a change in SAPA's constitution, and such a groundbreaking decision did cause serious "personal introspection, debate, and caution" among some members. But, as Dorward put it, "It set the course for the future" for the aging blinded veterans and their cherished association. According to Bill Mayne, SAPA members preferred a blind non-veteran to a sighted veteran, and only one unnamed voice was raised in protest at Sanders's appointment.

By the end of the year, Dorward was delighted to inform SAPA members that "it has been evident that the senior volunteers and management of CNIB unconditionally support the efforts and goals of our Association." It had been quite a turnaround in five years. Jim Sanders was made an honorary member of SAPA and Dorward heaped praise on him in the *SAPA Chronicle* and also on Pazdzior "for her tireless efforts on our behalf." He accurately described her as exhibiting "care and concern for people." Her position was funded by a VAC subsidy to the CNIB and she would stay in an administrative capacity with SAPA for the next two decades, liaising with members, handling the daily office needs of the association, and, ultimately, seeing SAPA through nearly to its close.[102]

Bill Mayne was enthusiastic about the historic appointment of a non-veteran to direct the affairs of SAPA. Mayne and the SAPA executive easily could "coach" Sanders along. In December 1988, Mayne and Dorward met with him to explain the SAPA-CNIB-VAC relationship, which Mayne described without exaggeration as "a complex and complicated set-up." In addition to being SAPA's executive director, Sanders's CNIB duties also included those of the former aftercare officer since, in 1989, the institute "reactivated" its War Blinded and Blinded Veterans Service Program. The CNIB had extended the war-blinded veterans a welcome and necessary lifeline. Perhaps more importantly, as Mayne put it, the "CNIB better appreciates our needs than does Veterans Affairs."[103] This statement implies that the war blinded, in later life, needed to be treated as blind Canadians more than as Canadian veterans. More than ever integrated into the "family" of Canada's blind population, they were home.

The Last Reunions

In 1970 the CNIB war-blinded aftercare budget included reunion expenses of $15 annually per blind veteran receiving aftercare services. As noted above, this amount doubled by the end of the decade. The money accumulated until it was needed to pay for the next reunion. Members' reunion transportation and accommodation were covered and, occasionally, additional financing was obtained through bequests to the CNIB with, according to Bill Mayne, "instructions [for it] to be used for the benefit of war-blinded veterans."[104] Mayne felt that the reunions were of incalculable morale benefit to the veterans and that every dollar expended was well spent. Helping SAPA helped the veterans directly, as he wrote to a DVA official: "The Association provides a sense of identity together with a voice whereby members

may criticize and help shape the Aftercare program and make representation to and negotiate with ... the Government of Canada with
respect to veterans' pensions and benefits." He viewed participation
at a reunion as a right, not a benefit, insisting that "it is an integral
part of the Aftercare program. To my knowledge it has been recognized as such by the CNIB, by the war-blinded veterans, by the former
Department of Soldiers' Civil Re-establishment, and the present
Department of Veterans Affairs."[105]

The 19-23 June 1972 reunion held in Toronto celebrated
SAPA's fiftieth anniversary. The Canadian Legion Concert Band led
the medal-bedecked war-blinded veterans, wearing their SAPA
berets and carrying white canes, during their traditional parade to
the cenotaph, a reprise of the emotive 1957 event. They marched in
ranks of three with an air cadet in the centre to act as escort. The city
and the armed forces offered strong support to the veterans, who
engaged in the usual visits and luncheons, though perhaps fewer
than in previous years, and all in Toronto. Some hundred members
and their escorts attended, and the gathering cost $35,000, roughly
the amount that had accumulated in the reunion fund since the last
gathering in 1965.[106]

Bill Mayne, a Manitoba native, might have influenced the
selection of Winnipeg as the site of the 20-24 June 1977 reunion. By
1975, the reunion account had accumulated more than $49,000 in
DVA funding, and SAPA's Manitoba branch, the event organizer,
reckoned that the amount would rise to more than $62,000 by the
reunion date, enough to cover members' anticipated travel and accommodation expenses, even given the hyperinflationary times. The
Manitoba offices of the CNIB and local DVA officials assisted with the
arrangements.[107]

As usual, the reunion succeeded. There were CNIB demonstrations of the sonic guide and laser beam cane, a tour of the mint, a
reception at Government House with the lieutenant governor, the
Honourable F.L. Jobin, and a dinner cruise on the Red River. Mayor

Stephen Juba proclaimed 19-24 June 1977 "The Sir Arthur Pearson Association of War Blinded Week" and urged all citizens to offer SAPA "a warm welcome during this their first reunion in Winnipeg." As had become customary, the reunion attracted a mix of corporate, institutional, civic, and benevolent group sponsorships and participation. For example, in addition to acknowledging the CNIB, DVA, and the Department of National Defence, SAPA warmly thanked the city of Winnipeg, the Royal Canadian Legion, Simpsons-Sears, Burns Foods, Ltd., Saan Stores, the United Grain Growers, the Bank of Montreal, Great West Life, the St. John Ambulance, and Manitoba Hydro, among others.[108]

The reunions were no longer as large as previously, but they still mattered enormously to the veterans. The following year, SAPA's president, Mervyn Carlton, wrote that "in our travels in Quebec and Ontario, we have met many of our SAPA members and there is one thing that they wish to discuss and that is the wonderful time they had at the reunion in Winnipeg. They not only enjoyed the friendships of their comrades of so many years, but also the friendliness of the Winnipeg people ... even after 14 and a half months, our members are still talking about that great reunion."[109]

The 16-20 June 1980 reunion was held at the Park Plaza Hotel in Toronto. For the first time, all associate members, numbering more than one hundred (i.e., DVA-sanctioned aftercare recipients who were not war-blinded veterans according to SAPA's strict interpretation) were invited to attend, and the reunion proved an excellent opportunity for the old hands to "get acquainted" with the newcomers. This experience no doubt helped SAPA members vote at that reunion's AGM to elevate the associate members to full active membership in the association. The reunion fund was able to cover transportation costs and half the hotel costs for any active or associate member resident in Canada, but, for the first time, could not afford to pay for their escorts.[110] The associate members proved expensive at this reunion, but additional DVA funds based on their active membership would help enormously in the future. By the time of the 26-29 June 1983 gathering in St. John, New Brunswick, the reunion fund had grown to more than $105,000 and SAPA was able to pay all transportation and hotel costs for the 180 attendees, including escorts.[111]

The 5-9 May 1986 reunion at the downtown Holiday Inn in Montreal was organized by a Quebec branch committee chaired by Beatrice Sigouin, the energetic wife of member Robert Sigouin. Once again, SAPA was able to pay hotel accommodation, transportation, luncheons, and entertainments for the sixty-nine members present and their escorts. The Quebec branch picked up a lot of tabs, including a lunch at the Longue Pointe army depot and another at the armoury of the Fusiliers Mont-Royal. The queen, Prime Minister Brian Mulroney, and Premier Robert Bourassa all sent their best wishes.[112]

As Winnipeg had done in 1977, the city of Montreal declared that week War Blinded Week. Mayne stated, "There are no words ... with which to adequately describe our recent Montreal Reunion." He raved about the "gracious welcome, the warm hospitality and the from-the-heart friendliness of our Quebec Members and the people of Montreal ... I am sure all of us left Montreal with warm and pleasant feelings in our hearts for these wonderful people." David Dorward stated categorically that the Montreal reunion was "a happy, inspiring and restorative occasion which we will long remember as a high point in our membership in the SAPA family."[113] Certainly the Quebec branch, ably and faithfully assisted by standout volunteers like Stu Christie and VAC's Bob Baker, had long been an enthusiastic bunch, meeting frequently in convivial surroundings and maintaining an active schedule of social activities. Their vibrant, positive outlooks had animated the entire reunion.

Writing in the *Chronicle* following the Montreal reunion, Mayne recalled a conversation that he had had with Edwin Baker and Bill Dies at the home of Lady Kemp during the 1957 reunion in Toronto. Dies had remarked that the war-blinded veterans attending were

being "restrengthened" and "tuned up," that the gathering was building their confidence and, as such, constituted a form of therapy for
the members. Being blind was not an easy life. "We meet, we compare notes, and we gain strength and confidence from our peers,"
Mayne wrote. But this privilege would subsequently come at a hefty
financial price as a result of SAPA's diminishing membership.

The reunion costs rapidly outstripped the shrinking overall
amount allotted by VAC, which by the early 1990s was exhibiting less
and less interest in funding the veterans' social activities, especially
since no other veterans' group was similarly favoured. The long-
standing personal contacts and friendships that had animated SAPA-
DVA relations in previous decades no longer existed, replaced by a
more strictly business relationship. The demonstrably important
psychological benefits to members provided by the reunions would
not induce even sufficient, never mind greater, VAC funding. According to Mayne, the previous understanding with respect to funding
was not a written obligation, and in 1986 he announced that "Veterans Affairs has stated that there will be no further financing of
National reunions." SAPA members were disappointed, some outraged, but Mayne insisted that "we must be prepared to raise money
by other means and we must be prepared to make personal contributions. Some members are already doing that." After all, "we are
older and we are not as tough as we were. Aging, and our disabilities,
tend to isolate us from general society, and our need for the association of our peers becomes greater and more essential."[114]

A special reunion fund was established at the AGM held in
Montreal for the next gathering, to be held in London, Ontario, in
1989; the executive deemed Toronto, the original choice, too expensive. But as late as March 1989, members had contributed only
$23,000 against the estimated costs of $90,000. In the end, the CNIB
and VAC assisted financially. The reunion was held 15-19 May, partly
at Wolseley Barracks, Canadian Forces Base London. Colonel W.J.

Aitchison, the base commander, wrote a word of welcome for the reunion program in which he stated, "It is an honour for all of us to host you who sacrificed so much that we might continue to enjoy our Canadian way of life." As usual, military authorities offered the disabled veterans their fullest co-operation.[115]

The 8-10 May 1992 reunion in Ottawa marked the seventieth anniversary of SAPA's founding. VAC's acting deputy minister, J.D. Nicholson, wrote SAPA that "economic restraint" prevented his department from helping fund the reunion that year, notwithstanding the "very special" services SAPA provided to the war blinded.[116] This appears to have been the only reunion without specific VAC funding. About seventy members attended, including five from the First World War and a contingent of about twenty who had lost their sight while in Japanese captivity. As usual, the CNIB hosted various displays of technology to assist the blind, and VAC offered seminars on veterans' benefits and programs. On Sunday, 10 May, the SAPA members gathered wearing their SAPA berets, medals, and white canes for an especially poignant 11 a.m. ceremony at the National War Memorial, followed by a Remembrance luncheon at the Chateau Laurier and a reception at the Army Officers' Mess. Colin Beaumont-Edmonds, president of St. Dunstan's, attended and "participated in all reunion activities" while Senator Jack Marshall, a tireless worker on behalf of veterans, was the guest of honour at the banquet. Cliff Chadderton, SAPA's honorary president and an occasional personal financial contributor to SAPA, was present, as were General John de Chastelain, chief of the defence staff, and Euclid Herie, president and CEO of the CNIB. The reunion succeeded again, helped by a long list of volunteers and donors, including local businesses, a very receptive media, local military units, and fifteen individual Legion branches, most from Quebec.[117]

Well-known *Ottawa Citizen* columnist Dave Brown, highly sympathetic to veterans and their causes, attended the reunion and felt that being in the presence of these war-blinded veterans proved "an odd mix of horror and humour" as the SAPA members recounted their tales in self-deprecating tones. For example, Brown described Jimmy Hunter, living in Winnipeg, but originally from Brooklyn, New York, as having a "fascinating face. It looks as if it was welded together by somebody with a good sense of humour. A large portion of the upper lip is missing, giving him a permanent wry smile." A veteran of Montreal's famed Royal Highland Regiment of Canada (the Black Watch), which he joined in 1940, Hunter, a sergeant, was severely injured by a German anti-tank shell explosion in the Netherlands in October 1944. "I was knocked down, but not knocked out," recalled Hunter. "I got up right away. At first I thought I was blind because there was blood in my eyes. I wiped with my hands and discovered I didn't have eyes." Despite his grade 5 education, Canada's Veterans Charter allowed him to attend university. While living at Baker Hall, he earned a master's degree in social work from the University of Toronto. A self-taught hobbyist furniture maker, Hunter still used power tools, including chainsaws, well into his seventies. By remarkable, though ghastly, coincidence, Warren Scott, from British Columbia, was also blinded in the same engagement, his last sight being the horrible wounding of Sergeant Hunter. As an eighteen-year-old raw replacement helping fill the Black Watch's depleted ranks, this was Scott's first action; his face needed major reconstruction surgery. Nearly five decades later, both men attended the Ottawa reunion and both wore their disfigurement with stoicism. As Brown noted, deeply impressed, "SAPA members continue, by example, to show young blind persons they can live relatively normal lives." Brown enjoyed being in their company. "These men laugh a lot," he wrote with a mixture of surprise and awe. One blind veteran, using a microphone, reminded the group that they were to board buses outside the front door. He then quipped, "if anybody knows where that is." Everyone roared with laughter.[118] The scenes Brown described epitomized the spirit that had animated SAPA over seven decades and demonstrated the reunions' importance to this remarkable group of Canadian veterans.

Bill Mayne reflected on the idea that SAPA members commonly hailed every reunion as the "best ever." These views implied "that the enjoyment and satisfaction members were deriving from participating in reunion activities was growing with every reunion. We were SAPA members assembled in the company of our peers to renew old friendships, to chat and compare notes, to review the well-being of our Association and the members and ... to generally enjoy ourselves."[119] But everyone was getting older with each passing three-year reunion period, and Mayne's views might have reflected the pleasant reality that SAPA was still vibrant and relevant, even as attrition decreased membership with alarming regularity.

Due to an anticipated lack of funds, the 1-4 June 1995 reunion in Gimli, Manitoba, was planned to be "less traditional and formal" than previous affairs. Government cutbacks and financial restraint meant that government subsidies would be difficult to obtain. Yet, as with most reunions (save 1992), some last-minute VAC funding materialized. Minister of Veterans Affairs Lawrence MacAuley agreed to contribute ten thousand dollars. Despite the fact that it was "not our policy to provide funding to veterans' organizations' reunions," MacAuley decided to "make an exception in this case."[120] This gesture demonstrated the department's commitment to the war blinded; SAPA and VAC had a unique relationship. Although sponsors were solicited for dinners and special activities, participants would be expected to pay for their own travel and accommodations.[121] Perhaps partly owing to this, the 1995 reunion was somewhat restrained, with just seventy-two attendees, including members and escorts. Activities included the veterans' parade and a wreath-laying ceremony at the Gimli cenotaph. The Air Command band from Winnipeg supplied the music at the banquet.[122]

Following this gathering, Mayne penned an article for the *SAPA Chronicle* entitled "The Best Reunion Ever." "I believe," he wrote, "that each of us left the reunion feeling a bit stronger, a bit more content and better able to face life and what it may offer." He noted wistfully that there occurred a "first in the history of our Association. Liquor was returned to the liquor store. Alas, the ravages of age."[123] The next reunions would be more frequent, every two years, despite the personal expenses involved.

SAPA's seventy-fifth anniversary reunion was held in Aurora, Ontario, 21-26 May 1997, with the local Royal Canadian Legion branch offering enormous assistance in planning the event. The reunion fund swelled with members' contributions, indicating a remarkable desire to be in each other's company. SAPA treasurer John Chatwell felt their generosity was "tremendous."[124] Two years later Edmonton hosted the reunion from 6 to 10 May 1999. Everyone had to pay their own way again, and it was a low-key affair. The co-operation of the Legion's Kingsway Branch 175 proved essential, and VAC, CNIB, the Edmonton Transit System, the city of Edmonton, and local businesses donated money or assistance.[125] The Legion had proven a good friend to the war blinded over the years.

In 2000 Anne Michielin, SAPA's Alberta-based president since 1995 and the first woman to hold this position, noted that recent reunions had seen "a considerable drop in donations and a large increase in expenses." VAC's financial support had dried up and the smaller number of attendees made group discounts difficult to obtain. The CNIB helped as much as it could, but members' donations remained essential. The time had come to plan the last gathering.[126]

Fittingly, Bill Mayne organized the eighteenth and final formal SAPA reunion held in Belleville, Ontario, 3-7 May 2001. Concerning costs, he noted that the previous four reunions had averaged $35,000. However, the average amount of dwindling VAC aftercare funding to the CNIB and members' donations had been only $20,000. Accordingly, the ever-generous CNIB had been disbursing some $15,000 on average to cover costs. This could no longer be sustained. And so Mayne made a strong appeal to remaining members to donate to help make the final reunion a memorable one.[127]

With Cliff Chadderton and VAC deputy minister Larry Murray serving as guests of honour at the closing banquet at CFB Trenton, the Belleville reunion acted as a closing ceremony for nearly eighty years of SAPA members' service and comradeship. It was not a wake, but there was an unmistakable sadness underpinning the event. Michielin referred to it as "emotionally packed."[128] SAPA members had endured so much, and now they would probably only infrequently be in each other's company, perhaps in sparsely attended branch meetings, which themselves were occurring less often as members passed away. Mayne, the driving force behind the reunions for half a century, wrote that "this reunion will recognize and honour everyone's hard work and their contributions to the great history of the Association, to the benefit of all veterans, and to the future of blind and visually impaired Canadian children." Perhaps to mark the significance of the event, not only were Chadderton and Murray present, but so, too, were St. Dunstan's Colin Beaumont-Edmonds, Fran Cutler, the CNIB's national chair, and Euclid Herie, its president.[129]

In an important symbolic touch linking past and present, veteran with civilian, and members' self-help with their overwhelming desire to help others, one of the 2001 scholarship winners, Jennifer Challenger, was a special guest at the reunion luncheon. Bill Mayne presented her with her cheque. It was an important moment: even as the association had begun its unavoidable winding down, Challenger's presence crystallized the war-blinded veterans' legacy to other blind Canadians. There were other poignant moments as the aging veterans danced "for the first time in years" at a reunion to such well-chosen songs as "Sentimental Journey" and "We'll Meet Again." Those present were keenly aware that their gathering would be the last in SAPA's proud history.[130]

There were only sixty-seven SAPA members left, and just sixteen were present at the reunion, sixty people in all including escorts and family members. They were well looked after by the military community in the Belleville-Trenton area. They visited the RCAF Memorial Museum in Trenton after solemnly celebrating Battle of the Atlantic Sunday and the anniversary of VE Day. As ever, VAC, CNIB, military authorities, and the Legion did all they could to help. Deputy Minister Larry Murray closed his remarks with the simple observation, "You really are a very special organization which has made a huge difference for many deserving people."[131] This is what the war-blinded veterans had known for decades and it is how they wished to be remembered.

SAPA's "Crowning Glory"

As Canada's war-blinded veterans aged, their interest in the notion of a lasting SAPA legacy began to take shape. The scholarship fund had always fulfilled one of SAPA's mandates, which was to assist all blinded Canadians overcome their handicaps and start out on career paths leading to rewarding lives. The evolution of the fund into a successful legacy project advanced incrementally and took two decades to achieve. But the results proved startling and allowed the name of the association to be linked in perpetuity to its goal of helping the young civilian blind.

Until 1971 SAPA awarded fifty-dollar scholarships to nominated high-school students attending each of Canada's five schools for the blind, with twenty-five-dollar awards made to students at lower levels at each school. One fifty-dollar bursary was awarded annually to a student in Ceylon. The fund was self-sustaining from interest earnings. But that year members of the SAPA Scholarship Committee felt that the time had come to extend eligibility to the hundreds of blind Canadian children and youths attending sighted schools. Their courage and travails, too, were important to recognize and reward. For example, in Ontario alone, 452 blind students attended sighted schools, 31 more were enrolled in preschool programs, and 138 studied in blinded schools. There were 59 attending sighted schools in Manitoba, 101 in British Columbia plus 76 at Vancouver's Jericho Hill School for the Blind, 67 in Alberta, 76 in Saskatchewan, and 53 in the Atlantic provinces. (SAPA could not immediately obtain statistics for Quebec.) Mervyn Carlton, who chaired the Scholarship Committee, hoped that, in the future, financial need would be considered alongside scholastic achievement in selecting scholarship recipients. Accordingly, SAPA's national executive decided to establish a new fifty-dollar scholarship to be awarded in each of the eight CNIB geographic divisions to students in regular schools, and that financial need be the primary factor followed by scholarly merit. Local CNIB officials would select candidates, and high school students in grade 10 or above would have priority.[132]

The veterans' money made a difference. Upon winning his fifty-dollar award, high school student Tom Cisar wrote Carlton of his intention of becoming a radio broadcaster. "Therefore, a good microphone and amplifier would be useful for developing a good, strong, healthy voice," he wrote. The CNIB's Ontario division recommended, on the basis of need, grade 11 student Melvin Bellefontaine, attending a sighted school, who had lost his sight to retinoblastoma, and whose eyes were enucleated. His father had recently died, his mother was ill, and an older brother had predeceased him at the age of eight. The only source of family income was a small pension received by his mother. Bellefontaine received a fifty-dollar scholarship from SAPA.[133]

In 1974 Ginette Chouinard and Guylaine Pimparé, both grade 7 students attending Montreal's Institut Nazareth, jointly sent SAPA a letter in which they wrote, "This generous gesture inspires us to pursue our studies with even more courage and perseverance and your gift makes our task as blind students easier." That year's scholarship to a student in Sri Lanka (the name by which Ceylon became known in 1971) went to B.A. Jothihamy, totally blind since the age of three as a result of malnutrition. Her mother was dead and her father too old and feeble to work; her family was destitute. She attended high school, taking courses in weaving. The fifty dollars would get her started with a weaving machine and the necessary yarn.[134] One 1975 recipient from Oakland, Ontario, William Linington, wrote of his bursary that "thinking about future education, this gift makes me more excited and enthusiastic ... it will give [me] a good morale boost." His mother, Joan Linington, wrote her own note: "As William's mother, I would just like to add my thanks and appreciation for the gift. It really has given him encouragement. He works hard at school and we are very proud of him."[135]

These sorts of letters encouraged SAPA members and friends of the association to donate to the fund. In 1971 long-time CNIB volunteer and honorary SAPA vice-president Elsie Gorman passed away, bequeathing a hefty two thousand dollars to the scholarship fund. Despite the difficult economic climate, with spiralling inflation and high unemployment, members' contributions remained stable: in 1975 seventy-five donated, representing a good percentage of SAPA members. The popularity of the fund was confirmed the next year when ninety-eight donors contributed nearly three thousand dollars. Half of this money was in the form of "gifts in memory of deceased persons" – an important means of financing the fund.[136] In 1977 the fund stood at nearly twenty-four thousand dollars. SAPA founder Harvey Lynes wrote, "Each June since 1966, my wife and I have spent a pleasant afternoon on Awards Day at the Jericho Hill School for the Blind ... The children and some parents gathered in one room eagerly awaiting the announcement of the awards ... pupils would come up smiling to receive the award amid enthusiastic applause from the other students ... After a chat with the winner ... we'd come away confident that our awards were serving a useful purpose."[137]

In December 1977, Lynes and his wife organized a dinner at the Grosvenor Hotel in Vancouver for six local SAPA scholarship winners from previous years as well as for members of the SAPA BC

Mainland branch. A local VAC representative also attended. The recipients recalled how they had spent their scholarship money (e.g.,
tape recorders, typewriters, Braille writers) and spoke of what they
were doing at that time. Two worked in darkrooms, and one had
graduated from the University of British Columbia with a BA.[138] This
sort of follow-up demonstrated the degree to which the scholarships
had become important to SAPA members and how, as they aged,
they increasingly sought to boost those similarly afflicted with blindness. As J.J. Doucet, chairman of the Scholarship Committee, wrote
in 1976, "We feel that in these days of inflation, cutbacks and job in-
security, it is more important than ever for blind children to be educated to their full limits in order to live and compete in a sighted
world."[139]

      But changes to tax regulations soon imposed a pressing need
for more donations and stimulated serious discussion about the
fund's future. Effective 1 January 1977, changes to Canada's Income
Tax Act obliged charitable organizations to disburse, that calendar
year, at least 50 percent of their contributions received in 1976 for
which income-tax receipts were issued. The disbursement level was
to rise to 80 percent by 1980. To comply, SAPA needed to significantly increase the value of its scholarships. In 1977, the association had
to award at least $2,200. Accordingly, the revised amounts and num-
ber of scholarships rose to fourteen worth $150 and four worth $75,
for a total of $2,400.[140] Their number and their value continued to rise
regularly in the coming years. But if donations decreased as SAPA's
membership declined, disbursements would eventually exceed income and either the fund would begin to deplete or the program
would have to be scaled back – both undesirable outcomes. For example, the $3,200 disbursed in scholarships in 1978 was $500 less
than the amount donated that year.[141] A plan had to be put in place
if the fund was to survive beyond the life of the association itself
and bloom into the lasting legacy that was becoming increasingly
attractive to SAPA members. Lynes referred to the scholarships as

"the life blood of our organization" and the "star in our crown." Members responded generously and by the early 1980s, despite the large sum of $9,400 awarded in 1983, for example, donations were increasing apace and the fund remained healthy. In 1980, at the instigation of Bill Mayne, the Association's national executive formally renamed the fund the F.J.L Woodcock-SAPA Scholarship Fund, in honour of the long-serving SAPA executive secretary who had initiated the project in the first place.[142]

In 1985 a total of forty-eight scholarships were allotted worth $10,800. The Scholarship Committee reported that "the fact that a blind student is selected for a scholarship has tremendous psychological impact. The student gains in self worth and is encouraged to pursue higher education, despite obstacles ... We, who have been through the mill, can appreciate how an education opens many doors for the blind." One young blind Montrealer, Steve Bell, on receiving a scholarship, wrote, "I must admit [that] I did not know about your association of war blinded. I am so pleased to learn that there is someone who cares about us. I will always remember you."[143] This was the sort of intergenerational, veteran-civilian bond that had always motivated SAPA members to give. For the first time, and indicative of the growing importance of this undertaking, SAPA's executive agreed to receive donations from other than members of SAPA and their immediate entourage.

In 1987 Bill Mayne, who chaired the Scholarship Committee, felt that the fund was at a crossroads and that an important decision was needed respecting its future course. One option was to allow the fund to deplete and die, along with SAPA, since it was "assumed that there will be no more wars and SAPA will cease to exist." The alternative was to create a separate self-sustaining foundation to maintain the fund beyond the lifespans of SAPA members and of the organization. At the end of 1986, the fund was valued at more than $48,000. If a foundation was to be created, Mayne estimated that the capital fund needed a minimum of $150,000 to maintain the same value of the scholarships then being awarded using interest earnings as a means of perpetual financing. Accordingly, donations to the fund would have to increase dramatically over the coming ten years, averaging more than $11,000 per annum – double the then-prevailing rate.[144] It seemed daunting.

In 1989 SAPA established a committee under the vigorous leadership of Beatrice Sigouin to investigate the future of the SAPA bursary program. That year Sigouin's committee recommended that the scholarship fund be converted into "a permanent foundation." According to her report, "This recommendation is based upon the fact that SAPA has directly and indirectly influenced the lives of blind Canadians for almost seven decades. A permanent foundation could continue to keep the torch alive and touch the lives of people in the decades to come."[145] Before such a foundation could come into being, money had to be found, and lots of it. Still, the idea was accepted with great enthusiasm by SAPA members, relatively few in number by this point, and, in the first three months of 1990, $15,000 was collected for the proposed foundation.[146] The capable Sigouin organized the ambitious fundraising drive, which solicited donations from SAPA members, their families and friends, and even further afield. In stimulating people to give, Sigouin mentioned SAPA's undeniably "rich heritage" and noted proudly that a scholarship foundation long outliving the association would prove to be SAPA's "crowning glory."[147]

By the summer of 1990, John Chatwell, SAPA's national treasurer, announced that the fundraising results were "gratifying" and that $35,000 had been invested in guaranteed investment certificates (GICs) paying a whopping 13 percent interest. The goal was to have the proposed foundation self-sustaining by 1995.[148] At the end of 1990, SAPA's president, David Dorward, was delighted to note that fundraising had "surpassed even the most optimistic projections." The embryonic fund already had $50,000 invested in GICs. Donors came from all quarters, including several bequests. SAPA's Quebec branch had also been successful in soliciting the financial support of numerous Royal Canadian Legion and Lions Club branches across the province. By the end of 1991, more than eighty Legion branches and more than forty Lions Club chapters nationwide had made donations, some of them substantial.[149] The foundation was well on pace to realization.

At this point, this legacy project took over as the focus and driving goal of SAPA. It provided aging members with a sense of permanence. Perhaps in creating and contributing to the planned foundation, their war service, painful rehabilitation process, and proven ability to carry on would not only be remembered to posterity, but would actually prove of some tangible benefit to others. Beatrice Sigouin, herself a donor to the fund, asked appropriately, "What better heritage to leave behind than education for blind children?"[150]

On 10 May 1992, at the Delta Hotel in Ottawa, SAPA's executive met to transform the existing SAPA scholarship program into a formal, self-sustaining foundation separate from the association itself. The F.J.L. Woodcock/SAPA Scholarship Foundation came into being. This meeting effectively reorganized SAPA into two distinct functional entities: a war-blinded veterans' social and advocacy group and a charitable foundation that would survive the former and perpetuate its name.[151] The foundation was established three years ahead of schedule with a capital fund exceeding $150,000. The greatest single donation, nearly $31,000, had come from the Order of the Eastern Star upon that organization's dissolution. Remaining monies in the scholarship fund were to be transferred by 1994.[152]

The new foundation was guided by a board of directors chaired by SAPA's national president and composed of Beatrice Sigouin, who would also serve as its chief fundraiser and public relations officer, John Chatwell, and SAPA executive director Jim Sanders. Mayne listed the objectives of the foundation as providing scholarships to blind students, perpetuating the memory of Sir Arthur Pearson and of SAPA, and paying tribute to "an outstanding member" of the association,

Fred Woodcock. Echoing the pride so many of Canada's war-blinded veterans felt, Mayne said of SAPA and the foundation, "We are few in number and yet we have achieved something which is very important. We have reached out to help other disabled persons. That is a fine illustration of the maturity of our association and our members."[153]

In 1993, the foundation awarded thirty-two scholarships totalling nearly $10,000. The winners were selected through a nomination process co-ordinated by local schools, regional CNIB officials, and SAPA branch presidents. Alexandre Dubois, of Blainville, Quebec, who was preparing to enter a community college, received $400. He wrote, "I find it very encouraging that an organization such as yours thinks of helping young students to continue their studies, especially handicapped students who cannot always obtain a summer job or even a part-time job. The sad thing is that these students can succeed as well as other students, given the right opportunities."[154] The returned veterans had had their opportunities, had made the most of them, and sought to return the favour to those who would follow.

On 18 May 1993, David Dorward and John Chatwell signed a letter of agreement with the CNIB whereby, upon the inevitable dissolution of SAPA, the institute agreed to manage the foundation in accordance with SAPA's by-laws and intentions. For SAPA, "perpetuity" was drawing closer. The CNIB agreed that the foundation's investments would "always be conservative in nature, never speculative." A 1999 addendum stipulated that the CNIB would not charge for the management of the foundation. Although the foundation boasted a capital amount of $165,000, falling interest rates dictated a renewed appeal for money to maintain the existing bursaries. The new target for sustainability was set at $200,000, and this objective was met in 1994. Among the donors to the foundation were Anne Michielin, Bill Mayne, and John Chatwell, all leading by example.[155]

By 1998 SAPA's associate executive director, Krysia Pazdzior, had sent invitations for applications to more than 100 interested groups, organizations, and individuals nationwide (a number rising to 150 by

2002). This included all CNIB offices across Canada, boards of education, and schools for the blind. The foundation had built up a strong reputation, and about 100 inquiries and applications were received at the SAPA national office. Winners continued to be highly appreciative. In 1999 Jesse Pozzo of Calgary wrote, "I am writing to thank you for the scholarship I received. I used it to upgrade my computer speech package which reads me exactly what I type as I type it. I also use it to surf the internet. When I finish grade twelve, I hope to go to university and learn how to design computer software which will make computers easier for blind people to use. Your organization is wonderful."[156]

In the meantime, the foundation's capital base remained solid. The deaths of David Dorward in June and John Chatwell in July 1997 prompted a flood of donations to the foundation in their memory. Dozens of members, widows, and friends donated tens of thousands of dollars. The same occurred following Fred Woodcock's death in July 1998.[157] In 2000 one Mrs. Roberts, daughter of deceased SAPA member Robert Marsh, established a $100,000 endowment fund under the auspices of the foundation, the interest from which would be used annually for scholarships. By the spring of that year the foundation had amassed capital of more than $300,000. In 2003, in a gesture typical of the association's members and their guiding philosophy, Neil Hamilton, blinded on active service with the RCAF, donated the $3,000 proceeds from his autobiography, *Wings of Courage*, to the foundation.[158]

The SAPA executive proposed to the members attending the 1999 reunion a draft constitution for the foundation to legally separate it from SAPA. The association and the foundation conducted different types of activities, and Revenue Canada insisted on two separate financial reports and constitutions. Moreover, given that SAPA was winding down while the foundation would continue, the latter needed to be firmly established on independent ground. This development also symbolized the final crossroads in SAPA's eighty-year history. The foundation's name would remain the same in perpetuity; all investments would remain highly conservative in nature; the fund's capital would always remain intact; and, if ever circumstances dictated the dissolution of the fund's capital base, all of it would be disbursed in the form of scholarships.[159] This would protect what the war blinded had achieved in their lifetimes and ensure that those for whom the monies had originally been generated obtained the fruits of the veterans' labours. SAPA members could now prepare to stand down.

Conclusion

In 1994 and 1995, alarming news reports appeared regarding the development in the United States, China, and elsewhere of high-technology military laser beams, or "dazzlers," adapted for simple mounting on rifles or vehicles and designed specifically to damage eyesight or permanently blind their victims. Some lasers were designed to transmit megawatts of energy in wavelengths that would irreparably damage the retinal system at ranges up to three kilometres. The International Committee of the Red Cross (ICRC) issued a 1994 information backgrounder on the subject expressing the committee's belief that "blinding is much more debilitating than most battlefield" wounds and that it considered the weapons to "cause superfluous injuries and ... suffering" and to be a "particularly cruel and unacceptable form of warfare." "The silence and invisibility of laser beams," the report continued, "which can blind in a millionth of a second, means that victims will not usually know of an attack until damage to the eye has already occurred." In late 1994, the ICRC and a group of thirteen nations, led by Sweden, sought to prohibit the use of these weapons through an amendment to the United Nations' 1980 Inhumane Weapons Convention.[1] This protocol was adopted in October 1995 and successfully banned, in the words of one report, the "use and transfer of weapons designed to cause permanent blindness to the naked eye." However, lasers could still be employed against an enemy's optical and range-finding devices, potentially causing blindness for their operators.[2]

The Sir Arthur Pearson Association of War Blinded (SAPA), of course, immediately announced its vehement opposition to such weapons.[3] For war-blinded veterans who had endured decades of personal and social challenges in overcoming their affliction, the notion that blindness would be purposefully inflicted upon soldiers seemed too horrible to contemplate. Those responsible for developing such weapons surely had no knowledge of what being blind meant to individuals and their families. The second generation of Canadian war blinded did not want to witness the creation of a third.

In 1998 Canada ratified the United Nations protocol prohibiting the use of laser weapons intended to cause blindness. Yet, a decade later, the introduction of seemingly less harmful lasers – intended to "flash" or temporarily disable an enemy's vision – reopened the debate about the actual harm that these weapons might cause. Beginning in 2006, some American troops fighting in Iraq were issued these less dangerous lasers, attached to their rifles, to disable potentially hostile civilians approaching their positions.[4] In 2007, Canada, too, earmarked ten million dollars for the acquisition of similar technology for use by its forces serving in Afghanistan. The idea apparently was to limit the number of Afghan civilian casualties by having troops temporarily blind potential assailants rather than shooting them outright. The controversial purchase was put in abeyance, however, pending further study and to ensure that Canada was abiding by its international agreements. Meetings had earlier been held between Canadian military and diplomatic representatives and the ICRC to discuss the testing of the weapons, or "warning devices," as some industry sources preferred to call them.[5]

In February 2009, Canadian military authorities once again expressed interest in acquiring the weapons for use in Afghanistan. But officials acknowledged that, if used improperly, or at too close a range, permanent eye damage could result.[6] Despite the Canadian government's nearly century-long commitment to care for its war-blinded veterans, to honour and privilege the Sir Arthur Pearson Association of War Blinded, as it had done for no other veterans' group, and to encourage greater social integration for its blind citizens, the nation might resort to the use of potentially blinding weapons in combat. If Canadian troops were ever to intentionally blind an enemy or a presumed enemy, it would prove a difficult pill for Canada's blind and war-blinded population to swallow. Will the painful lessons of sightlessness be lost on others? Time will tell.

In 1995 Anne Michielin, from Drumheller, Alberta, was elected SAPA's president, the first woman and first westerner to occupy that position. She went on to head SAPA for the next fifteen years (and was still president at the time of writing), taking on the unwelcome task of winding down the organization. Michielin had served with the 16th Company, Canadian Women's Army Corps, in Calgary during the war, and her macular degeneration was due to the wartime aggravation of an existing visual impairment. Upon her election, Michielin stated, "I'm proud and ... filled with humility that these men have chosen me as their national leader."[7] Nevertheless, being based in Alberta had some disadvantages, as she fully recognized, and Jim Sanders, SAPA's executive director, remained heavily involved in the day-to-day operations of the association and seeing to the needs of its members.

In 1997 Sanders moved from Ottawa to the Canadian National Institute for the Blind headquarters in Toronto to assume his duties as the CNIB's vice-president of client services and international relations. He advanced quickly through a string of increasingly senior positions to become the institute's president and CEO in November 2001.[8] His accession to the CNIB's top position was no doubt beneficial to SAPA as the association prepared to draw down with dignity. Sanders carried on as SAPA's executive director – a position he took enormously seriously and to which he often referred with evident pride. He also regularly reconfirmed the CNIB's commitment to underwrite SAPA's administrative expenses, including maintaining its national office in Ottawa and paying the salary of Krysia Pazdzior, who worked part-time as SAPA's associate executive director.[9]

Pazdzior, too, cared deeply about the SAPA members on whose behalf she worked. Regularly in contact with the war-blinded veterans, their families, and an ever-growing number of widows, she served for nearly two decades as the institutional linchpin linking the CNIB to SAPA and dealing with a host of outside authorities including Veterans Affairs Canada and the National Council of Veteran Associations. In 1995 she was made an honorary member of SAPA, a proud moment for her. Pazdzior noted that her affiliation with the war blinded constituted "the most rewarding work I have done." What struck her in particular was that the SAPA veterans "believe that the sacrifices they made and the suffering they experienced were nothing in relation to the resulting benefits to humanity."[10] The blinded soldier quoted in Chapter 1 who remarked in 1918 that "if as the result of our blindness the public will become interested in and have sympathy for the civilian blind, the affliction will have been well worth while"[11] also displayed the same sense of selflessness. While perhaps not every SAPA member would have fully agreed with that unnamed veteran, he spoke for the *spirit* of the war blinded in a sentiment that prevailed nearly nine decades on.

At the turn of the century, SAPA's declining membership obliged several of the association's branches to cease operations. Attrition made it more difficult for members to meet, let alone reach a quorum. In 1995 the Ottawa-Hull branch voted to dissolve given its tiny membership. By 1999, the Quebec, Manitoba, and Vancouver Island branches had been thinned to the bone, the last-named having but two members "able to get around and participate." The Manitoba branch, with only three members left, wound up its activities and transferred its assets to the final 2001 reunion fund. Anne Michielin's 2001 message to members in the *SAPA Chronicle* reminded the remaining veterans that although there could no longer be any reunions, there were still a couple of branches in operation, the *Chronicle* to keep members abreast of each other's activities, Paz-dzior's cheerfully rendered assistance, and, as always, the CNIB to support their needs. By the middle of 2005, there were only forty-three members nationwide, most in Ontario and some in rapidly de-clining health. At the time of writing, fewer than thirty remained.[12]

In March 2005, Michielin wrote to the organization's Executive Committee, "Our SAPA is currently facing an unavoidable and most regrettable circumstance: the demise of the Association as an active entity." The average age of members was eighty-three. The Maritime branch, too, had by this time become inactive with the remainder soon to follow, if not formally then in practice. "It is a sad time which we knew was inevitable," wrote Michielin. "However, the years of fellowship, sharing, support and great times were what kept us strong and united for so long. It is the spirit of SAPA and of every Canadian, and will live on in history and stand many in good stead in the future." Few, if any, war blinded would have disagreed. In addition to seizing the reins of their destinies and carving out productive lives from the discouraging lot consigned them through the fortunes of war, the veterans needed their experiences to serve as models for what the blind could achieve. They wanted to be remembered, and to *matter*.

The 9 May 1999 addendum to the 1993 letter of agreement be-tween SAPA and the CNIB regarding the scholarship foundation also established that, in the event of a future conflict involving Canadians resulting in large-scale eye casualties, SAPA would be "reactivated." Michielin's 23 March 2005 "Plan of Action" noted that the time had arrived to ensure that the members continued to obtain all the care to which they were entitled, that the association's name be main-tained and its cherished archives safeguarded, and that these be transferred into the custody of the CNIB, which henceforth would become the formal reporting authority for SAPA's affairs. The associa-tion would shortly formally move to dormant status. An "agreement

to transfer" document, outlining the process of orderly and respectful cession of SAPA operations to the CNIB was signed in April 2005.
Fittingly, perhaps, Bill Mayne signed on behalf of Michielin, putting
"his" association to rest. An "agreement of trust" was signed at the
same time whereby the CNIB solemnly agreed to execute SAPA's
wishes following the demise of the last member – an event that will
double as SAPA's final act. Michielin described this process as "extremely difficult." But, finding opportunity in crisis, she also remarked
on the importance of ensuring that "we continue to benefit from
being a member of SAPA as long as we are of this world, and that
we will be well remembered in perpetuity through our Scholarship
Foundation."[13]

SAPA's final years as a vibrant and influential veterans' organization were fulfilling ones in the sense that these war-blinded men and
women could look back with enormous pride at their personal successes and also with deeply rooted satisfaction that their lives, their
experiences, their hardships, and their association itself had helped
forge ties among all veterans, between veterans' groups and government, between blinded veterans and blinded civilians, and among
the war blinded of all nations. Their wartime sacrifices and highly
successful postwar rehabilitation and social reintegration had gone
a long way in obliging sighted Canadians to revise their stigmatized
views of the nation's blind. It was an enduring legacy as important as
any other.

This was also a time for recognition and honours. In 2002 Veterans Affairs Canada established the Minister's Commendation Award
"to recognize individuals who have made an outstanding contribution
to the care and well-being of veterans or who have been instrumental in raising awareness of veterans' contributions, sacrifices and
achievements." At two ceremonies held 7 November 2002 and 31
March 2003, fifty-two veterans or individuals supporting veterans
and their memories received the commendation. Among them was
Bill Mayne, for a lifetime of service to blind, disabled, and, in fact, all

veterans.[14] In addition, former CNIB president and fellow war-blinded Hong Kong veteran Ross Purse, Jim Sanders, Beatrice Sigouin, and Anne Michielin received the Queen's Golden Jubilee Medal. They were among thirteen SAPA members, honorary members, and widows to receive this award, a significant proportion of the association's remaining membership and "extended family."[15]

In 2004 Jim Sanders was named a member of the Order of Canada, like SAPA giants Edwin Baker, Fred Woodcock, and Bill Mayne before him. A "driving force" behind CNIB and SAPA, according to the *Chronicle,* Sanders "has studied the history of war-blinded veterans and understands their needs completely. He has worked tirelessly to protect veterans' rights and benefits. He has made a long-term commitment ... to the continuity of the Scholarship Foundation for decades to come."[16] Sanders was a blind civilian carrying forward SAPA's needs with a dedication and pride until then found only within the community of the war blinded itself. He symbolized the passing of the torch between war veteran and civilian and between active operations and legacies. But, in the end, they were *all* veterans of a sort, veterans of blindness, joined together in a lifetime relationship of mutual understanding.

In the 1990s St. Dunstan's undertook the massive task of compiling a list of all Commonwealth St. Dunstan's-trained, war-blinded veterans deceased up to 30 June 1995. The resulting Books of Remembrance were intended one each for Britain, Canada, Australia, New Zealand, and South Africa. The British volume contained 4,410 names, Australia's 668, New Zealand's 243, and South Africa's 116. The Canadian volume, delayed until 2000 because of St. Dunstan's and SAPA's difficulties in gaining access to government-controlled personal and service-related information on deceased veterans, contained 354 names. This number is less than half the total number of Canadian war blinded since, as a result of the existence of the CNIB, many of the Second World War casualties did not attend St. Dunstan's and neither did the vast majority of delayed or attributable

Canadian cases of war blindness stemming from both world wars. Compiling the Canadian volume was a major research effort lasting five years and involving SAPA, the CNIB, VAC, and the National Archives of Canada.[17] It was also a means of honouring the veterans as soldiers, and not only blinded ones, and of listing them as a group, reinforcing the notion of their lifetime of solidarity.

In addition to the honours and commemorative efforts others bestowed upon the war blinded, they, too, had thanks to give. In probably the most moving document the author discovered while researching this study, Bill Mayne recorded with emotion and sincerity his appreciation for the rich legacy of co-operation and unflinching devotion that individuals and institutions had provided the war blinded over the decades. Without this help, their challenges would have been difficult to bear, perhaps too difficult for many. In a five-page piece entitled "We Are Most Grateful," published in the 1992 SAPA reunion program, Mayne expressed his and fellow members' thanks, and neatly conveyed, sometimes between the lines, decades of mixed experiences to which all war blinded could relate. He also highlighted the manner in which Canada's war-blinded veterans from both world wars endured and, ultimately, beat blindness.

In offering thanks to the CNIB, he wrote that "the relationship between SAPA and the CNIB is one of co-operation, mutual respect, and friendship. We are most grateful to the CNIB for its involvement in our lives." He also paid tribute to Veterans Affairs Canada employees who "supported the veterans ... and their submissions," even providing "guidance in the framing of them. Without their assistance, our negotiations would have been more difficult and our successes fewer." Many other institutions and friends helped along the way. Mayne singled out the St. John Ambulance and Red Cross Voluntary Aid Detachment workers (VADs), and instructors at the rehabilitation facilities "who made that extra effort to ensure that we were properly trained." Similarly, he remembered with profound admiration "the women of the Pearson Hall and Baker Hall house committees who worked so diligently to make our training days so pleasant." These people had altered the lives of hundreds of war-blinded veterans since the closing days of the First World War. Hundreds of volunteers, from various organizations or serving as individuals, also greatly facilitated SAPA's many social and branch activities over the years. These were "true and sincere friends."

But Mayne reserved his most heartfelt tribute to "our ladies." "We come now to that very special group: our mothers, sisters, and wives, especially our wives. Theirs was the greatest of all contributions to our well-being," he wrote. Bill Mayne's own wife, Celia or "Bicky," passed away in October 1987 after a lifetime assisting war-blinded veterans. At first working as a VAD at St. Dunstan's during the Second World War, upon her return to Canada she exercised the same role at Baker Hall before joining the CNIB. This is how Mayne met her, and they were married a short time later.[18] He obviously had her in his mind's eye as he wrote; his readers no doubt thought of their own spouses. Mayne powerfully summed up in honest terms what being blinded in war had meant for him, for Bicky, and for his fellow veterans and their spouses and families:

> When the training and rehabilitation was finished and we were part of the working world, they were the ones who gave us that daily understanding, encouragement, and support. Somehow they were able to soothe our frustrations, abate our anger, and raise us from our despondency. They were tactful, understanding, and strong, encouraging when necessary, but not hesitating to be critical if circumstances so dictated. Without formal training or degrees in social work or psychology, they guided, cajoled and led us to the successes we achieved. They did it with patience, understanding, loyalty, and love. Without them all other assistance, encouragement, and support extended by others would have counted for little. There are no words with which we can adequately express to these

wonderful women our appreciation for the magic they have performed in our lives. We can but say, "We offer you our gratitude and our love."[19]

We in Canada know so little of the history of our war wounded. And so no one can argue with Bill Mayne's assessment of the world of the war blinded. Still, he might also have recognized and expressed gratitude to perhaps the most important players in this large-scale defeat of blindness: the veterans themselves, men like him, bonded in mutual assistance lasting a lifetime, and displaying courage few of us who are sighted will ever be able to understand. This was *their* victory.

Notes

Introduction

1 Dr. Keith Gordon, Vice-President Research, CNIB, email to author, 16 March 2009.

2 Frances A. Koestler, *The Unseen Minority: A Social History of Blindness in the United States* (New York: David McKay, 1976), 45.

3 Euclid Herie, *Journey to Independence: Blindness – The Canadian Story* (Toronto: Dundurn and CNIB, 2005), 15.

4 Koestler, *Unseen Minority*, 191.

5 Ibid., 1, 3.

6 Ibid., 9.

7 Ibid., 7.

8 Gabriel Farrell, *The Story of Blindness* (Cambridge, MA: Harvard University Press, 1956), 174.

9 Desmond Morton and Glenn Wright, *Winning the Second Battle: Canadian Veterans and the Return to Civilian Life, 1915-1930* (Toronto: University of Toronto Press, 1987), 14-15.

10 David A. Gerber, "Introduction: Finding Disabled Veterans in History," in David A. Gerber, ed., *Disabled Veterans in History* (Ann Arbor: University of Michigan Press, 2000), 8.

11 Ibid., 11-12.

12 Farrell, *Story of Blindness*, 173.

13 Koestler, *Unseen Minority*, 245.

14 Ibid., 7.

15 Herie, *Journey to Independence,* 48-52.

16 Susanne Commend, *Les Instituts Nazareth et Louis-Braille: Une histoire de coeur et de vision* (Ste-Foy, QC: Septentrion, 2001), 239.

17 Gerber, "Introduction," *Disabled Veterans,* 14.

18 Mary Tremblay, "Lieutenant John Counsell and the Development of Medical Rehabilitation and Disability Policy in Canada," in Gerber, *Disabled Veterans,* 322-46.

19 Gerber, "Introduction," *Disabled Veterans,* 14-15.

20 Herie, *Journey to Independence;* Marjorie Wilkins Campbell, *No Compromise: The Story of Colonel Baker and the CNIB* (Toronto: McClelland and Stewart, 1965).

21 William Mayne, "The Sir Arthur Pearson Association of War Blinded 1922-1997," n.d. [1997], file 820, "History," SAPA Archives.

22 Robert Weldon Whalen, *Bitter Wounds: German Victims of the Great War, 1914-1939* (Ithaca, NY: Cornell University Press, 1984), 117-19.

23 Gerber, "Introduction," *Disabled Veterans,* 6.

24 Gerber, ibid., 4-5, also makes this point with respect to the American war blinded.

25 Ibid., 2.

26 Koestler, *Unseen Minority,* 287. One senses from her criticisms of the American veterans' re-establishment programs, and to some extent the war-blinded community itself, that the Canadians were more cohesive, perhaps the result of superb leadership, allowing greater social bonding and successful advocacy.

27 A similar though less structured situation developed in the United States. See Gerber, "Introduction," *Disabled Veterans,* 25.

28 For the First World War, see Morton and Wright, *Winning the Second Battle,* and two articles by Morton: "'Noblest and the Best': Retraining Canada's War Disabled," *Journal of Canadian Studies* 16, 3-4 (1981): 75-85, and "Resisting the Pension Evil: Democracy, Bureaucracy, and Canada's Board of Pension Commissioners, 1916-1933," *Canadian Historical Review* 68, 2 (1987): 199-224. See also W.E. Segsworth, *Retraining Canada's Disabled Soldiers* (Ottawa: King's Printer, 1920). Desmond Morton's excellent study, *Fight or Pay: Soldiers' Families in the Great War* (Vancouver and Toronto: UBC Press, 2004), is also useful. For the Second World War, see Peter Neary and J.L. Granatstein, eds., *The Veterans Charter and Post-World War II Canada* (Montreal and Kingston: McGill-Queen's University Press, 1998), especially the article by Mary Tremblay, "Going Back to Main Street: The Development and Impact of

Casualty Rehabilitation for Veterans with Disabilities, 1945-1948," 160-78. See also Tremblay's essay cited earlier, "Lieutenant John Counsell"; Robert England, *Discharged: A Commentary on Civil Re-establishment of Veterans in Canada* (Toronto: Macmillan, 1943); Walter S. Woods, *Rehabilitation: A Combined Operation* (Ottawa: Queen's Printer, 1953); and Barry Broadfoot, *The Veterans' Years: Coming Home from the War* (Vancouver and Toronto: Douglas and McIntyre, 1985). Important international studies include Deborah Cohen, *The War Come Home: Disabled Veterans in Britain and Germany, 1914-1939* (Berkeley: University of California Press, 2001); Antoine Prost, *In the Wake of War: 'Les Anciens Combattants' and French Society 1914-1939* (Oxford: Berg, 1992); and Whalen, *Bitter Wounds.* For the CNIB and blindness in general, see Herie, *Journey to Independence.*

29 Gerber, "Introduction," *Disabled Veterans,* 1, 4-5.
30 Clifford Bowering, *Service: The Story of the Canadian Legion 1925-1960* (Ottawa: Canadian Legion, 1960); James Hale, *Branching Out: The Story of the Royal Canadian Legion* (Ottawa: Royal Canadian Legion, 1995); Jonathan Vance, "'Today They Were Alive Again': The Canadian Corps Reunion of 1934," *Ontario History* 87, 4 (1995): 327-44.
31 *SAPA Chronicle*, June 1997, 17.

Chapter 1: Canada's First War Blinded, 1899-1918

1 Jack Schecter, "The Achievements of Trooper Mulloy," *Canadian Military History* 11, 1 (2002): 71-74. This article is the most complete published account of Mulloy's life. See also Canadian Patriotic Fund Executive Committee Minutes, 10 February 1910, RG 7 G-21, vol. 365, Governor General's files, vol. 2425, 1910-1939, Library and Archives Canada (LAC).
2 Carman Miller, *Painting the Map Red: Canada and the South African War 1899-1902* (Montreal and Kingston: McGill-Queen's University Press and the Canadian War Museum, 1993), 429.
3 Schecter, "Achievements of Trooper Mulloy," 75.
4 Morton, *Fight or Pay,* 53; Miller, *Painting the Map Red*, 431.
5 Schecter, "Achievements of Trooper Mulloy," 74-75.
6 Ibid., 77-78.
7 Morton and Wright, *Winning the Second Battle,* 11.
8 Ibid., x-xi, 13.
9 Ibid., 5.

10 Ibid., xi.

11 G.W.L. Nicholson, *Canadian Expeditionary Force 1914-1919* (Ottawa: Queen's Printer, 1964), 548.

12 Ibid., 49-55.

13 A.G. Viets, Personnel File, RG 150, box 9947-88, accession 1992-93/166, LAC.

14 Born in Britain in 1873, Scammell proved to be "one of those officials a wise organization cherishes." Morton and Wright, *Winning the Second Battle,* 7-8. See also Segsworth, *Retraining Canada's Disabled Soldiers,* 10.

15 For more on Canadian military medicine during the First World War, see Sir Andrew Macphail, *The Medical Services. Official History of the Canadian Forces in the Great War 1914-19* (Ottawa: King's Printer, 1925), and G.W.L. Nicholson, *Seventy Years of Service: A History of the Royal Canadian Army Medical Corps* (Ottawa: Borealis Press, 1977).

16 In 1934 more than 77,000 Canadian veterans still received disability pensions. Morton and Wright, *Winning the Second Battle,* 9-10, 44.

17 Ibid., 14-15.

18 Quoted ibid., 15-16.

19 Ibid., 24, 247n31.

20 Macphail, *Medical Services,* 280.

21 Ibid., 280-81.

22 Ibid., 281; Tim Cook, *No Place to Run: The Canadian Corps and Gas Warfare in the First World War* (Vancouver and Toronto: UBC Press, 1999), 151, 156.

23 Mary G. Thomas, *The Royal National Institute for the Blind, 1868-1956* (London: Royal National Institute for the Blind, 1957), 35; Sidney Dark, *The Life of Sir Arthur Pearson* (London: Hodder and Stoughton, [1922?]), 16, 127.

24 Thomas, *Royal National Institute for the Blind,* 35.

25 David Castleton, *Blind Man's Vision: The Story of St. Dunstan's in Words and Pictures* (London: St. Dunstan's, 1990), 2-3.

26 Ibid., 3, 5; Lord Fraser of Lonsdale, *My Story of St Dunstan's* (London: George G. Harrap, 1961), 29; James H. Rawlinson, *Through St. Dunstan's to Light* (Toronto: Thomas Allen, 1919), 24-25. The name derived from the existence on the property of an old clock tower originally from the church of St.-Dunstan-in-the-West, Fleet Street, London. (The clock tower has since been restored to Fleet Street.) St. Dunstan is the patron saint of goldsmiths and silversmiths, having nothing to do with blindness or the blind. Castleton, *Blind Man's Vision,* 6, 8.

27 Castleton, *Blind Man's Vision,* 10.
28 Sir Arthur Pearson, *Victory over Blindness* (New York: George H. Doran, 1919), 13-14.
29 Lonsdale, *My Story of St Dunstan's,* 23; see also Castleton, *Blind Man's Vision,* 25.
30 Castleton, *Blind Man's Vision,* 11, 21; Pearson, *Victory over Blindness,* 28.
31 Sir Ian Fraser, *Whereas I Was Blind* (London: Hodder and Stoughton, 1943), 41, 50. British Captain Angus Buchanan was the only recipient of the Victoria Cross blinded during the First World War.
32 Pearson to Dr. C.R. Dickson, President, CNIB, 29 June 1918, MG 28 I 233, CNIB Papers, vol. 2, file 17, "Blinded Soldiers 1916-21," LAC; E.A. Baker to Emilia Houlton, 21 October 1918, CNIB Papers, vol. 7, file 17, "Department of Soldiers' Civil Re-establishment 1918-1920." In 1919, the Canadian government arranged to reimburse St. Dunstan's for the costs of training Canadians. See E.A. Baker to S.T.J. Fryer, Vocational Officer for Toronto, Department of Soldiers' Civil Re-establishment (DSCR), 29 April 1919, CNIB Papers, "Department of Soldiers' Civil Re-establishment 1918-1920."
33 Pearson, *Victory over Blindness,* 26; Castleton, *Blind Man's Vision,* 10; Lonsdale, *My Story of St Dunstan's,* 29.
34 Third Annual Report of St. Dunstan's Hostel for Blinded Soldiers and Sailors (year ending 31 March 1918) (hereafter St. Dunstan's Annual Report 1918), 4-5, CNIB Archives.
35 Fraser, *Whereas I Was Blind,* 89.
36 St. Dunstan's Annual Report 1918, 5; Pearson, *Victory over Blindness,* 205; Lonsdale, *My Story of St Dunstan's,* 58.
37 Lonsdale, *My Story of St Dunstan's,* 130-31.
38 Castleton, *Blind Man's Vision,* 14, 16-17.
39 Lonsdale, *My Story of St Dunstan's,* 41.
40 St. Dunstan's Annual Report 1918, 23.
41 Captain F. Russell Roberts, Adjutant, St. Dunstan's, to Director Medical Services, 8 May 1919, RG 9, series III, vol. 2697, file C-33-33, "Casualties – Disposal of Blind Soldiers," LAC.
42 Strome Galloway, *The White Cross in Canada 1883-1983: A History of the St. John Ambulance,* centennial edition (Ottawa: St. John Ambulance, 1983), 52-53.
43 Thomas, *Royal National Institute for the Blind,* 32.

44 Pearson, *Victory over Blindness,* 202-5; Dr. C.R. Dickson, Canadian Free Library for the Blind (CFLB), to Noel Marshall, Canadian Red Cross Society, Toronto, 17 October 1916, CNIB Papers, "Blinded Soldiers 1916-21."

45 Rawlinson, *Through St. Dunstan's to Light,* 1-3.

46 Ibid., 6-8. See also Lonsdale, *My Story of St Dunstan's,* 90.

47 Rawlinson, *Through St. Dunstan's to Light,* 9.

48 Ibid., 16, 19.

49 Ibid., 20-21, 29, 85; Segsworth, *Retraining Canada's Disabled Soldiers,* 140.

50 Rawlinson, *Through St. Dunstan's to Light,* 29, 44; Viets quoted in Castleton, *Blind Man's Vision,* 27.

51 Lonsdale, *My Story of St Dunstan's,* 206.

52 Rawlinson, *Through St. Dunstan's to Light,* 61-62, 79-82, 84.

53 George Eades to Dickson, 24 November 1918, CNIB Papers, "Blinded Soldiers 1916-21."

54 Rawlinson, *Through St. Dunstan's to Light,* 86.

55 E.A. Baker, Personnel File, RG 150, box 367-23, accession 1992-93/166, LAC; E.A. Baker, "Memorandum Covering Formation and Establishment of the CNIB," CNIB Papers, "Blinded Soldiers 1916-21"; E.A. Baker, "Captain E.A. Baker," [1917?], MG 30 C 103, Edwin Albert Baker Papers (hereafter "Baker Papers"), vol. 2, file "Biographical Material 1960," LAC.

56 Typescript recollections – E.A. Baker, n.d., CNIB Papers, vol. 26, file 8, "Mr. Harris Turner – 1937-39"; Campbell, *No Compromise,* 2-4. Baker's medical board findings of 24 July 1916 stated "that this officer was wounded by a rifle bullet which entered the right side of the orbit, passing through the left globe and then to the right, completely destroying both sights. Blindness is permanent." He was struck off strength "unfit for further service" 1 August 1916. E.A. Baker, box 367-23, accession 1992-93/166.

57 Campbell, *No Compromise,* 7-10.

58 Ibid., 14, 16, 21, 24, and passim; Pearson noted that Baker would be the second Canadian officer to join them, seemingly contradicting the commonly held view that Baker was the first Canadian officer blinded in the war. Pearson to Mrs. Baker, 15 November 1915, Baker Papers, vol. 2, file "Casualty E.A. Baker – Correspondence 1915-1917."

59 Pearson to Mrs. Baker, 21 December 1915, 12 January and 4 March 1916, 19 September 1918, Baker Papers, "Casualty E.A. Baker – Correspondence 1915-1917." On the other hand, Pearson noted in June 1916 that Baker was

occasionally prone to "fits of depression." Pearson to Mrs. Baker, 16 June 1916.

60 Campbell, *No Compromise,* 29.

61 Ibid., 39-40.

62 Dickson to Noel Marshall, 17 October 1916, CNIB Papers, "Blinded Soldiers 1916-21"; Campbell, *No Compromise,* 36, 42.

63 Dickson to R.A. Payne, Ontario Government Office, London, England, 26 September 1916, CNIB Papers, "Blinded Soldiers 1916-21."

64 Campbell, *No Compromise,* 43.

65 Ernest Scammell, Secretary, Military Hospitals Commission (MHC), to Sherman Swift, CFLB, 15 November 1915, CNIB Papers, vol. 13, file 6, "Military Hospitals Commission 1915-18."

66 T.B. Kidner, Vocational Secretary, MHC, to Dickson, CFLB, 25 March 1916, CNIB Papers, "Military Hospitals Commission 1915-18."

67 Kidner to Dickson, 12 June 1916, CNIB Papers, "Military Hospitals Commission 1915-18."

68 Kidner to Swift, 18 July 1916, CNIB Papers, "Military Hospitals Commission 1915-18."

69 Dickson to Frederick Fraser, Halifax School for the Blind (HSB), 6 December 1916, CNIB Papers, vol. 4, file "CNIB – Formation and Early History 1916-37; 1968."

70 Dickson to Noel Marshall, 17 October 1916, CNIB Papers, "Blinded Soldiers 1916-21"; Herie, *Journey to Independence,* 41.

71 Miscellaneous material on Dr. Charles Rea Dickson, "Journey to Independence" fonds, box 3, CNIB Archives, Toronto.

72 Dickson to R.A. Payne, Ontario Government Office, London, England, 26 September 1916, CNIB Papers, "Blinded Soldiers 1916-21."

73 Dickson to W.F. Moore, MHC, Discharge Depot, Quebec, 25 October 1916, CNIB Papers, "Blinded Soldiers 1916-21."

74 Fraser to Dickson, 17 July 1917, CNIB Papers, "CNIB – Formation and Early History 1916-37; 1968."

75 Dickson to Mrs. A.E. Gooderham, President, Imperial Order Daughters of the Empire, Toronto, 1 October 1917, CNIB Papers, "CNIB – Formation and Early History 1916-37; 1968."

76 Swift to Sir James Lougheed, MHC, 22 October 1917; Swift to Lougheed, [October?] 1917, CNIB Papers, "Military Hospitals Commission 1915-18."

77 Swift to Lougheed, 22 October 1917; Swift to Lougheed, [October?] 1917; Scammell to Dickson, 2 November 1917, CNIB Papers, "Military Hospitals Commission 1915-18."

78 Swift to Scammell, 14 November 1917, and reply, 16 November 1917, CNIB Papers, "Military Hospitals Commission 1915-18."

79 Dickson circular letter to various boards of trade in Ontario, December 1916, CNIB Papers, "Blinded Soldiers 1916-21."

80 Swift to J.D. Todd, Board of Pension Commissioners (BPC), 29 December 1916, CNIB Papers, "Military Hospitals Commission 1915-18."

81 Morton and Wright, *Winning the Second Battle,* 43, 45-46.

82 Dickson to BPC, 10 December 1916, CNIB Papers, vol. 19, file 4, "Pensions for War Blinded, 1916-1934."

83 Morton, *Fight or Pay,* 159. Although other veterans had assisted the French-speaking Poirier to communicate with the English-speaking federal bureaucracy, he felt language difficulties had contributed to his claim's rejection.

84 Dickson to Lieutenant-Colonel Panet, Pensions and Claims Board, 28 May 1918, CNIB Papers, "Blinded Soldiers 1916-21"; Dickson to N.W. Rowell, Chairman, Special Committee on Pensions, 20 April 1918, CNIB Papers, "Pensions for War Blinded, 1916-1934."

85 Quoted in Morton, "Resisting the Pension Evil," 206. Turner was elected by Saskatchewan's soldiers in the autumn of 1917 to represent them in the legislature. The provincial government had made special provisions for the troops to be represented by one of their own. Turner's official designation was "the Honourable Member for France." These overseas constituencies were discontinued in the 1921 election, though Turner was re-elected in Saskatoon for another term. He was defeated in 1925. After *Turner's Weekly,* he edited the *Western Producer,* the organ of the Wheat Pool. In addition, he was for two years an alderman in Saskatoon. CNIB Papers, "Mr. Harris Turner – 1937-39."

86 C.F. Fraser, Superintendent, HSB, to Dickson, 11 December 1917, CNIB Papers, vol. 10, file 10-8, "Halifax Explosion and Relief Commission, 1917-1928."

87 Fraser to Swift, 27 December 1917, CNIB Papers, "Halifax Explosion and Relief Commission, 1917-1928."

88 Laura M. Mac Donald, *Curse of the Narrows: The Halifax Explosion 1917* (Toronto: HarperCollins, 2005), 234; Baker to Dickson, 13 August 1918, CNIB Papers, "Department of Soldiers' Civil Re-establishment 1918-1920."

89 G.W. Theakston, North End Mission, to Swift, 11 December 1917, CNIB
    Papers, "Halifax Explosion and Relief Commission, 1917-1928." See Herie,
    Journey to Independence, 43-52, for the details surrounding this bitter
    rivalry.

90 H.M. Coyle, "The Sir Arthur Pearson Association of War Blinded," from the
    Report of the 1957 Reunion, file 820, "History," SAPA Archives.

91 Swift to Miss F.J. Bowes, Halifax, 25 January and 20 February 1918, CNIB
    Papers, "Halifax Explosion and Relief Commission, 1917-1928."

92 Press release, 20 December 1917, CNIB Papers, "Military Hospitals Commission
    1915-18."

93 Sergeant Alexander Graham, Royal Canadian Garrison Artillery, to Dickson,
    22 February 1918, CNIB Papers, "CNIB – Formation and Early History 1916-37;
    1968."

94 Ibid.

95 Corporal Abel Knight to Dickson, 20 February 1918, CNIB Papers, "CNIB –
    Formation and Early History 1916-37; 1968."

96 Swift to Edward M. Van Cleve, Principal, New York Institute for the Education
    of the Blind, 2 March 1918, CNIB Papers, "CNIB – Formation and Early History
    1916-37; 1968."

97 Swift to Scammell, 25 and 27 February 1918, CNIB Papers, "Military Hospitals
    Commission 1915-18."

98 Lewis Wood to Arthur Pearson, 25 March 1918, CNIB Papers, "CNIB – Formation
    and Early History 1916-37; 1968."

99 CNIB information sheet, [summer 1918?], CNIB Papers, "CNIB – Formation
    and Early History 1916-37; 1968."

100 Herie, *Journey to Independence,* 56-57.

101 Holmes to Dickson, 29 July 1918, CNIB Papers, "Blinded Soldiers 1916-21."

102 Pearson to Dickson, 5 April 1918, CNIB Papers, "Blinded Soldiers 1916-21."

103 Dickson to Pearson, 24 April 1918, CNIB Papers, "Blinded Soldiers 1916-21."

104 Pearson to Dickson, 13 May 1918, CNIB Papers, "Blinded Soldiers 1916-21."

105 Secretary, Overseas Military Forces of Canada, to Director of Medical Services,
     OMFC, 9 May 1918, RG 9, series III, vol. 2697, file C-33-33, "Casualties – Disposal
     of Blind Soldiers," LAC.

106 Morton and Wright, *Winning the Second Battle,* 92; Dickson to Segsworth,
     20 April 1918, CNIB Papers, "Department of Soldiers' Civil Re-establishment
     1918-1920"; Segsworth, *Retraining Canada's Disabled Soldiers,* 17.

107 Segsworth to Dickson, 31 May 1918, CNIB Papers, "Department of Soldiers' Civil Re-establishment 1918-1920"; Dickson to Pearson, 6 June 1918, CNIB Papers, "Blinded Soldiers 1916-21."

108 Dickson to Mrs. W.R. Riddell, Imperial Order Daughters of the Empire, Toronto, 23 May 1918, CNIB Papers, "CNIB – Formation and Early History 1916-37; 1968"; Dickson to Wood, 13 August 1918, CNIB Papers, "Blinded Soldiers 1916-21."

109 Undated speech by Sir James Lougheed [1918], Baker Papers, vol. 2, file "Department of Soldiers' Civil Re-establishment – Correspondence 1919-1960."

110 CNIB information sheet, n.d. [summer 1918?], CNIB Papers, "CNIB – Formation and Early History 1916-37; 1968."

111 Unidentified newspaper clipping, [August?] 1918, Baker Papers, "Department of Soldiers' Civil Re-establishment – Correspondence 1919-1960"; Campbell, *No Compromise*, 46-47.

112 C.W. Holmes to Baker, 4 October 1918, CNIB Papers, "Department of Soldiers' Civil Re-establishment 1918-1920."

113 Baker, "Rehabilitation of Canadian Blinded Soldiers"; Segsworth, *Retraining Canada's Disabled Soldiers*, 128, 133-34, 138.

114 Baker to Holmes, 16 November 1918 and 16 January 1919, CNIB Papers, "Department of Soldiers' Civil Re-establishment 1918-1920"; Segsworth, *Retraining Canada's Disabled Soldiers*, 139.

115 Baker to Holmes, 16 January 1919, CNIB Papers, "Department of Soldiers' Civil Re-establishment 1918-1920"; CNIB *Bulletin* 15, 1 December 1919, CNIB Papers, vol. 5, file 5, "CNIB Bulletins 1918-1922." All *Bulletins* referenced subsequently are from this file.

116 Segsworth, *Retraining Canada's Disabled Soldiers*, 136, 140.

117 Ibid., 140-41, 144.

118 *SAPA Chronicle*, June 1976, 4-5.

119 Baker to F.R. Sexton, DSCR Vocational Officer, Halifax, 18 October 1918, CNIB Papers, "Military Hospitals Commission 1915-18"; Capt. E.A. Baker, "Rehabilitation of Canadian Blinded Soldiers," n.d. [October 1918], Baker Papers, "Department of Soldiers' Civil Re-establishment – Correspondence 1919-1960."

120 Baker, "Rehabilitation of Canadian Blinded Soldiers"; Segsworth, *Retraining Canada's Disabled Soldiers*, 128, 133-34, 138.

121 Report of the General Secretary [Dickson] to the CNIB Executive Committee, 16 September 1918, CNIB Papers, "Blinded Soldiers 1916-21."

122 S.C. Swift, "The CNIB, Its Necessity, Its Ideal, Its Practice," [December?] 1918, CNIB Papers, "CNIB – Formation and Early History 1916-37; 1968."

123 CNIB Executive Committee Minutes, 16 and 23 September 1918, CNIB Papers, "CNIB – Formation and Early History 1916-37; 1968."

124 Scammell to Wood, 30 December 1919, unfiled correspondence, CNIB Archives.

125 CNIB Annual Report, 31 May 1919, 17; Segsworth, *Retraining Canada's Disabled Soldiers,* 130. Following the opening of Bakerwood, the CNIB's new Toronto headquarters, the city of Toronto purchased Pearson Hall from the CNIB in 1956 for the sum of $200,000. It became a learning centre for mentally disabled children and is now a heritage site administered by the province of Ontario, rented out as a conference or meeting venue. See *SAPA Chronicle*, Christmas 1989, 6.

126 *St. Dunstan's Review*, February 1919, 3 (reprinted article from an unnamed Toronto newspaper, 7 January 1919). All issues of the *St. Dunstan's Review* cited are located in the SAPA Archives.

127 CNIB *Bulletin* 24, December 1921.

128 Campbell, *No Compromise,* 48.

129 "Public Testimonial" programme, file 802, "Events 1919," SAPA Archives; Pearson's account of his trip to Toronto (provided by St. Dunstan's), unfiled, CNIB Archives; speech by E.A. Baker, CNIB Papers, vol. 23, file 145, "Sir Arthur Pearson Club 1918-1919"; Campbell, *No Compromise,* 48.

130 Dickson to Holmes, General Secretary, CNIB, 2 July 1919, CNIB Papers, vol. 8, file 8-9, "Blinded Soldiers' Fund 1917-1939"; D.A. Sutherland, Chief Steward, S.S. *Assiniboia,* to Pearson Hall, 29 June 1921; additional correspondence and material located in the same file.

131 Swift, "The CNIB, Its Necessity, Its Ideal, Its Practice," [December?] 1918; Report from Dickson to CNIB Council, 6 December 1918, both in CNIB Papers, "CNIB – Formation and Early History 1916-37; 1968"; CNIB *Bulletin* 2, 1 November 1918; CNIB Annual Report, 31 May 1919, 22, 25.

132 Jean Graham, *The Story of the Canadian National Institute for the Blind,* booklet (Toronto: CNIB 1920), 18; CNIB Annual Report, 31 May 1919, 10, 18; E.A. Baker, "Pearson Hall," February 1957, file 850, "Pearson Hall History," SAPA Archives; Segsworth, *Retraining Canada's Disabled Soldiers,* 138.

133 Herie, *Journey to Independence,* 52, 55; Campbell, *No Compromise,* 47; CNIB
     Annual Report, 31 May 1919, 18.
134 Segsworth, *Retraining Canada's Disabled Soldiers,* 130.
135 Typescript recollections – Bill Dies, n.d., CNIB Papers, "Mr. Harris Turner –
     1937-39."
136 Dickson to Edith (his cousin), 29 November 1918, CNIB Papers, "CNIB –
     Formation and Early History 1916-37; 1968."
137 CNIB Annual Report, 31 May 1919, 9.
138 Segsworth, *Retraining Canada's Disabled Soldiers,* 141.
139 William Mayne, "The Sir Arthur Pearson Association of War Blinded 1922-
     1997," n.d. [1997], file 820, "History," SAPA Archives; CNIB Annual Report, 31
     May 1919, 9; "Treatment and Care of Blinded Soldiers of the Present War," 6
     December 1939, CNIB Papers, vol. 22, file 16, "St. Dunstan's – General 1937-
     40"; Baker to Capt. (Rev.) W.A. Cameron, Toronto, 15 December 1921, CNIB
     Papers, vol. 25, file 1, "Sir Arthur Pearson Memorial 1921-1923."
140 Baker to Holmes, 16 January 1919, CNIB Papers, "Department of Soldiers'
     Civil Re-establishment 1918-1920."
141 Dickson to Pearson, 13 February 1919, CNIB Papers, "Sir Arthur Pearson Club
     1918-1919"; Segsworth, *Retraining Canada's Disabled Soldiers,* 140.

Chapter 2: The Sir Arthur Pearson Club of War Blinded Soldiers and Sailors, 1919-29

  1 Pearson, *Victory over Blindness,* 26.
  2 Ibid., 207.
  3 Fraser, *Whereas I Was Blind,* 55-56.
  4 Baker to Captain W.C. Nicholson, 1 July 1919, and reply, 14 July 1919, Baker
     Papers, "Department of Soldiers' Civil Re-establishment – Correspondence
     1919-1960"; Campbell, *No Compromise,* 50.
  5 F.G.J. McDonagh to Canadian Pension Commission, 12 September 1960,
     F.J.L. Woodcock Papers, Box 1, file "Attendance Allowance," CNIB Archives.
  6 Baker to Mrs. A.T. Barnard, 16 February 1920, CNIB Papers, "Department of
     Soldiers' Civil Re-establishment 1918-1920."
  7 Memorandum of Agreement, 26 June 1919, CNIB Papers, "Department of
     Soldiers' Civil Re-establishment 1918-1920."

8 Baker to Captain McPhun, 10 June 1920, CNIB Papers, vol. 9, file 15, "Department of Soldiers' Civil Re-establishment – Grants 1920-1923," and miscellaneous material in the same file.

9 Herie, *Journey to Independence,* 46, 58, 65; CNIB *Bulletin* 10, 1 July 1919.

10 Captain W.C. Nicholson to Baker, 14 July 1919, Baker Papers, "Department of Soldiers' Civil Re-establishment – Correspondence 1919-1960."

11 CNIB Second Annual Report for year ending 31 May 1920, 22.

12 CNIB *Bulletin* 21, 2 January 1921.

13 "Care of the Blind," 1922 Departmental Report, CNIB Papers, vol. 7, file 18, "Department of Soldiers' Civil Re-establishment 1921-1928."

14 "Names and Addresses of Men in After-Care," April 1921; list from Captain W.B. Powell, June 1921; both in CNIB Papers, "Department of Soldiers' Civil Re-establishment 1921-1928."

15 Baker's biographer states there were 329 Canadian war blinded of the First World War, though it is not clear how this number was derived. Campbell, *No Compromise,* 67.

16 Baker to Major A.M. Wright, DSCR, 16 December 1924 and 6 February 1925; 1924 report "Blinded Soldiers"; all in CNIB Papers, "Department of Soldiers' Civil Re-establishment 1921-1928."

17 "Blinded Soldiers Eligible for DSCR Aftercare," 20 February 1925, CNIB Papers, "Department of Soldiers' Civil Re-establishment 1921-1928."

18 Baker to Major A.M. Wright, 15 June 1926, CNIB Papers, "Department of Soldiers' Civil Re-establishment 1921-1928."

19 CNIB *Bulletin* 24, December 1921.

20 W.B. Powell, "After-Care Tour July to September 1921"; Baker, General Secretary, CNIB, to Mrs. E.M.C. Bates, St. Dunstan's, 11 October 1921; "Pearson Hall After-care Tour 1921"; all in CNIB Papers, "Department of Soldiers' Civil Re-establishment 1921-1928."

21 "Statement 1: Arguments in Favour of Permanent Pension on and after September 1924," CNIB Papers, vol. 23, file 16, "Sir Arthur Pearson Club 1922-1927."

22 "Blinded Soldiers' Training and Aftercare – General Remarks," CNIB Papers, "Department of Soldiers' Civil Re-establishment 1921-1928."

23 *Manitoba Free Press*, 16 April 1920, clipping in CNIB Papers, "Department of Soldiers' Civil Re-establishment – Grants 1920-1923."

24 Powell, "After-Care Tour July to September 1921," CNIB Papers, "Department of Soldiers' Civil Re-establishment 1921-1928."

25 C.W. Holmes to E.A. Baker, 5 February 1920, CNIB Papers, "Department of Soldiers' Civil Re-establishment 1921-1928."

26 "Supplies Given to Blinded Soldiers," CNIB Papers, vol. 7, file 15, "Department of Pensions and National Health 1928-1939."

27 Baker to Wright, 8 January 1927, and reply, 19 February 1927, CNIB Papers, "Department of Soldiers' Civil Re-establishment 1921-1928."

28 CNIB *Bulletin* 19, 1 July 1920; CNIB *Bulletin* 18, 1 April 1920.

29 Campbell, *No Compromise,* 54-55.

30 Ibid., 56; CNIB *Bulletin* 18, 1 April 1918; Lougheed to Baker, 13 September 1920; Flexman to Baker, 8 September 1920; N.F. Parkinson to Baker, 10 September 1920; G. Hulbert, DSCR, to Baker, 15 December 1920; all in CNIB Papers, "Department of Soldiers' Civil Re-establishment 1918-1920."

31 CNIB *Bulletin* 4, 2 January 1919; Segsworth, *Retraining Canada's Disabled Soldiers,* 135.

32 Segsworth, *Retraining Canada's Disabled Soldiers,* 140.

33 Lewis Wood to Arthur Pearson, 25 March 1918, CNIB Papers, "CNIB – Formation and Early History 1916-37; 1968."

34 Baker to Dickson, 13 August 1918; CNIB Executive Committee Minutes, 16 September 1918; both in CNIB Papers, "Department of Soldiers' Civil Re-establishment 1918-1920."

35 Segsworth, *Retraining Canada's Disabled Soldiers,* 134-35; Morton and Wright, *Winning the Second Battle,* 93; Baker to Holmes, 16 January 1919, CNIB Papers, "Department of Soldiers' Civil Re-establishment 1918-1920."

36 Segsworth, *Retraining Canada's Disabled Soldiers,* 134-35, 140; CNIB *Bulletin* 3, 2 December 1918.

37 Baker to Holmes, 16 January 1919, CNIB Papers, "Department of Soldiers' Civil Re-establishment 1918-1920."

38 Lieutenant-Colonel Robert Wilson, Consultant, Military School of Ortho-paedic Surgery and Physiotherapy, Hart House, Toronto, to Dr. Dickson, CNIB, 6 December 1918, CNIB Papers, "Blinded Soldiers 1916-21."

39 CNIB *Bulletin* 6, 1 March 1919.

40 CNIB *Bulletin* 14, 1 November 1919.

41 CNIB *Bulletin* 21, 2 January 1921.

42 CNIB *Bulletin* 10, 1 July 1919; "D.J. McDougall (Canadian)," St. Dunstan's Archives, welfare cards, located in CNIB Archives.

43 CNIB *Bulletin* 22, 2 May 1921; "Care of the Blind," 1922 Departmental Report, CNIB Papers, "Department of Soldiers' Civil Re-establishment 1921-1928."

44 CNIB *Bulletin* 22, 2 May 1921; CNIB *Bulletin* 21, 2 January 1921.

45 Baker to J.W. McKee, Assistant Deputy Minister, Department of Pensions and National Health (DPNH), 14 and 30 September 1929; E.H. Scammell, DPNH, to Baker, 20 November 1929; all in CNIB Papers, "Department of Pensions and National Health, 1928-1939"; Morton and Wright, *Winning the Second Battle,* 135.

46 SAPA Minutes, 15 September 1925, SAPA Archives; "D.J. McDougall (Canadian)," St. Dunstan's Archives, welfare cards. "Aided by his remarkable wife [Agnes]," wrote Desmond Morton, "McDougall continued at the university [of Toronto] as a crusty but effective professor of history." Morton, *Fight or Pay,* 271n30. McDougall died on 29 January 1978.

47 Sam Hughes, *Steering the Course: A Memoir* (Montreal and Kingston: McGill-Queen's University Press, 2000), 29. I am indebted to Dr. Tim Cook for this reference.

48 CNIB *Bulletin* 17, 2 February 1920; CNIB Second Annual Report for year ending 31 May 1920, 6; CNIB Annual Report for year ending 31 March 1922, 12, 20; E. Flexman, Director of Vocational Training, DSCR, to L.M. Wood, President, CNIB, 25 November 1919, CNIB Papers, "Department of Soldiers' Civil Re-establishment 1918-1920." Millionaire James Carruthers, a CNIB founder, appears to have granted the $35,000 from a fund he had set aside for Ottawa's use for the postwar re-establishment of disabled veterans. See Morton and Wright, *Winning the Second Battle,* 192.

49 Baker to E.H. Scammell, DPNH, 19 June 1928, and various other correspondence, CNIB Papers, "Department of Pensions and National Health, 1928-1939"; CNIB Annual Report for Year Ending March 31, 1929, 9.

50 Baker to E.H. Scammell, DPNH, 19 June 1928, CNIB Papers, "Department of Pensions and National Health, 1928-1939."

51 Herie, *Journey to Independence,* 56, 58, 98.

52 Powell to Baker, 11 January 1921, CNIB Papers, "Department of Soldiers' Civil Re-establishment 1921-1928."

53 CNIB *Bulletin* 12, 1 September 1919.

54 CNIB *Bulletin* 24, December 1921.

55 CNIB *Bulletin* 13, 1 October 1919.

56 CNIB Second Annual Report for year ending 31 May 1920, 17, 23.

57 CNIB *Bulletin* 20, 1 October 1920.

58 CNIB Second Annual Report for year ending 31 May 1920, 22.
59 Baker to Dr. Graham, DSCR Vocational Officer for Ontario, 1 May 1919, CNIB Papers, "Department of Soldiers' Civil Re-establishment 1918-1920."
60 J.P. Lynes, Honorary Secretary, SAPA, untitled reminiscences, n.d. [1989?], file 820, "History," SAPA Archives.
61 CNIB *Bulletin* 24, December 1921.
62 N.F. Parkinson to Pearson, 10 January 1921, CNIB Papers, "Department of Soldiers' Civil Re-establishment 1921-1928."
63 CNIB *Bulletin* 25, June 1922.
64 CNIB Annual Report for Year Ending March 31, 1922, 9.
65 CNIB Annual Report for Year Ending March 31, 1929, 12; Baker to Parkinson, 17 and 22 December 1921, CNIB Papers, "Department of Pensions and National Health 1921-28."
66 CNIB Annual Reports for years ending 31 March 1925-30.
67 CNIB Second Annual Report for year ending 31 May 1920, 17; W.B. Powell, Superintendent, Pearson Hall, to Baker, 11 January 1921, CNIB Papers, "Department of Soldiers' Civil Re-establishment 1921-1928."
68 CNIB Annual Reports for years ending 31 March 1924-32.
69 CNIB Annual Report for year ending 31 March 1924, 15.
70 CNIB *Bulletin* 24, December 1921.
71 Lonsdale, *My Story of St Dunstan's,* 80.
72 Baker to Lady Pearson, 9 December 1921, CNIB Papers, "Sir Arthur Pearson Memorial 1921-1923."
73 CNIB *Bulletin* 24, December 1921.
74 Fraser, *Whereas I Was Blind,* 66-67.
75 Dark, *Life of Sir Arthur Pearson*, 214-15; Fraser, *Whereas I Was Blind,* 68.
76 Dark, *Life of Sir Arthur Pearson,* 225; Lonsdale, *My Story of St Dunstan's,* 80; Fraser, *Whereas I Was Blind,* 68.
77 "Memorial Service," poster, file 802, "Events 1921," SAPA Archives. See also Baker to Captain (Rev.) W.A. Cameron, Toronto, 15 December 1921, CNIB Papers, "Sir Arthur Pearson Memorial 1921-1923." The Amputations Association of the Great War was occasionally referred to at the time as the Amputations Association of Canada.
78 CNIB *Bulletin*, Christmas edition, December 1922; SAPA Minutes, 2 February 1923; *St. Dunstan's Review*, November 1922, 19.
79 Castleton, *Blind Man's Vision*, 27-31.

80 In 1942 the name was shortened to the Sir Arthur Pearson Association of War Blinded, with the acronym SAPA, which is used throughout this work for simplicity.

81 CNIB Second Annual Report for year ending 31 May 1920, and for year ending 31 March 1922.

82 Lonsdale, *My Story of St Dunstan's,* 90.

83 J. Harvey Lynes to David Dorward, 18 October 1982, "History," SAPA Archives. See also "J.H. Lynes (Canadian)," St. Dunstan's Archives, welfare cards, located in CNIB Archives; Coyle, "Sir Arthur Pearson Association of War Blinded."

84 "J.H. Lynes (Canadian)," St. Dunstan's Archives, welfare cards.

85 Lynes to Dorward, 18 October 1982, "History," SAPA Archives.

86 Constitution of the Sir Arthur Pearson Club," n.d. [1922?], file 101, "Governance-Constitution," SAPA Archives; CNIB *Bulletin* 25, June 1922.

87 SAPA Minutes, 7 April 1922; Lynes to Dorward, 18 October 1982, "History," SAPA Archives.

88 SAPA Minutes, 20 April 1922.

89 William Mayne, "The Sir Arthur Pearson Association of War Blinded 1922-1997," n.d. [1997], file 820, "History," SAPA Archives.

90 CNIB *Bulletin* 25, June 1922.

91 Morton and Wright, *Winning the Second Battle,* 185-86.

92 Campbell, *No Compromise,* 78-79.

93 Lynes to Dorward, 18 October 1982, "History," SAPA Archives. See also SAPA Minutes, 20 April 1922.

94 Bill Mayne, CNIB Aftercare Services Officer and SAPA Executive Secretary, to D.S. Parr, Department of Veterans Affairs, 17 December 1974, extract updated in 1979, "History," SAPA Archives.

95 Mayne to D.S. Parr, 17 December 1974, extract updated in 1979, "History," SAPA Archives.

96 CNIB *Bulletin* 25, June 1922.

97 Lynes to Dorward, 18 October 1982, "History," SAPA Archives. See also SAPA Minutes, 20 April 1922.

98 CNIB Second Annual Report for year ending 31 May 1920, 10.

99 Ibid., 9 and 13; CNIB Annual Report for year ending 31 March 1922, 12 and 20.

100 CNIB Annual Reports for years ending 31 March; 1927, 28; 1928, 30; 1929, 40; 1930, 65.

101 SAPA Minutes, 11 August 1922.

102 SAPA Minutes, 30 September 1922.

103 "J.H. Lynes (Canadian)," St. Dunstan's Archives, welfare cards.

104 SAPA Minutes, 8 and 9 September 1923.

105 SAPA Minutes, 10 September 1926.

106 SAPA Minutes, 11 September 1924, 15 September 1925.

107 SAPA Minutes, 15 September 1925.

108 Miscellaneous material, file 850, "Pearson Hall Events," SAPA Archives.

109 SAPA Minutes, 10 September 1926.

110 SAPA Minutes, 9 September 1927.

111 Fraser, *Whereas I Was Blind,* 57; Castleton, *Blind Man's Vision,* 49.

112 CNIB *Bulletin* 24, December 1921; Baker to Parkinson, 10 December 1925, CNIB Papers, "Department of Soldiers' Civil Re-establishment 1921-1928."

113 DSCR Report 1923, CNIB Papers, "Department of Soldiers' Civil Re-establishment 1921-1928." Baker seems to have been the principal author of, or at least the source of information for, these reports.

114 CNIB *Bulletin* 24, December 1921.

115 CNIB *Bulletin,* Christmas edition, 1922.

116 Miscellaneous material in file 310, "Reunions 1923-31," SAPA Archives.

117 DSCR Report 1923, CNIB Papers, "Department of Soldiers' Civil Re-establishment 1921-1928."

118 1926 Reunion program and miscellaneous material in file 310, "Reunions 1923-31," SAPA Archives.

119 "Blinded Soldiers," 1927 report, CNIB Papers, "Department of Soldiers' Civil Re-establishment 1921-1928."

120 Miscellaneous material in "Reunions 1923-31," SAPA Archives; "List of Blinded Soldiers and their Escorts Attending Reunion 1931," file 850, "Pearson Hall Events," SAPA Archives.

121 Miscellaneous material in "Reunions 1923-31," SAPA Archives.

122 Castleton, *Blind Man's Vision,* 31, 35-39.

123 Lonsdale, *My Story of St Dunstan's,* 142-44, 189; Bund der Kriegsblinden Deutschlands E.V., *Kriegsblinden Jahrbuch 1993* (Bonn: self-published, 1993), 16, 24-27; Whalen, *Bitter Wounds,* 55, 134, 137.

124 Farrell, *Story of Blindness,* 175.

125 Ibid., 175-76.

126 Prost, *In the Wake of War,* 30, 39.

127　Ishbel Ross, *Journey Into Light: The Story of the Education of the Blind* (New York: Appleton-Century-Crofts, 1951), 279; Winifred Holt, *The Light Which Cannot Fail* (New York: E.P. Dutton, 1925), 60.

128　For a broad discussion of the American war blinded of the First World War, see Koestler, *Unseen Minority,* 245-57.

129　Morton and Wright, *Winning the Second Battle,* 201.

130　Ibid., 133.

131　Ibid., 166.

132　Ibid., 130-32.

133　Ottawa *Citizen,* undated clipping [1920], CNIB Papers, "Department of Soldiers' Civil Re-establishment 1918-1920"; Campbell, *No Compromise,* 97-98.

134　Turner to Baker, 4 July 1919, Baker Papers, "Department of Soldiers' Civil Re-establishment – Correspondence 1919-1960."

135　D.J. McDougall, President, SAPA, to Secretary, Canadian Patriotic Fund, 13 February 1923, CNIB Papers, "Sir Arthur Pearson Club 1922-1927."

136　Morton and Wright, *Winning the Second Battle,* 155.

137　Ibid., 169-70.

138　SAPA Minutes, 20 January 1923.

139　SAPA Minutes, 2 February 1923.

140　SAPA Minutes, 8 September 1923; Baker, DSCR, to BPC, 7 July 1920, CNIB Papers, "Department of Soldiers' Civil Re-establishment 1918-1920."

141　"Statement 2: Arguments in Favour of Permanent Pension on and after September 1924," CNIB Papers, "Sir Arthur Pearson Club 1922-1927."

142　Ibid.

143　Ibid.

144　"Blinded Soldiers," 1927 report, CNIB Papers, "Department of Soldiers' Civil Re-establishment 1921-1928."

145　SAPA Minutes, 15 September 1925.

146　Baker to Scammell, 17 April 1923; DSCR Report 1923; both in CNIB Papers, "Department of Soldiers' Civil Re-establishment, 1921-1928."

147　Second annual report of the SAPA Special Permanent Committee on Pensions and Re-establishment, SAPA Minutes, 15 September 1925.

148　Ibid.

149　Coyle, "Sir Arthur Pearson Association of War Blinded."

150　SAPA Minutes, 7 September 1928.

151 Lonsdale, *My Story of St Dunstan's,* 135, 139.

152 Coyle, "Sir Arthur Pearson Association of War Blinded."

153 Ibid.

154 Ibid.

155 SAPA Minutes, 6 September 1929.

156 Lonsdale, *My Story of St Dunstan's,* 65; *Sussex Daily News*, clipping, 10 July 1929, Baker Papers, vol. 12, file "Conference of St. Dunstan's Delegates."

157 E.A. Baker to C.W. Holmes, 6 May 1920, CNIB Papers, "Department of Soldiers' Civil Re-establishment 1918-1920."

158 Morton and Wright, *Winning the Second Battle,* 223.

159 Ibid., 224-25.

160 Ibid., 198-201; Bowering, *Service,* 5, 16, 27, 46-49; Hale, *Branching Out,* 20.

161 Lonsdale, *My Story of St Dunstan's,* 181-82.

162 "Souvenir of a Conference of St. Dunstan's Delegates Representing the War-Blinded Men of the Empire, London, July 1929," Baker Papers, "Conference of St. Dunstan's Delegates"; *St. Dunstan's Review*, July 1929, 6; SAPA Minutes, 6 September 1929.

Chapter 3: The Years of Struggle, 1930-39

 1 SAPA Minutes, 17 November 1934.

 2 CNIB, 1936 Annual Report, 17, 1939 Annual Report, 27, Baker Papers, vol. 9, file "CNIB Annual Reports."

 3 SAPA Minutes, 29 September 1933, 17 November 1934.

 4 Baker, "Statement of Facts," CNIB Papers, "Department of Soldiers' Civil Re-establishment, 1918-1920"; SAPA Minutes, 2 February 1934.

 5 SAPA Minutes, 7 March 1936.

 6 Clara Sutherland, Convenor, 1938 House Committee Report, file 850, "Pearson Hall Committee Reports," SAPA Archives.

 7 SAPA Minutes, 14 September 1931.

 8 CNIB, 1939 Annual Report, 27, Baker Papers, "CNIB Annual Reports"; "Pearson Hall V.A.D.s," "Pearson Hall Committee Reports," SAPA Archives.

 9 CNIB, 1937 Annual Report, 12, Baker Papers, "CNIB Annual Reports."

10 CNIB, 1939 Annual Report, 6, Baker Papers, "CNIB Annual Reports."

11 Lonsdale, *My Story of St Dunstan's,* 161-63.

12 SAPA Minutes, 14 September 1931.

13 *St. Dunstan's Review,* October 1934, 1; SAPA Minutes, 17 November 1934; "Memorandum News Sheet," November 1934, CNIB Papers, vol. 24, file 5, "Sir Arthur Pearson Club, 1934."

14 SAPA Minutes, 17 November 1934; "Memorandum News Sheet," November 1934, CNIB Papers, "Sir Arthur Pearson Club, 1934"; Lonsdale, *My Story of St Dunstan's,* 199.

15 *St. Dunstan's Review,* October 1934, 1.

16 *St. Dunstan's Review,* December 1936, 7; SAPA Minutes, 21 November 1936.

17 SAPA Minutes, 11 September 1937; CNIB Papers, vol. 2, file 5, "Australian Blinded Soldiers Association, 1930-41."

18 SAPA Minutes, 30 September 1932, 29 September 1933.

19 File 351, "Special Events – Memorial Service 1934," SAPA Archives; SAPA Minutes, 7 March 1936; "The Toronto Women's Auxiliary to the Canadian National Institute for the Blind 1917-1967," 11, CNIB Papers, vol. 19, file 4, "Pensions for War Blinded, 1916-1934."

20 SAPA Minutes, 14 September 1931.

21 CNIB, 1939 Annual Report, 5, 27, Baker Papers, "CNIB Annual Reports"; SAPA Minutes, 3 September 1938.

22 Morton and Wright, *Winning the Second Battle,* 207, 214.

23 SAPA Minutes, 11 September 1924, 7 September 1928. In 1924, in recognition of their vital roles, SAPA allowed members' widows to become honorary members of the association if they so chose.

24 SAPA Minutes, 14 September 1931, 30 September 1932, 29 September 1933, 1 March 1937, 9 April 1938, 3 September 1938, 29 October 1938, 5 December 1939; CNIB, 1937, 1938, and 1939 Annual Reports, Baker Papers, "CNIB Annual Reports."

25 SAPA Minutes, 11 September 1936, 23 October 1937.

26 SAPA Minutes, 9 April, 3 September, and 29 October 1938; CNIB, 1937, 1938, and 1939 Annual Reports, Baker Papers, "CNIB Annual Reports."

27 SAPA Minutes, 29 September 1933.

28 CNIB, 1933 Annual Report, 21, CNIB Papers, "Department of Pensions and National Health 1928-1939."

29 E.A. Baker, "Memo on the Interpretation of Membership Clauses," 1934, CNIB Papers, "Sir Arthur Pearson Club, 1934"; SAPA Minutes, 2 February and 13 April 1934.

30 SAPA Minutes, 2 February 1934.

31 E.A. Baker, "Memo on the Interpretation of Membership Clauses," 1934, CNIB Papers, "Sir Arthur Pearson Club, 1934."
32 SAPA Minutes, 13 April 1934.
33 E.A. Baker, "Memo on the Interpretation of Membership Clauses," 1934, CNIB Papers, "Sir Arthur Pearson Club, 1934."
34 SAPA Minutes, 2 February, 3 March, and 13 April 1934.
35 SAPA Minutes, 14 September 1931.
36 SAPA Minutes, 3 September 1938; CNIB, 1937 Annual Report, Baker Papers, "CNIB Annual Reports."
37 SAPA Minutes, 21 November 1936, 3 September 1938.
38 News of the World (Britain), undated clipping [August 1934], CNIB Papers, "Pensions for War Blinded, 1916-1934"; Lonsdale, My Story of St Dunstan's, 191, 222.
39 SAPA Minutes, 5 December 1939.
40 William Mayne, "The Sir Arthur Pearson Association of War Blinded 1922-1997," n.d. [1997], file 820, "History," SAPA Archives; Hand Book of General Information for Ex-Service Men (Toronto: Soldiers' Aid Commission of Ontario, 1935), 46; SAPA Minutes, 31 October 1936.
41 Globe and Mail, clipping, 5 July 1948, CNIB Papers, vol. 92, file 8, 1 of 2, "War Amputations of Canada, 1940-1953."
42 SAPA Minutes, 14 September 1931. See also "The E.A. Baker Foundation for the Prevention of Blindness," booklet, 1962, file 802, "E.A. Baker Foundation," SAPA Archives.
43 CNIB, 1936 Annual Report, 18, Baker Papers, "CNIB Annual Reports."
44 SAPA Minutes, 23 October 1937.
45 SAPA Minutes, 14 September 1931; Morton and Wright, Winning the Second Battle, 211.
46 SAPA Minutes, 30 September 1932.
47 Bowering, Service, 72; England, Discharged, 30, 32; SAPA Minutes, 14 September 1931.
48 SAPA Minutes, 7 March 1936.
49 SAPA Minutes, 11 September 1936.
50 SAPA Minutes, 29 September 1933.
51 Major A.M. Wright to Baker, 14 May 1934; A.H. Ward, DPNH, to Baker, 27 July 1934; and attached lists; all in CNIB Papers, "Department of Pensions and National Health, 1928-1939."
52 SAPA Minutes, 29 September 1933.

53 SAPA Minutes, 17 November 1934.

54 SAPA Minutes, 7 March 1936.

55 SAPA Minutes, 17 November 1934.

56 SAPA Minutes, 29 September 1933.

57 Baker to Wright, 29 April 1932; Baker to A. Gulvin, DPNH, 16 May 1932; Wright to Baker, 19 May 1932, and Baker marginal notation thereon of 20 May 1932; all in CNIB Papers, "Department of Pensions and National Health, 1928-1939."

58 SAPA Minutes, 29 September 1933, 17 November 1934.

59 SAPA Minutes, 3 March 1934.

60 SAPA Minutes, 17 November 1934.

61 Hale, *Branching Out,* 39. King wrote in his diary of his participation at the veterans' convention, noting with glee that Prime Minister Bennett, who did not even speak, and Minister of Pensions and National Health Murray McLaren made very poor impressions on the veterans, while he, King, gave a warm speech in support of the returned men. See William Lyon Mackenzie King Diaries, March 12 and 15, 1934, available online at LAC, http://www.collectionscanada.gc.ca/databases/king.

62 James Melville to Bill Mayne, 18 May 1977, reprinted in *SAPA Chronicle,* September 1977, 5-6.

63 SAPA Minutes, 17 November 1934.

64 E.A. Baker to Deputy Minister, DPNH, "Memorandum Reference Artificial Eyes, Eye Glasses and Supplies," [1934], CNIB Papers, "Department of Pensions and National Health, 1928-1939."

65 Ibid.

66 Ibid.

67 Ibid.

68 SAPA Minutes, 13 April 1934.

69 SAPA Minutes, 17 November 1934, 7 March 1936, 11 September 1936.

70 Bowering, *Service,* 70-71; Hale, *Branching Out,* 38.

71 SAPA Minutes, 5 September 1930, 11 September 1937, 11 December 1937; Bowering, *Service,* 71.

72 SAPA Minutes, 17 November 1934; SAPA "Memorandum News Sheet," November 1934, CNIB Papers, "Sir Arthur Pearson Club, 1934." See also Vance, "Today They Were Alive Again," 327-44.

73 SAPA Minutes, 17 November 1934.

74 SAPA Minutes, 29 September 1933, 3 September 1938.

75 See the correspondence in Baker Papers, vol. 2, file "Canadian Legion of the BESL 1930-1938, Correspondence and Memoranda."

76 SAPA Minutes, 7 March 1936. The 1935 AGM was held in March 1936 and the 1936 AGM was held in September 1936.

77 SAPA Minutes, 11 September 1936.

78 SAPA Minutes, 11 December 1937.

79 SAPA Minutes, 14 and 23 February 1938.

80 SAPA Minutes, 23 February 1938.

81 SAPA Minutes, 5 December 1939.

82 For a discussion of these pilgrimages see David W. Lloyd, *Battlefield Tourism: Pilgrimage and the Commemoration of the Great War in Britain, Australia and Canada, 1919-1939* (Oxford: Berg, 1998).

83 SAPA Minutes, 5 September 1930, 14 September 1931.

84 J.R. Bowler, General Secretary, Canadian Legion, to Baker, 6 November 1934, and reply, 4 December 1934; Ben Allen, "The Vimy and Battlefields Pilgrimage, July 1936," 5 July 1935; all in CNIB Papers, vol. 4, file 2, "Canadian Legion Vimy Ridge Pilgrimage, 1934-37"; Bowering, *Service,* 85.

85 Baker to SAPA membership, 19 August 1935; Baker to Sir Ian Fraser, 25 October 1935; Baker to Bertram Mayell, 18 February 1936; all in CNIB Papers, "Canadian Legion Vimy Ridge Pilgrimage, 1934-37."

86 See for example, Baker to R.S. Morland, 18 January 1935; Baker to SAPA membership, 19 August 1935; both in CNIB Papers, "Canadian Legion Vimy Ridge Pilgrimage, 1934-37."

87 Baker to Ben Allen, 28 April 1936, CNIB Papers, "Canadian Legion Vimy Ridge Pilgrimage, 1934-37."

88 Baker to Messrs. Heming Bros., Hamilton, Ontario, 2 July 1936, CNIB Papers, "Canadian Legion Vimy Ridge Pilgrimage, 1934-37." E.S. Palmer, travelling without an escort, voyaged on the *Ascania*, for unknown reasons. "Blinded Soldiers Attending the Pilgrimage," 28 July 1936, CNIB Papers, "Canadian Legion Vimy Ridge Pilgrimage, 1934-37."

89 SAPA Minutes, 11 September 1936; W.W. Murray, *The Epic of Vimy* (Ottawa: Legion, 1937), 11.

90 *Mail and Empire* (Toronto), 27 July 1936, clipping, CNIB Papers, "Canadian Legion Vimy Ridge Pilgrimage, 1934-37."

91 SAPA Minutes, 11 September 1936; Baker to Sir Ian Fraser, telegram, 29 June 1936, CNIB Papers, "Canadian Legion Vimy Ridge Pilgrimage, 1934-37." Still

the fullest source on the subject of the 1936 Vimy pilgrimage is Murray, *Epic of Vimy*.

92 SAPA Minutes, 11 September 1936. See also CNIB, 1937 Annual Report, Baker Papers, "CNIB Annual Reports."

93 "The E.A. Baker Foundation for the Prevention of Blindness," booklet, 1962, "E.A. Baker Foundation," SAPA Archives.

94 Ian Mackenzie to Baker, 10 January 1938 and reply 21 January 1938; extract from *Canada Gazette*, 19 February 1938; all in Baker Papers, vol. 4, file "Promotion to Rank of Lieutenant-Colonel, Correspondence 1938"; Herie, *Journey to Independence,* 65.

95 SAPA Minutes, 3 September 1938.

96 SAPA Minutes, 4 February and 5 July 1939; CNIB, 1939 Annual Report, 6, Baker Papers, "CNIB Annual Reports."

97 SAPA Minutes, 1 September 1939.

98 CNIB, 1939 Annual Report, 27, Baker Papers, "CNIB Annual Reports."

Chapter 4: Rehabilitating the Blinded Casualties of the Second World War, 1939-50

1 "Assistance offered by St. Dunstan's for the Service of those Blinded in a Future War," 1 November 1938, RG 25, G-1, vol. 1939, file 1939-1171, "Offer of St. Dunstan's for Canadians Blinded during War," LAC.

2 Ibid.

3 Report from Vincent Massey, High Commissioner for Canada in Britain, to Secretary of State for External Affairs, 14 November 1939, RG 25, G-1, vol. 1939, file 1939-1171, "Offer of St. Dunstan's for Canadians Blinded during War," LAC. See also "Treatment and Care of Blinded Soldiers of the Present War," CNIB Memorandum [written by Baker], 6 December 1939, 4, CNIB Papers, "St. Dunstan's – General 1937-40."

4 "Treatment and Care of Blinded Soldiers of the Present War," 8, CNIB Papers, "St. Dunstan's – General 1937-40."

5 R.E. Wodehouse, MD, Deputy Minister, DPNH, to O.D. Skelton, Under-Secretary of State for External Affairs, 30 November 1939, and H. DesRosiers, Acting Deputy Minister (Militia), Department of National Defence (DND), to Skelton, 2 and 19 December 1939, RG 25, G-1, vol. 1939, file 1939-1171, "Offer of St. Dunstan's for Canadians Blinded during War," LAC.

6 Skelton to Vincent Massey, 9 January 1940, RG 25, G-1, vol. 1939, file 1939-1171, "Offer of St. Dunstan's for Canadians Blinded during War," LAC.

7 "Treatment and Care of Blinded Soldiers of the Present War," 4, CNIB Papers, "St. Dunstan's – General 1937-40."

8 Ibid., 5-7.

9 Castleton, *Blind Man's Vision*, 71, 73; Fraser, *Whereas I Was Blind*, 42. The London headquarters of St. Dunstan's was destroyed in a German bombing raid, and Ovingdean was taken over by the British Admiralty during the war and returned to St. Dunstan's in 1945. St. Dunstan's entire operations moved to Church Stretton and Stoke Mandeville. See "Fourth General Reunion June 16-21, 1957 and History of The Sir Arthur Pearson Association of War Blinded," booklet, 2-3, file 310 "Reunions 1957," SAPA Archives.

10 "Treatment and Care of Blinded Soldiers of the Present War," 9, CNIB Papers, "St. Dunstan's – General 1937-40." See also CNIB, 1944 Annual Report, 7, CNIB Archives.

11 "Treatment and Care of Blinded Soldiers of the Present War," 10-11, CNIB Papers, "St. Dunstan's – General 1937-40."

12 Ibid., 5.

13 Baker to Lieutenant-Colonel A.C. Arnold, Royal Canadian Army Medical Corps, Medical Services Branch, DND, 16 October 1940, Baker Papers, vol. 2, file 17, "Department of National Defence Correspondence 1941-45"; SAPA Minutes, 29 February 1940, 3 January 1941.

14 Baker, Memorandum to the Inter-Departmental Sub-committee on Major Disabilities, 26 October 1940, CNIB Papers, vol. 85, file 4, "Rehabilitation War Blinded 1940."

15 CNIB, 1940 Annual Report, 6-7; 1944 Annual Report, 7.

16 Baker, Memorandum to the Inter-Departmental Sub-committee on Major Disabilities, 26 October 1940, CNIB Papers, "Rehabilitation War Blinded 1940."

17 Ibid.; Dr. Ross Millar, Chairman, Subcommittee of the General Advisory Committee on Demobilization and Rehabilitation, to Brigadier H.F. McDonald, Chairman of the General Advisory Committee on Demobilization and Rehabilitation, 31 January 1940, and subcommittee meeting report, 27 November 1940, CNIB Papers, vol. 85, file 6, "Rehabilitation War Casualties 1940-43."

18 "Supplemental Agreement," 28 February 1944, CNIB Papers, vol. 68, file 15, "Government of Canada and CNIB Agreement on Aftercare 1944."

19 SAPA Minutes, 13 October 1942; and CNIB, 1942 Annual Report, 13.

20 Baker to Brigadier R.M. Gorssline, Director General, Medical Services, DND, 14 September 1942, Baker Papers, "Department of National Defence Correspondence 1941-45"; SAPA Minutes, 13 October 1942.

21 Ross Millar to Gorssline, 12 February 1943, Baker Papers, "Department of National Defence Correspondence 1941-45."

22 Walter Thornton, *Cure for Blindness* (London: Hodder and Stoughton, 1968), 13.

23 Major-General H.F.G. Letson, Adjutant General, to Baker, 24 May 1943, Baker Papers, "Department of National Defence Correspondence 1941-45."

24 SAPA Minutes, 3 April 1944 and 18 January 1947.

25 Fraser, *Whereas I Was Blind,* 77; "General Reunion June 1947," booklet, 13, file 310, "Reunions 1947," SAPA Archives; CNIB, 1943 Annual Report, 14, CNIB Archives; "Pearson Hall Committee Reports," 1944 and 1945, file 850, SAPA Archives; Campbell, *No Compromise,* 125-26; SAPA Minutes, 13 October 1942.

26 CNIB, 1943 Annual Report, 14; SAPA Minutes, 5 April 1941, 13 October 1942.

27 Coyle, "Sir Arthur Pearson Association of War Blinded," 13.

28 SAPA Minutes, 5 April 1941.

29 SAPA Minutes, 1 November 1941, 30 January 1943.

30 CNIB, 1942 Annual Report, 16, CNIB Archives.

31 SAPA Minutes, 10 January and 13 October 1942, 12 March 1943.

32 Baker to SAPA Members, 19 November 1943, appended to SAPA Minutes, 17 November 1943.

33 SAPA Minutes, 22 January 1944.

34 SAPA Minutes, 4 September 1945, 2 April 1946.

35 SAPA Minutes, 4 November 1946, 7 January and 4 November 1947, 12 January 1948; "General Reunion June 1947," "Reunions 1947," SAPA Archives.

36 SAPA Minutes, 3 June 1947, 24 January 1948; "General Reunion June 1947," "Reunions 1947," SAPA Archives.

37 SAPA Minutes, 2 November 1948, 29 January 1949, 28 January 1950.

38 CNIB, 1942 Annual Report, 11, 16, 31.

39 Ibid., 12.

40 Ibid., 11.

41 SAPA Minutes, 1 November 1941, 13 October 1942; CNIB, 1942 Annual Report, 11, 16, 31.

42 CNIB, 1943 Annual Report, 11; SAPA Minutes, 13 October 1942.

43 SAPA Minutes, 12 March, 11 June, 17 November 1943; SAPA Archives, War-Blinded Training Committee (WBTC) Minutes, 21 February 1944.

44 "Treatment of Blinded Prisoners of War," Vincent Massey to Secretary of State for External Affairs, telegram, 5 January 1942, and Lieutenant-Colonel H.N. Straight, Commissioner of Internment Operations, Department of the Secretary of State, to Dr. A. Rive, Department of External Affairs, 6 January 1942, RG 25, series A-3-b, vol. 2766, file 621-AH-40, LAC.

45 *Daily Star* (Montreal), 25 June 1942, clipping in "Treatment of Blinded Prisoners of War."

46 Castleton, *Blind Man's Vision,* 78, 81, 83; *New Beacon* (Royal National Institute for the Blind) 78, 921 (1994).

47 Lonsdale, *My Story of St Dunstan's,* 291-93.

48 *New Beacon* 78, 921 (1994).

49 SAPA Minutes, 12 March 1943.

50 *New Beacon* 78, 921 (1994); Castleton, *Blind Man's Vision,* 83. See also F.J.L. Woodcock, "To You from Failing Hands We Toss the Torch," speech prepared 20 April 1989 for the SAPA Annual Reunion in London, Ontario, 15-19 May 1989, file 820, "History," SAPA Archives.

51 W.R. Feasby, *Official History of the Canadian Medical Services 1939-1945,* vol. 2, *Clinical Subjects* (Ottawa: Queen's Printer, 1953), 308; SAPA Minutes, 27 January 1945.

52 Feasby, *Canadian Medical Services,* 310-12.

53 Ibid., 313-15.

54 Farrell, *Story of Blindness,* 188-89.

55 SAPA Minutes, 12 March and 11 June 1943.

56 SAPA Minutes, 17 November 1943, and attached memorandum, Baker to SAPA members, 19 November 1943.

57 SAPA Minutes, 11 June and 17 November 1943.

58 In the Royal Canadian Ordnance Corps, this rank is the equivalent of a warrant officer.

59 SAPA Minutes, 17 November 1943, 22 January, 4 April, and 19 September 1944.

60 The totals are cumulative annually. CNIB, 1940-49 Annual Reports; Feasby, *Canadian Medical Services,* 312.

61 Feasby, *Canadian Medical Services,* 312.

62 SAPA Minutes, 22 January 1944.

63 SAPA Minutes, 22 January 1944; CNIB, 1944 Annual Report, 7.

64 CNIB, 1944 Annual Report, 7.
65 Baker to Major-Chaplain P.J. Dykes, 15 July 1944, Baker Papers, "Department of National Defence Correspondence 1941-45."
66 CNIB, 1944 Annual Report, 7.
67 Baker to Dykes, 15 July 1944, Baker Papers, "Department of National Defence Correspondence 1941-45."
68 Ibid.
69 SAPA Minutes, 3 April and 18 May 1944; individual case files, file 210, SAPA Archives.
70 SAPA Minutes, 19 September 1944, 27 January 1945.
71 Baker to Brigadier W.P. Warner, Acting Director General, Medical Services, DND, 10 January 1945, Baker Papers, "Department of National Defence Correspondence 1941-45."
72 November 1943 Report, file 850, "Pearson Hall Committee Reports," SAPA Archives. In 1953, one paralyzed blinded veteran of the First World War died who had spent the final thirty-five years of his life on his back in a government medical facility. Visiting committee members had read to him daily for the previous decade. See Women's Auxiliary to the CNIB, 1953 Annual Report, CNIB Archives.
73 November 1944 Report, file 850, "Pearson Hall Committee Reports," SAPA Archives.
74 November 1945 and November 1946 Reports, file 850, "Pearson Hall Committee Reports," SAPA Archives; Woodcock, "To You from Failing Hands We Toss the Torch," "History," SAPA Archives; SAPA Minutes, 18 January 1947.
75 SAPA Minutes, 18 May, 19 September, and 25 October 1944; CNIB, 1945 Annual Report, 2.
76 WBTC Minutes, 7 January and 7 February 1944; SAPA Minutes, 22 January 1944.
77 WBTC Minutes, 7 February 1944.
78 Toronto Daily Star, 28 February 1946, clipping, Woodcock Papers, box 1, CNIB Archives.
79 Elsinore Burns, "Baker Hall: Residence for War Blinded Toronto 1944-1950," booklet, June 1950, 14, file 801, "Baker Hall," SAPA Archives.
80 November 1944 Report, file 850, "Pearson Hall Committee Reports," SAPA Archives.
81 Burns, "Baker Hall," 14-15; CNIB, 1947 Annual Report, 8.
82 WBTC Minutes, 28 February and 6, 15, 22, and 27 March 1944.

83 CNIB, 1945 Annual Report, 8.
84 WBTC Minutes, 27 March, 8 May, and 6 November 1944; William Mayne, "The Sir Arthur Pearson Association of War Blinded 1922-1997," n.d. [1997], file 820, "History," SAPA Archives.
85 Burns, "Baker Hall," 14-15.
86 SAPA Minutes, 29 February 1940, 19 September 1944; WBTC Minutes, 6 March, 12 June, 20 November, and 11 December 1944, 19 March 1945; Herie, *Journey to Independence,* 114; CNIB, 1946 Annual Report, 7-8.
87 CNIB, 1945 Annual Report, 8; and WBTC Minutes, 20 November 1944.
88 Unidentified, undated newspaper clippings, Woodcock Papers, box 1, CNIB Archives.
89 CNIB, 1948 Annual Report, 9.
90 Burns, "Baker Hall," 14-15.
91 "Second Supplemental Agreement 24 August 1944," CNIB Papers, "Government of Canada and CNIB Agreement on Aftercare 1944."
92 David M. Dorward, *The Gold Cross: One Man's Window on the World* (Toronto: Canadian Stage and Arts Publication, 1978), 1, 58-60, and back cover.
93 Ibid., 61, 73.
94 WBTC Minutes, 12 June 1944, 17 October 1945; SAPA Minutes, 22 October 1945; Dorward, *Gold Cross,* 76, 86, 90, 92.
95 Barney Danson, *Not Bad for a Sergeant* (Toronto: Dundurn, 2002), 20, 50-51.
96 Neil R. Hamilton, *Wings of Courage: A Lifetime of Triumph over Adversity* (Calgary: Nacelles, 2000), 208-9.
97 John Windsor, *Blind Date* (Sidney, BC: Gray's Publishing Canada, 1963), 48, 54.
98 Ibid., 68-69, 98.
99 Ibid., 94, 103-5; WBTC Minutes, 24 September 1945.
100 *Toronto Daily Star*, 28 February 1946, clipping, Woodcock Papers, box 1, CNIB Archives.
101 WBTC Minutes, 17 January 1949.
102 CNIB client questionnaire, Norman Daniel, 24 October 1945, SAPA Archives.
103 Serge Durflinger, *Fighting from Home: The Second World War in Verdun, Quebec* (Vancouver: UBC Press, 2006), 196, 249n27.
104 CNIB, 1948 Annual Report, 7.
105 E.A. Baker, response to "Questionnaire on the War Blinded of Canada," 10 June 1952, 3, unfiled correspondence, CNIB Archives.
106 Bill Mayne, interview, 31 May 2006; WBTC Minutes, 18 November 1946.
107 WBTC Minutes, 18 November 1946.

108 WBTC Minutes, 2 April 1945.

109 WBTC Minutes, 29 May and 11 September 1944; 22 January, 19 March, 16 April, and 9 July 1945; and 18 December 1948; Woodcock, "To You from Failing Hands"; Bill Mayne, interview by author, Toronto, 31 May 2006.

110 WBTC Minutes, 18 and 25 June 1945.

111 CNIB, 1948 Annual Report, 15-16.

112 WBTC Minutes, 18 December 1950.

113 WBTC Minutes, 12 January, 1 March, and 14 June 1948; Burns, "Baker Hall," 19.

114 WBTC Minutes, 6 May, 8 July, and 4 November 1946; SAPA Minutes, 5 January 1949; Burns, "Baker Hall," 16.

115 Woods, *Rehabilitation,* 350.

116 Ibid., 351.

117 Tremblay, "Going Back to Main Street," 160-61, and Woods cited 165-66; Woods, *Rehabilitation,* 350; SAPA Minutes, 19 September 1944; WBTC Minutes, 8 May 1944.

118 Tremblay, "Going Back to Main Street," 166. See also Jeffrey A. Keshen, *Saints, Sinners, and Soldiers: Canada's Second World War* (Vancouver: UBC Press, 2004), 279-80.

119 Woods, *Rehabilitation,* 288.

120 WBTC Minutes, 24 September 1945.

121 Woods, *Rehabilitation,* 287-88.

122 Ibid., 289, 304-5. Woods reprints the entire agreement on pp. 301-6.

123 November 1944 Report, file 850, "Pearson Hall Committee Reports," SAPA Archives.

124 CNIB Council Minutes, extract 28 September 1943, and Minutes of the Residence and Training Centre for the War Blinded Committee, 8 October 1943, CNIB Papers, vol. 47, file 14, "Baker Hall – 78 Admiral Road 1943-47."

125 Minutes of the Residence and Training Centre for the War Blinded Committee, 8 and 28 October 1943, and L. Henderson, of Elmes, Henderson, and Son, to H.W. Shapely, KC, 12 January 1944, CNIB Papers, "Baker Hall – 78 Admiral Road 1943-47."

126 SAPA Minutes, 17 November 1943; "News of the Blind," CNIB newsletter, n.d. [1954], clipping, file "Lady Kemp," CNIB Archives; CNIB, 1944 Annual Report, 8; James W. Somers, City Clerk, City of Toronto, to Baker, 6 December 1943, and L. Henderson to H.W. Shapely, KC, 12 January 1944, CNIB Papers, "Baker Hall – 78 Admiral Road 1943-47."

127 L. Henderson to H.W. Shapely, KC, 12 January 1944, CNIB Papers, "Baker Hall – 78 Admiral Road 1943-47."

128 James W. Somers, City Clerk, City of Toronto, to Baker, 6 December 1943, CNIB Papers, "Baker Hall – 78 Admiral Road 1943-47."

129 *Globe and Mail*, 4 December 1943, clipping, CNIB Papers, "Baker Hall – 78 Admiral Road 1943-47."

130 Ibid.

131 *Globe and Mail*, 4 December 1943, *Toronto Daily Star*, 3 December 1943, clippings, CNIB Papers, "Baker Hall – 78 Admiral Road 1943-47."

132 *Globe and Mail*, 6 December 1943, clipping, CNIB Papers, "Baker Hall – 78 Admiral Road 1943-47."

133 Toronto *Daily Star*, 3 December 1943, clipping, CNIB Papers, "Baker Hall – 78 Admiral Road 1943-47."

134 *Globe and Mail*, 14 December 1943 and 22 January 1944, clippings, CNIB Papers, "Baker Hall – 78 Admiral Road 1943-47."

135 *Globe and Mail*, 22 and 25 January 1944, clippings, CNIB Papers, "Baker Hall – 78 Admiral Road 1943-47."

136 *Globe and Mail*, 22 January 1944, clipping, CNIB Papers, "Baker Hall – 78 Admiral Road 1943-47"; Campbell, *No Compromise,* 134.

137 "Baker Hall Dedicated by Athlone," clipping from unidentified Toronto newspaper, n.d. [23 or 24 March 1944], Baker Papers, vol. 9, file 5, "Baker Hall Residence for War Blinded"; SAPA Minutes, 3 April 1944.

138 Herie, *Journey to Independence,* 101; Mackenzie & Saunderson, Barristers, to CNIB, 4 September 1946, CNIB Papers, "Baker Hall – 78 Admiral Road 1943-47."

139 Burns, "Baker Hall," 4.

140 Herie, *Journey to Independence,* 133-34; Burns, "Baker Hall," 4, 16-19; Mayne, "Sir Arthur Pearson Association of War Blinded 1922-1997"; WBTC Minutes, 16 October 1944.

141 "Baker Hall House Committee," n.d., and "Baker Hall," 30 August 1944, CNIB Papers, "Baker Hall – 78 Admiral Road 1943-47."

142 CNIB, 1946 Annual Report, 8.

143 Burns, "Baker Hall," 1.

144 *All Clear: Chronicle of Baker Hall*, vol. 1, no. 1, December 1944, 5, CNIB Papers, "Baker Hall – 78 Admiral Road 1943-47."

145 *SAPA Chronicle*, June 1976, 10-11.

146 Bill Mayne, Toronto, 31 May 2006.

147 "Fourth General Reunion," 17, "Reunions 1957," SAPA Archives.
148 *All Clear: Chronicle of Baker Hall*, vol. 1, No. 1, December 1944, 2, CNIB Papers, "Baker Hall – 78 Admiral Road 1943-47."
149 Burns, "Baker Hall," 8.
150 *SAPA Chronicle*, June 1976, 10-11.
151 Galloway, *White Cross in Canada,* 91-92, 94, 100.
152 Burns, "Baker Hall," 8-9.
153 *Evening Telegram* (Toronto), clipping, 5 June 1946, and loose, unidentified Toronto-area newspaper clippings, Woodcock Papers, box 1, CNIB Archives; CNIB, 1946 Annual Report, 8.
154 *Telegram* (Toronto), 4 July 1950, clipping, CNIB Papers, vol. 47, file 15, "Baker Hall – 78 Admiral Road 1947-52."
155 Unidentified Toronto-area newspaper clippings, Woodcock Papers, box 1, CNIB Archives; Burns, "Baker Hall," 17.
156 Burns, "Baker Hall," 10-11.
157 Ibid.
158 Ibid., 7, 12.
159 Baker Hall Stag Night Committee to SAPA members of the First World War, 24 September 1945, CNIB Papers, "Baker Hall – 78 Admiral Road 1943-47."
160 *Veterans' Advocate*, 1 January 1949, clipping, file "Lady Kemp," CNIB Archives.
161 Burns, "Baker Hall," 1; Herie, *Journey to Independence,* 133-34; A.V. Weir to J.C. Smith, CNIB, 7 June 1951, CNIB Papers, "Baker Hall – 78 Admiral Road 1947-52."
162 CNIB, 1948 Annual Report, 16; and WBTC Minutes, 31 March 1947, and 30 March 1950.
163 WBTC Minutes, 30 March and 29 November 1950; and CNIB, 1951 Annual Report, 5.
164 CNIB, 1951 Annual Report, 5.
165 Burns, "Baker Hall," 16-19.
166 Ibid.
167 WBTC Minutes, 8 November 1948, 18 April 1951.
168 WBTC Minutes, 18 April 1951; John Chatwell, "The Sir Arthur Pearson Association of War Blinded 1922-1997," one-page document, n.d. [1997], file 820, "History," SAPA Archives.
169 CNIB, 1948 Annual Report, 16.

Chapter 5: Older and Wiser: Canada's War Blinded, 1945-70

1 "History," n.d. [1972 ?], 1, file 840, "National Council of Veteran Associations in Canada," SAPA Archives.
2 SAPA Minutes, 22 January 1944.
3 Ibid.
4 Ibid.; "History," 2, "National Council of Veteran Associations in Canada," SAPA Archives.
5 Coyle, "Sir Arthur Pearson Association of War Blinded," 16.
6 E.A. Baker, Chairman, National Council of Veteran Associations (NCVA), to A. Rukmini, Office of the High Commissioner for India, Ottawa, 28 April 1952, unfiled correspondence, CNIB Archives.
7 Ibid.
8 SAPA Minutes, 22 January 1944.
9 SAPA Minutes, 12 March and 17 November 1943, 27 January 1945.
10 SAPA Minutes, 22 January 1944. See also Bowering, *Service,* 162-64.
11 SAPA Minutes, 24 January 1948.
12 E.A. Baker, Chairman, NCVA, to Milton Gregg, Minister of Veterans Affairs, 20 January 1948, letter appended to SAPA Minutes, 24 January 1948.
13 Ibid. See also "General Reunion June 1947," "Reunions 1947," SAPA Archives.
14 Baker to Gregg, 20 January 1948, letter appended to SAPA Minutes, 24 January 1948.
15 Ibid.
16 Ibid.; "History," 2, "National Council of Veteran Associations in Canada," SAPA Archives.
17 E.A. Baker, response to "Questionnaire on the War Blinded of Canada," 10 June 1952, 1, unfiled correspondence, CNIB Archives; "Duties of the War Blinded Office," Woodcock Papers, box 4, CNIB Archives; Herie, *Journey to Independence,* 132-33.
18 SAPA Minutes, 28 January, 10 May, and 3 October 1956.
19 SAPA Minutes, 18 June 1957, 11 February 1961.
20 House of Commons, Standing Committee on Veterans Affairs, Minutes of Proceedings and Evidence, 16 March 1959, 157, copy in file 862, "Submissions: Standing Committee on Veterans Affairs, 1959," SAPA Archives. See also page 166.
21 SAPA Minutes, 8 February 1958.

22 December 1968 submission, 5, "Submissions – Parliament 1969," SAPA Archives.

23 SAPA Minutes, 14 February 1959.

24 SAPA Minutes, 13 and 14 February 1959.

25 Standing Committee on Veterans Affairs, Minutes of Proceedings and Evidence, 16 March 1959, 155-56, 159-60, 171.

26 SAPA Minutes, 30 January 1960.

27 SAPA Minutes, 14 February 1959, 30 January 1960.

28 SAPA Minutes, 22 February 1960.

29 SAPA Minutes, 21 March 1960; Woodcock to E. Norman Brannen, 31 May 1961, case file "Brannen, E. Norman," SAPA Archives.

30 SAPA Minutes, 2 November 1960, 11 February 1961.

31 SAPA Minutes, 8 July 1965.

32 SAPA Minutes, 11 February and 5 June 1961, 15 February 1963.

33 SAPA Minutes, 29 February 1964.

34 December 1968 submission, 4, "Submissions – Parliament 1969," SAPA Archives.

35 SAPA Minutes, 29 February 1964.

36 SAPA Minutes, 29 February and 22 September 1964.

37 SAPA Minutes, 8 July 1965, 26 March 1966.

38 December 1968 submission, 4, "Submissions – Parliament 1969," SAPA Archives.

39 Woodcock to Justice Mervyn Woods, 31 May 1967, copy appended to SAPA Minutes, 17 November 1967.

40 SAPA Minutes, 14 October 1970; House of Commons, *Debates*, 14 April 1969, 7513-15; Woodcock to all members of the House of Commons and Senate, 15 April 1969, "Submissions – Parliament 1969," SAPA Archives.

41 SAPA Minutes, 26 June 1968, 16 October 1969, 22 April and 14 October 1970.

42 SAPA Minutes, 14 October 1970; "History," 3, "National Council of Veteran Associations in Canada," SAPA Archives.

43 SAPA Minutes, 14 October 1970.

44 SAPA Minutes, 22 January 1944; Koestler, *Unseen Minority,* 258, 260-61.

45 SAPA Minutes, 22 January 1944; WBTC Minutes, 15 April 1945; Lonsdale, *My Story of St Dunstan's,* 288; Koestler, *Unseen Minority,* 258.

46 Lonsdale, *My Story of St Dunstan's,* 289; Koestler, *Unseen Minority,* 263, 265-66. Baker toured Old Farms in January 1945, though his impressions, if

recorded, have not been found. WBTC Minutes, 2 February and 17 October 1945.

47 SAPA Minutes, 27 January 1945.

48 Lonsdale, *My Story of St Dunstan's,* 289; Koestler, *Unseen Minority,* 280.

49 Koestler, *Unseen Minority,* 258. See also Robert Brown and Hope Schutte, *Our Fight: A Battle Against Darkness* (Washington, DC: Blinded Veterans Association, n.d. [1991?]).

50 Ibid., 266-69.

51 Ibid., 275-76.

52 C. Warren Bledsoe, ed., *War Blinded Veterans in a Postwar Setting* (Washington, DC: Veterans Administration, 1958), 27, 32, 34.

53 SAPA Minutes, 18 January 1947.

54 Koestler, *Unseen Minority,* 282-83.

55 SAPA Minutes, 10 February 1962.

56 See Robert L. Robinson, ed., *Blinded Veterans of the Vietnam Era* (New York: American Foundation for the Blind, 1973), 1-5, 21.

57 SAPA Minutes, 30 January 1960, 29 February 1964, 17 November 1967.

58 Lonsdale, *My Story of St Dunstan's,* 357.

59 Ibid., 243, 287, 352-53; SAPA Minutes, 8 July 1965.

60 Lonsdale, *My Story of St Dunstan's,* 313, 342.

61 Ibid., 65; Castleton, *Blind Man's Vision,* 110-11.

62 CNIB, 1940 Annual Report, 2-3 and 8.

63 "Duties of the War Blinded Office," Woodcock Papers, box 4, CNIB Archives.

64 SAPA Minutes, 30 January 1960.

65 E.A. Baker, response to "Questionnaire on the War Blinded of Canada," 2, 10 June 1952, unfiled correspondence, CNIB Archives; Regulations under the Department of Veterans Affairs Act, amended 10 September 1957, 3, marginal notation, file 121, "Agreements – Veterans Affairs," SAPA Archives.

66 SAPA Minutes, 16 February 1963.

67 SAPA Minutes, 14 February 1959.

68 A.V. Weir, General Manager, CNIB, to F.T. Mace, Financial Advisor, DVA, 7 December 1951, file "War Blinded Aftercare," CNIB Archives.

69 Baker, response to "Questionnaire on the War Blinded of Canada," 3-4, CNIB Archives; SAPA Minutes, 22 September 1964.

70 Bass Dawson, District Supervisor, Casualty Welfare, Veterans Welfare Services Branch, to G.L. Mann, Director, Casualty Welfare Services, 13 December

1956, case file, "Feasby, William Richard," CNIB Archives; E.A. Baker to Dr. Ross Millar, DPNH, 26 October 1942, RG 38, vol. 198, file "St. Dunstan's Training of Blinded Soldiers," LAC; *Toronto Star*, 26 November 1970.

71 Woodcock report, 11 September 1951, and Dawson to Mann, 13 December 1956, case file, "Feasby, William Richard," CNIB Archives.

72 For Feasby's role as an official historian, see Tim Cook, *Clio's Warriors: Canadian Historians and the Writing of the World Wars* (Vancouver and Toronto: UBC Press, 2006), 172-74.

73 Case file, "Hines, Harold B.," SAPA Archives.

74 Case file, "Latham, Merrill B.," SAPA Archives.

75 Case file, "Capson, Cecil E.," SAPA Archives.

76 Case file, "Friedman, Earl A.," SAPA Archives.

77 Case file, "Ashworth, J.," SAPA Archives.

78 Case file, "Blemkie, L.," SAPA Archives.

79 Ibid.

80 Case file, "Howard, Robert S.," SAPA Archives.

81 Ibid.

82 Case file, "Sheppard, G.A.," SAPA Archives.

83 Ibid.

84 Case file, "Arno, Frank," SAPA Archives.

85 SAPA Minutes, 13 October 1942.

86 CNIB, 1945 Annual Report, 16.

87 SAPA Minutes, 26 March 1966.

88 SAPA Committee on the Constitution and By-Laws Minutes, 7 December 1943; SAPA Minutes, 3 April 1944.

89 SAPA Membership Committee Minutes, 12 and 20 November 1952, 28 January 1954.

90 SAPA Minutes, 18 June 1957.

91 SAPA Minutes, 1 November 1961, 10 February 1962, 15 February 1963.

92 SAPA Minutes, 18 June 1957, 8 February 1958.

93 SAPA Minutes, 9 January and 14 February 1959, 5 June and 1 November 1961, 10 February 1962, 22 September 1964.

94 SAPA Membership Committee Minutes, 11 March 1957.

95 SAPA Minutes, 18 June 1957.

96 SAPA Minutes, 13 February 1959.

97 Fred Woodcock to Judge Frank McDonagh, 29 March 1960, case file, "Brannen, E. Norman," SAPA Archives; Woodcock to A.D. Reynolds, Secretary,

St. Dunstan's, 22 May 1963, case file, "Lovie, J.A.," SAPA Archives; SAPA Minutes, 15 February 1963.

98 SAPA Minutes, 2 November 1960, 5 June 1961, 11 July 1965.

99 SAPA Minutes, 28 October 1965.

100 Letter to members, 1966, Woodcock Papers, box 4, CNIB Archives.

101 SAPA Minutes, 6 May 1967.

102 Edwin Baker, "Summary of Address to Delegates, Canadian Corps Association, January 27th, 1943 – Royal York Hotel," Baker Papers, vol. 2, file 10, "Canadian Corps Association," LAC.

103 CNIB, 1945 Annual Report, 16.

104 CNIB, 1946 Annual Report, 16.

105 SAPA Minutes, Special Supplementary Report, 24 June 1947.

106 Coyle, "Sir Arthur Pearson Association of War Blinded," 16.

107 SAPA Minutes, 1 February 1944, 27 January 1945, 29 January 1949.

108 SAPA Minutes, 18 June 1957; Herie, *Journey to Independence,* 135.

109 Fraser, *Whereas I Was Blind,* 83; Lonsdale, *My Story of St Dunstan's,* 234-35.

110 SAPA Minutes, 29 February 1964, 23 November 1968.

111 SAPA Minutes, 29 February 1964.

112 SAPA Minutes, 28 January 1956, 18 June 1957.

113 SAPA Minutes, 18 June 1957.

114 SAPA Minutes, 30 January 1960.

115 SAPA Minutes, 4 February 1948; F.J.L. Woodcock, "Provision for Local Group Functions," 5 January 1949, located with SAPA Minutes of 2 March 1954.

116 SAPA Minutes, 4 February 1948, 5 and 29 January 1949; Woodcock, "Provision for Local Group Functions."

117 SAPA Minutes, 5 and 29 January 1949, 31 January and 26 May 1953, 28 January 1956, 8 February 1958.

118 SAPA Minutes, 26 March 1966.

119 Woodcock to Ivan White, president of the SAPA Vancouver Island Branch, 15 November 1967, appended to SAPA Minutes, 17 November 1967; David Dorward, "A Brief History," November 1979, file 801, "Bakerwood," SAPA Archives.

120 SAPA Minutes, 6 February 1954.

121 SAPA Minutes, 17 June 1959, 30 January 1960.

122 *National News of the Blind* (CNIB) 17, 2 (1957): 8, CNIB Archives; SAPA Minutes, 8 July 1965.

123 SAPA Minutes, 9 January 1959, 8 July 1965.

124 SAPA Minutes, 24 November 1966.

125 SAPA Minutes, 20 March and 6 May 1967, 27 April 1968.

126 SAPA Minutes, 17 November 1967.

127 CNIB, 1948 Annual Report, 18; "General Reunion June 1947," 16, "Reunions 1947," SAPA Archives. Ironically, Clara Sutherland's vision failed her late in life and she was registered as a client of the CNIB in June 1957. "Fourth General Reunion," 8, "Reunions 1957," SAPA Archives.

128 "War-Blinded Reunion Transportation," memorandum from CNIB to DVA, n.d. [1947], CNIB Papers, vol. 92, file 12, "War Blinded Training Programme, 1945-1949"; see also Baker to A. Rukmini, Office of the High Commissioner for India, Ottawa, 28 April 1952, unfiled correspondence, CNIB Archives.

129 CNIB, 1948 Annual Report, 18; "General Reunion June 1947," 13, "Reunions 1947," SAPA Archives.

130 "General Reunion June 1947," 2, "Reunions 1947," SAPA Archives.

131 Ibid., 9, 12.

132 Ibid., 12-13.

133 Baker to A.V. Weir, CNIB, 21 March 1956, file "War Blinded Aftercare," CNIB Archives.

134 SAPA Reunion Committee Meeting Minutes, 10 May 1957.

135 SAPA Minutes, 18 June 1957, 8 February 1958.

136 "Fourth General Reunion," 7, 18, "Reunions 1957," SAPA Archives; Herie, *Journey to Independence,* 134; *Toronto Daily Star*, 1 October 1957, clipping, unfiled, CNIB Archives.

137 SAPA Reunion Committee Meeting Minutes, 27 May 1957; "Fourth General Reunion," 10-11, "Reunions 1957," SAPA Archives.

138 *Telegram* (Toronto), 19 June 1957, and other unidentified press accounts, quoted from "Fourth General Reunion," 10-11, "Reunions 1957," SAPA Archives.

139 SAPA Minutes, 8 February 1958; "Fourth General Reunion," 18, "Reunions 1957," SAPA Archives.

140 Ibid.

141 SAPA Minutes, 10 and 18 June 1957; Coyle, "Sir Arthur Pearson Association of War Blinded," 12, 20-21.

142 "Fourth General Reunion," 18, "Reunions 1957," SAPA Archives.

143 General reunion booklet, file 310, "Reunions 1965," SAPA Archives; SAPA Minutes, 8 July 1965.

144 SAPA Minutes, 21 December 1964, 26 March 1966. So much did SAPA members appreciate Mann that he was made an honorary member of the association in 1968.

145 SAPA Minutes, 21 December 1964.

146 SAPA Minutes, 8 July 1965, 26 March 1966.

147 General reunion booklet, "Reunions 1965," SAPA Archives.

148 SAPA Minutes, 2 June 1954, 26 April, 30 May, and 12 October 1955.

149 See various material in File 801, "Bakerwood," SAPA Archives; Herie, *Journey to Independence,* 140.

150 SAPA Minutes, 8 February 1958.

151 Ibid.; Mayne, "Sir Arthur Pearson Association of War Blinded 1922-1997."

152 SAPA Minutes, 13 February, 17 June, 13 October 1959, 2 November 1960.

153 SAPA Minutes, 17 June and 13 October 1959.

154 SAPA Minutes, 2 November 1960.

155 SAPA Minutes, 19 January and 5 June 1961, 31 May 1962.

156 SAPA Minutes, 15 February 1963, 29 February 1964.

157 SAPA Minutes, 5 September 1963.

158 SAPA Minutes, 9 January 1964, 27 April and 26 June 1968, 14 October 1970.

159 SAPA Minutes, 8 July 1965; Woodcock to Ivan White, President, SAPA Vancouver Island Branch, 15 November 1967, appended to SAPA Minutes, 17 November 1967; SAPA Minutes, 27 April 1968.

160 SAPA Minutes, 1 June 1949; CNIB Papers, vol. 91, file 15, "Viets, A.G. 1949."

161 SAPA Minutes, 17 June 1959, 30 January 1960.

162 SAPA Minutes, 6 February 1954, 28 January 1956.

163 SAPA Minutes, 5 February 1955; 1949 Committee Report, file 850, "Pearson Hall Committee Reports," SAPA Archives.

164 SAPA Minutes, 26 September 1962, 16 February 1963.

165 "E.A. Baker Foundation," CNIB booklet, 4, file 802, "E.A. Baker Foundation," SAPA Archives.

166 Campbell to Baker, 8 July 1967 and reply 25 July 1967, Baker Papers, vol. 2, file "Companion of Order of Canada 1967-1968 Correspondence"; SAPA Minutes, 27 April 1968.

167 SAPA Minutes, 27 April 1968. The text of Neal's eulogy is appended to the minutes.

168 SAPA Minutes, 22 January 1970.

169 F.J.L. Woodcock, "William Dies," *St. Dunstan's Review*, February 1969, 7; *Veter-ans Advocate*, January 1960, clipping, case file, "W.C. Dies," CNIB Archives.
170 SAPA Minutes, 22 April 1970.

Chapter 6: Twilight, 1971-2002

1 This new "applied title" for the Department of Veterans Affairs came into use in the 1980s as a result of Ottawa's Federal Identity Program, which made mandatory the use of the word "Canada" to describe government depart-ments. Federal statutes continue to use "Department of Veterans Affairs."
2 SAPA Minutes, 23 February 1971.
3 SAPA Minutes, 30 October 1971.
4 SAPA Minutes, 20 June 1972.
5 Quoted in David M. Dorward, Director of War Blinded and Blind Veterans Services, CNIB, to C.L. Gibbery, Commissioner, Canadian Pension Commis-sion, 15 March 1982, Appendix B, file "VAC-EIA Exceptional Disability Allow-ance," SAPA Archives.
6 SAPA Minutes, 30 October 1971.
7 *SAPA Chronicle*, Summer 1993, 6.
8 SAPA Minutes, 30 October 1971.
9 SAPA Minutes, 27 March 1972, 12 July and 27 October 1973.
10 SAPA Minutes, 12 July and 27 October 1973.
11 SAPA Minutes, 27 October 1973.
12 Ibid.
13 Woodcock disability statement, August 1974, and Mayne to Woodcock, 27 August 1974, file 210, "Fred Woodcock," SAPA Archives.
14 Mayne to Dr. C.N. Brebner, Chief Medical Advisor, Canadian Pension Com-mission, 8 August 1974, file "VAC – Canadian Pension Commission," SAPA Archives; "Re: Brief from National War Blinded Aftercare Officer – Mr. W.M. Mayne, Exceptional Disability Allowance for Blindness," 25 November 1974, 1-2, file "VAC-EIA Exceptional Disability Allowance," SAPA Archives.
15 "Re: Brief from National War Blinded Aftercare Officer – Mr. W.M. Mayne, Exceptional Disability Allowance for Blindness," 25 November 1974, 3, file "VAC-EIA Exceptional Disability Allowance," SAPA Archives.
16 Mayne to Brebner, 31 January 1975, file "VAC-EIA Exceptional Disability Allowance," SAPA Archives.

17 "Exceptional Disability Allowance for Blindness, Review of Mr. Mayne's secondary submission of February 17, 1975," 11 March 1975, and A.O. Solomon, Chairman, CPC, to Mayne, 31 July 1975, file "VAC-EIA Exceptional Disability Allowance," SAPA Archives.

18 Solomon, Chairman, CPC, to Mayne, 31 July 1975, file "VAC-EIA Exceptional Disability Allowance," SAPA Archives; SAPA Minutes, 29 July 1975.

19 Mayne to MacDonald, 23 November 1977, and MacDonald to Andrew C. Clarke, Canadian Paraplegic Association, 23 March 1978 (copied to Mayne), file "VAC-EIA Exceptional Disability Allowance," SAPA Archives; *SAPA Chronicle*, March 1978, 12.

20 MacDonald to Clarke, Canadian Paraplegic Association, 23 March 1978 (copied to Mayne), file "VAC-EIA Exceptional Disability Allowance," SAPA Archives.

21 SAPA Minutes, 18 February 1982; Dorward to C.L. Gibbery, Commissioner, CPC, 15 March 1982, file "VAC-EIA Exceptional Disability Allowance," SAPA Archives.

22 *SAPA Chronicle*, August 1984, 1-2.

23 Dorward to L.M. Hanway, Chief Pensions Advocate, BPA, 21 May 1984, file "VAC-EIA Exceptional Disability Allowance," SAPA Archives.

24 *SAPA Chronicle*, June 1988, 1-2.

25 *SAPA Chronicle*, Christmas 1992, 20.

26 *SAPA Chronicle*, December 1991, 1; Dorward to Marcel Chartier, Chairman, CPC, 4 February 1992, and Dorward, letter to SAPA members, 19 February 1992, file "VAC Contract 1984-2000," SAPA Archives.

27 Senate of Canada, Standing Committee on Social Affairs, Science and Technology, *Proceedings of the Subcommittee on Veterans Affairs,* 17 August 1994, *Fourth Proceedings,* 23-32. See also *SAPA Chronicle*, Autumn 1994, 7-10.

28 SAPA Minutes, 5 October 1974.

29 SAPA Minutes, 25 October 1975.

30 *SAPA Chronicle*, March 1979, 9-13.

31 File 700, "Publications – General," SAPA Archives; SAPA Minutes, 12 July 1973.

32 SAPA Minutes, 25 October 1975.

33 *SAPA Chronicle*, 9 February 1976, 4-5; February 1977, 13; November 1977, 7.

34 *SAPA Chronicle*, November 1977, 8.

35 *SAPA Chronicle*, June 1978, 4-6.

36 *SAPA Chronicle*, December 1985, 2.

37 *SAPA Chronicle*, February 1977, 1, 4.
38 *SAPA Chronicle*, 12 February 1982, 4.
39 *SAPA Chronicle*, August 1984, 3.
40 SAPA Minutes, 1 June and 30 October 1971.
41 SAPA Minutes, 27 March 1972.
42 SAPA Minutes, 27 March, 6 June, and 20 June 1972.
43 SAPA Minutes, 22 June 1972. Eventually St. Dunstan's accepted any ex-service people having lost their effective vision from any cause.
44 SAPA Minutes, 27 October 1973.
45 SAPA Minutes, 27 May and 5 October 1974.
46 SAPA Minutes, 5 October 1974.
47 Ibid.
48 Ibid.
49 *SAPA Chronicle*, September 1977, 4; March 1978, 25; September 1978, 4.
50 *SAPA Chronicle*, March 1979, 1.
51 SAPA Membership Committee Minutes, 24 October 1979; "Report and Recommendations of the Ad Hoc Committee on Membership – Amendments to SAPA Constitution," file 201, "Members," SAPA Archives.
52 SAPA Minutes, 6 May 1983, 6-7 May 1986.
53 *SAPA Chronicle*, Summer 1994, 11, 14.
54 *SAPA Chronicle*, special supplement, Autumn 2001, 15.
55 *SAPA Chronicle*, December 1998, 8; Summer 2000, 8.
56 Krysia Pazdzior to Sanders, 28 July 1997, file 570, "SAPA Lounge," SAPA Archives.
57 *SAPA Chronicle*, November 1977, 3-4.
58 *SAPA Chronicle*, September 1985, 6-8.
59 *SAPA Chronicle*, November 1977, 5-6.
60 *SAPA Chronicle*, June 1986, 5.
61 *SAPA Chronicle*, 12 September 1982, 6-8; June 1985, 3.
62 *SAPA Chronicle*, September 1998, 4-5.
63 *SAPA Chronicle*, November 1977, 11-12.
64 *SAPA Chronicle*, June 1978, 18-19.
65 *SAPA Chronicle*, June 1979, 13-14.
66 *SAPA Chronicle*, reunion supplement, July 1995, 10.
67 SAPA Minutes, 5 November 1974. See Cyril Greenland, *Vision Canada: The Unmet Needs of Blind Canadians*, vol. 1 (Toronto: Leonard Crainford Associates for the CNIB, 1976).

68 Laura Buchanan to Bill Mayne, 10 March 1975, file "War-Blinded Steering Committee," CNIB Archives. This trend was noticeable in other countries as well, where the war blinded obtained a status well above that of the civilian blind. See Farrell, *Story of Blindness,* 173.

69 Mr. and Mrs. Charles E. Baker to Mayne[?], 12 February 1975, file "War-Blinded Steering Committee," CNIB Archives.

70 "CNIB National War Blinded Aftercare Services Administration Manual," July 1976, 4-5, file "VAC-EIA Exceptional Disability Allowance," SAPA Archives; *SAPA Chronicle*, 20 January 1983, 4; December 1987, 4; Summer 1990, 9-10; Summer 1991, 6.

71 SAPA Minutes, 25 October 1975.

72 SAPA Minutes, 12 July 1973.

73 Mayne to Ross C. Purse, Managing Director, CNIB, 9 February 1979, and Mayne to D.S. Parr, Chief, Budget and Administration, Welfare Services, DVA, 17 December 1974, file 123, "VAC Contract 1984-2000," SAPA Archives.

74 "CNIB National War Blinded Aftercare Services Administration Manual," 4-5.

75 *SAPA Chronicle*, September 1978, 7.

76 *SAPA Chronicle*, June 1979, 1.

77 SAPA Minutes, 18 November 1982.

78 *SAPA Chronicle*, December 1984, 1-2.

79 SAPA Minutes, 6 May 1983.

80 SAPA Minutes, 27-28 June 1983.

81 Ibid.

82 Ibid.

83 Brian MacGregor, Policy Analyst, Health Programs, Veterans Affairs Canada (VAC), to Jim Sanders, CNIB, 24 March 1997, file "VAC Contract 1984-2000," SAPA Archives.

84 SAPA Minutes, 27-28 June 1983.

85 Dorward to G.J. Parker, Director, Benefit Administration, VAC, 30 March 1984; M.H. Acker, Program Officer, VAC, "Concerns for Discussion," 1 August 1984; Dorward to Russ Comeau, Procurement Officer, Supply and Services Canada, 7 February 1986; all in file "VAC Contract 1984-2000," SAPA Archives.

86 Dorward to G.J. Parker, Director, Benefit Administration, VAC, 15 May 1984, file "VAC Contract 1984-2000," SAPA Archives.

87 SAPA Minutes, 20 August 1984, 6-7 May 1986.

88 Dorward to SAPA Executive, 10 August 1983, file 105, "Structure – Proposed Changes," SAPA Archives.

89 *SAPA Chronicle*, June 1985, 3.

90 Woodcock, "To You from Failing Hands We Toss the Torch," 4.

91 SAPA Minutes, 6-7 May 1986; Bill Mayne interview, 31 May 2006.

92 SAPA Minutes, 6-7 May 1986.

93 *SAPA Chronicle*, March 1986, 4; SAPA Minutes, 6-7 May 1986.

94 *SAPA Chronicle*, September 1986, 1.

95 Dorward to G.J. Parker, Director General, Health and Social Services Division, VAC, 14 December 1988; Bryson MacDonald, Senior Departmental Counsellor, VAC, to Dorward, 25 January 1988; both in file 121, "Agreements Veterans Affairs 1988," SAPA Archives; SAPA Minutes, 16 and 18 May 1989.

96 Bill Mayne interview, 31 May 2006.

97 Dorward to SAPA executive, 10 February 1987; Euclid Herie to Mayne, 11 January 1988; Herie and Dorward to George Hees, Minister of Veterans Affairs, 3 March 1988; all in file 105, "Structure – Proposed Changes," SAPA Archives; Mayne to Herie, 3 June 1989, file 204, "Honorary Members," SAPA Archives.

98 Herie, *Journey to Independence,* 203.

99 *SAPA Chronicle*, June 1989, 2; Sanders to Pat McEachran, Supply and Services Canada, 18 April 1990 and 4 May 1991, file "VAC Contract 1984-2000," SAPA Archives.

100 Bill Mayne interview, 31 May 2006.

101 *SAPA Chronicle*, June 1989, 2-3; Fall 1989, 1.

102 *SAPA Chronicle*, June 1989, 3; Christmas 1989, 1-2; Mayne to Herie, 3 June 1989, file 204, "Honorary Members," SAPA Archives; Bill Mayne interview, 31 May 2006.

103 *SAPA Chronicle*, June 1989, 2; Mayne to Sanders, 10 January 1989, "Honorary Members," SAPA Archives.

104 Bill Mayne, Aftercare Services Officer and Executive Secretary, SAPA, to D.S. Parr, DVA, 17 December 1974, file 820, "History," SAPA Archives.

105 Ibid.

106 General reunion booklet, file 310, "Reunions 1972," SAPA Archives; Mayne to Parr, 17 December 1974, "History," SAPA Archives; SAPA Minutes, 22 June 1972.

107 SAPA Minutes, 29 July 1975.

108 General reunion booklet, and City of Winnipeg, "Proclamation," "Reunions 1977," SAPA Archives.

109 *SAPA Chronicle*, September 1978, 1.

110 *SAPA Chronicle*, March 1979, 4.

111 *SAPA Chronicle*, 12 September 1982, 1; SAPA Minutes, 27-28 June 1983.

112 *SAPA Chronicle*, September 1986, 1; SAPA Minutes, 6-7 May 1986; 10th General Reunion Program, Montreal, May 5-8 1986, file 310, "Reunions 1986," SAPA Archives.

113 *SAPA Chronicle*, September 1985, 2; December 1985, 1; June 1986, 1-2.

114 *SAPA Chronicle*, June 1986, 2.

115 *SAPA Chronicle*, June 1986, 3; June 1987, 5-6; March 1989, 2-3.

116 J.D. Nicholson, Acting Deputy Minister, VAC, to Jim Sanders, SAPA executive director, 24 February 1992, file "VAC Contract 1984-2000," SAPA Archives.

117 *SAPA Chronicle*, Christmas 1992, 12-13; Dave Brown, "Brown's Beat," *Ottawa Citizen*, 3 April and 13 May 1992, clippings, file 310, "Reunions 1992," SAPA Archives; miscellaneous material from same file; Dave Brown, email to author, 3 May 2007.

118 Dave Brown, "Brown's Beat," *Ottawa Citizen*, 13 May 1992, clippings, file 310, "Reunions 1992," SAPA Archives; Dave Brown to author, 3 May 2007.

119 *SAPA Chronicle*, Christmas 1992, 15.

120 Lawrence MacAuley, Minister of Veterans Affairs, to Sanders, 6 March 1995, file "VAC Contract 1984-2000," SAPA Archives.

121 *SAPA Chronicle*, Autumn 1993, 17; April 1995, 4.

122 *SAPA Chronicle*, reunion supplement, July 1995, 6, 12-13.

123 Ibid., 6, 10-11.

124 *SAPA Chronicle*, March 1997, 4; September 1997, 5.

125 *SAPA Chronicle*, June 1999, 4-6.

126 *SAPA Chronicle*, Summer 2000, 1.

127 Ibid., 7.

128 *SAPA Chronicle*, Summer 2001, 1.

129 *SAPA Chronicle*, Christmas 2000, 6; Spring 2001, 3-4.

130 *SAPA Chronicle*, special supplement, Autumn 2001, 11, 13.

131 Ibid., 14; *Intelligencer* (Belleville), 7 May 2001.

132 SAPA Minutes, 23 February, 1 June, 18 August, and 30 October 1971.

133 Tom Cisar to Merv Carlton, 23 June 1971, file 320, "Annual 1971," SAPA Archives; SAPA Minutes, 20 June 1972.

134 Letters appended to SAPA Minutes, 5 October 1974 (translation provided in the minutes). The Chouinard-Pimparé letter is dated 21 June 1974. See also C.H. Gunawardena, Principal, Mount Lavinia School for the Blind, 4 July 1974, and reply from M.J. Carlton, 23 July 1974.

135 *SAPA Chronicle*, 9 February 1976, 10-11. Scholarships to blind Sri Lankan students were discontinued in 1996. SAPA Minutes, 6 May 1999.

136 SAPA Minutes, 18 August 1971, 25 October 1975; *SAPA Chronicle*, 9 February 1976, 10-11.

137 *SAPA Chronicle*, February 1977, 14.

138 *SAPA Chronicle*, March 1978, 17.

139 *SAPA Chronicle*, June 1976, 3.

140 *SAPA Chronicle*, April 1977, 14-15.

141 *SAPA Chronicle*, March 1979, 2.

142 SAPA Minutes, 18 February 1982, 27-28 June 1983; *SAPA Chronicle*, 10 October 1980.

143 *SAPA Chronicle*, March 1985, 1; September 1985, 4.

144 *SAPA Chronicle*, June 1987, 2.

145 *SAPA Chronicle*, Christmas 1989, 3.

146 *SAPA Chronicle*, April 1990, 6.

147 *SAPA Chronicle*, Summer 1990, 3.

148 Ibid., 3, 5.

149 *SAPA Chronicle*, Christmas 1990, 1, 14-15; Spring 1991, 14-15, Summer 1991, 11; Autumn 1991, 6.

150 *SAPA Chronicle*, Spring 1991, 11; December 1991, 12.

151 File 610, "Scholarship Program – Foundation 1992," SAPA Archives; Mayne, "Sir Arthur Pearson Association of War Blinded 1922-1997."

152 *SAPA Chronicle*, Autumn 1992, 1-2; file 610, "Scholarship Program – Foundation 1992," SAPA Archives.

153 *SAPA Chronicle*, Christmas 1992, 16.

154 *SAPA Chronicle*, Spring 1993, 10; Christmas 1993, 9.

155 *SAPA Chronicle*, Summer 1993, 3, 12-13; Christmas 1994, 1; March 1996, 14.

156 *SAPA Chronicle*, September 1999, 10.

157 *SAPA Chronicle*, September 1997, 10-11; September 1998, 11.

158 SAPA Minutes, 30 March 2000; *SAPA Chronicle*, Spring 2000, 5; Christmas 2003, 7.

159 SAPA Minutes, 6 May 1999.

Conclusion

1 ICRC, "Blinding Laser Weapons: Questions and Answers," 16 November 1994, http://www.icrc.org/Web/Eng/siteeng0.nsf/htmlall/57JMCZ, accessed 23 March 2009.

2 See Christopher Bellamy, "US Cancels Laser Weapon That Can Cause Blindness," *Independent* (London), 14 October 1995, http://www. independent.co.uk, accessed 23 March 2009.

3 *SAPA Chronicle*, October 1995, 5.

4 *Ottawa Citizen*, 19 November 2007.

5 *National Post*, 24 December 2007.

6 Shane Roberts, "Soldiers May Be Armed with Laser Weapons," *American Chronicle*, 26 February 2009, http://www.americanchronicle.com, accessed 23 March 2009.

7 *SAPA Chronicle*, July 1995, 1; Toronto *Star*, 6 May 2001.

8 SAPA Minutes, 27 May 1997; Herie, *Journey to Independence,* 203. Jim Sanders retired in March 2009.

9 See, for example, SAPA Minutes, 30 March 2000.

10 *SAPA Chronicle*, July 1995, 8, 10.

11 CNIB information sheet, n.d. [summer 1918?], CNIB Papers, "CNIB – Formation and Early History 1916-37; 1968."

12 *SAPA Chronicle*, October 1995, 3; Autumn 2001, 1; SAPA Minutes, 6 May 1999, 30 March 2000; Krysia Pazdzior, email to Bill Mayne, 30 June 2005, unfiled correspondence, SAPA Archives; Jim Sanders, email to author, 9 April 2009.

13 Michielin to SAPA executive, 23 March 2005, unfiled correspondence, SAPA Archives.

14 *SAPA Chronicle*, Spring 2002, 10; Spring-Summer 2003, 4.

15 *SAPA Chronicle*, Spring-Summer 2003, 17.

16 *SAPA Chronicle*, Christmas 2004, 9.

17 *SAPA Chronicle*, Autumn 2000, 5.

18 *SAPA Chronicle*, December 1987, 4.

19 Bill Mayne, "We Are Most Grateful," file 310, "Reunions 1992," SAPA Archives.

Select Bibliography

Archival Sources

Sir Arthur Pearson Association of Canada (SAPA) Archives, Ottawa
Canadian National Institute for the Blind (CNIB) Archives, Toronto
Library and Archives Canada (LAC)
    CNIB Papers MG 28 I 233
    Edwin Albert Baker Papers MG 30 C 103
    E.A. Baker RG 150, accession 1992-93/166
    A.G. Viets RG 150, accession 1992-93/166
    Department of Militia and Defence RG 9
    Department of External Affairs RG 25
    Department of Veterans Affairs RG 38

Other Sources

Ansell, Sir Mike. *Soldier On: An Autobiography.* London: Peter Davies, 1973.
Bledsoe, C. Warren, ed. *War Blinded Veterans in a Postwar Setting.* Washington, DC: Veterans Administration, 1958.
Bowering, Clifford. *Service: The Story of the Canadian Legion 1925-1960.* Ottawa: Canadian Legion, 1960.
Broadfoot, Barry. *The Veterans' Years: Coming Home from the War.* Vancouver and Toronto: Douglas and McIntyre, 1985.
Brown, Robert, and Hope Schutte. *Our Fight: A Battle against Darkness.* Washington, DC: Blinded Veterans Association, n.d. [1991?].
Campbell, Marjorie Wilkins. *No Compromise: The Story of Colonel Baker and the CNIB.* Toronto: McClelland and Stewart, 1965.

Castleton, David. *Blind Man's Vision: The Story of St Dunstan's in Words and Pictures*. London: St. Dunstan's, 1990.

Cohen, Deborah. *The War Come Home: Disabled Veterans in Britain and Germany, 1914-1939*. Berkeley: University of California Press, 2001.

Commend, Susanne. *Les Instituts Nazareth et Louis-Braille: Une histoire de coeur et de vision*. Ste-Foy, QC: Septentrion, 2001.

Cook, Tim. *Clio's Warriors: Canadian Historians and the Writing of the World Wars*. Vancouver and Toronto: UBC Press, 2006.

–. *No Place to Run: The Canadian Corps and Gas Warfare in the First World War*. Vancouver and Toronto: UBC Press, 1999.

Danson, Barney. *Not Bad for A Sergeant*. Toronto: Dundurn, 2002.

Dark, Sidney. *The Life of Sir Arthur Pearson*. London: Hodder and Stoughton, [1922?].

Dorward, David M. *The Gold Cross: One Man's Window on the World*. Toronto: Canadian Stage and Arts Publication, 1978.

England, Robert. *Discharged: A Commentary on Civil Re-establishment of Veterans in Canada*. Toronto: Macmillan, 1943.

–. *Twenty Million World War Veterans*. Toronto: Oxford University Press, 1950.

Farrell, Gabriel. *The Story of Blindness*. Cambridge, MA: Harvard University Press, 1956.

Feasby, W.R. *Official History of the Canadian Medical Services 1939-1945*. Vol. 2, *Clinical Subjects*. Ottawa: Queen's Printer, 1953.

Fraser, Sir Ian. *Whereas I Was Blind*. London: Hodder and Stoughton, 1943.

Galloway, Strome. *The White Cross in Canada 1883-1983: A History of the St. John Ambulance*. Centennial ed. Ottawa: St. John Ambulance, 1983.

Gerber, David A. "Blind and Enlightened: The Contested Origins of the Egalitarian Politics of the Blinded Veterans Association." In *The New Disability History: American Perspectives,* ed. Paul K. Longmore and Lauri Umansky, 313-34. New York: New York University Press, 2001.

–, ed. *Disabled Veterans in History*. Ann Arbor: University of Michigan Press, 2000.

–. "Disabled Veterans, the State and the Experience of Disability in Western Societies, 1914-1950," *Journal of Social History* 36, 4 (2002): 899-916.

Goodchild, George, ed. *Blinded Soldiers and Sailors Gift Book*. Toronto: Musson; London: Jarrold and Sons, [1916?].

Graham, Jean. *The Story of the Canadian National Institute for the Blind*. Booklet. Toronto: CNIB, 1920.

Greenland, Cyril. *Vision Canada: The Unmet Needs of Blind Canadians*, vol. 1.
    Toronto: Leonard Crainford Associates, for the CNIB, 1976.
Hale, James. *Branching Out: The Story of the Royal Canadian Legion*. Ottawa:
    Royal Canadian Legion, 1995.
Hamilton, Neil R. *Wings of Courage: A Lifetime of Triumph over Adversity*.
    Calgary: Nacelles, 2000.
Herie, Euclid, *Journey to Independence: Blindness – The Canadian Story*.
    Toronto: Dundurn and CNIB, 2005.
Holt, Winifred. *The Light Which Cannot Fail*. New York: E.P. Dutton, 1925.
Keshen, Jeffrey A. *Saints, Sinners, and Soldiers: Canada's Second World War*.
    Vancouver: UBC Press, 2004.
Koestler, Frances A. *The Unseen Minority: A Social History of Blindness in the
    United States*. New York: David McKay, 1976.
Lloyd, David W. *Battlefield Tourism: Pilgrimage and the Commemoration of the
    Great War in Britain, Australia and Canada, 1919-1939*. Oxford: Berg, 1998.
Longmore, Paul K., and Lauri Umansky, eds. *The New Disability History:
    American Perspectives*. New York: New York University Press, 2001.
Lonsdale, Lord Fraser of. *My Story of St Dunstan's*. London: George G. Harrap,
    1961.
Mac Donald, Laura M. *Curse of the Narrows: The Halifax Explosion 1917*.
    Toronto: HarperCollins, 2005.
Macphail, Sir Andrew. *The Medical Services. Official History of the Canadian
    Forces in the Great War 1914-19*. Ottawa: King's Printer, 1925.
McDonagh, Frank G.J. "The Vision of Eddie Baker." In *In Search of Canada*,
    118-123. Montreal: Reader's Digest, 1971. Originally published in
    Reader's Digest, February 1970.
McIntosh, Dave. *Hell on Earth: Aging Faster, Dying Sooner, Canadian Prisoners
    of the Japanese during World War II*. Toronto: McGraw-Hill Ryerson, 1997.
Miller, Carman. *Painting the Map Red: Canada and the South African War
    1899-1902*. Montreal and Kingston: McGill-Queen's University Press and
    the Canadian War Museum, 1993.
Morton, Desmond. "The Canadian Veterans' Heritage from the Great War." In
    The Veterans Charter and Post-World War II Canada, ed. Peter Neary and
    J.L. Granatstein, 15-31. Montreal and Kingston: McGill-Queen's
    University Press, 1998.
–. *Fight or Pay: Soldiers' Families in the Great War*. Vancouver and Toronto:
    UBC Press, 2004.

–. "'Noblest and the Best:' Retraining Canada's War Disabled," *Journal of Canadian Studies* 16, 3-4 (1981): 75-85.

–. "Resisting the Pension Evil: Democracy, Bureaucracy, and Canada's Board of Pension Commissioners, 1916-1933," *Canadian Historical Review* 68, 2 (1987): 199-224.

Morton, Desmond, and Glenn Wright. *Winning the Second Battle: Canadian Veterans and the Return to Civilian Life, 1915-1930*. Toronto: University of Toronto Press, 1987.

Murray, W.W. *The Epic of Vimy*. Ottawa: Legion, 1937.

Neary, Peter, and J.L. Granatstein, eds. *The Veterans Charter and Post-World War II Canada*. Montreal and Kingston: McGill-Queen's University Press, 1998.

Nicholson, G.W.L. *Canadian Expeditionary Force 1914-1919*. Ottawa: Queen's Printer, 1964.

–. *Seventy Years of Service: A History of the Royal Canadian Army Medical Corps*. Ottawa: Borealis Press, 1977.

Pearson, Sir Arthur. *Victory over Blindness*. New York: George H. Doran, 1919.

Prost, Antoine. *In the Wake of War: 'Les Anciens Combattants' and French Society 1914-1939*. Oxford: Berg, 1992.

Rawlinson, James H. *Through St. Dunstan's to Light*. Toronto: Thomas Allen, 1919.

Robinson, Robert L., ed., *Blinded Veterans of the Vietnam Era*. New York: American Foundation for the Blind, 1973.

Ross, Ishbel. *Journey into Light: The Story of the Education of the Blind*. New York: Appleton-Century-Crofts, 1951.

Rusalem, Herbert. *Coping with the Unseen Environment: An Introduction to the Vocational Rehabilitation of Blind Persons*. New York: Teachers College Press, 1972.

Schecter, Jack. "The Achievements of Trooper Mulloy," *Canadian Military History* 11, 1 (2002): 71-79.

Segsworth, W.E. *Retraining Canada's Disabled Soldiers*. Ottawa: King's Printer, 1920.

Thomas, Mary G. *The Royal National Institute for the Blind 1868-1956*. London: Royal National Institute for the Blind, 1957.

Thornton, Walter. *Cure for Blindness*. London: Hodder and Stoughton, 1968.

Tremblay, Mary. "Going Back to Main Street: The Development and Impact of Casualty Rehabilitation for Veterans with Disabilities, 1945-1948." In

The Veterans Charter and Post-World War II Canada, ed. Peter Neary and
   J.L. Granatstein, 160-78. Montreal and Kingston: McGill-Queen's
   University Press, 1998.
−. "Lieutenant John Counsell and the Development of Medical Rehabilitation
   and Disability Policy in Canada." In *Disabled Veterans in History*, ed.
   David A. Gerber, 322-46. Ann Arbor: University of Michigan Press, 2000.
Turner, John Frayn. *The Blinding Flash*. London: George G. Harrap, 1962.
Vance, Jonathan F. *Death So Noble: Memory, Meaning, and the First World War*.
   Vancouver: UBC Press, 1997.
−. "'Today They Were Alive Again': The Canadian Corps Reunion of 1934,"
   Ontario History 87, 4 (December 1995): 327-44.
Whalen, Robert Weldon. *Bitter Wounds: German Victims of the Great War,
   1914-1939*. Ithaca, NY: Cornell University Press, 1984.
Windsor, John. *Blind Date*. Sidney, BC: Gray's Publishing Canada, 1963.
Woods, Walter S. *Rehabilitation: A Combined Operation*. Ottawa: Queen's
   Printer, 1953.

Index

Bold type indicates a photographic plate occurring after page 104 (plates 1-23) or after page 200 (plates 24-54).

Studies in Canadian Military History

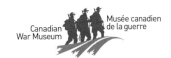

John Griffith Armstrong, *The Halifax Explosion and the Royal Canadian Navy: Inquiry and Intrigue*

Andrew Richter, *Avoiding Armageddon: Canadian Military Strategy and Nuclear Weapons, 1950-63*

William Johnston, *A War of Patrols: Canadian Army Operations in Korea*

Julian Gwyn, *Frigates and Foremasts: The North American Squadron in Nova Scotia Waters, 1745-1815*

Jeffrey A. Keshen, *Saints, Sinners, and Soldiers: Canada's Second World War*

Desmond Morton, *Fight or Pay: Soldiers' Families in the Great War*

Douglas E. Delaney, *The Soldiers' General: Bert Hoffmeister at War*

Michael Whitby, ed., *Commanding Canadians: The Second World War Diaries of A.F.C. Layard*

Martin Auger, *Prisoners of the Home Front: German POWs and "Enemy Aliens" in Southern Quebec, 1940-46*

Tim Cook, *Clio's Warriors: Canadian Historians and the Writing of the World Wars*

Serge Marc Durflinger, *Fighting from Home: The Second World War in Verdun, Quebec*

Richard O. Mayne, *Betrayed: Scandal, Politics, and Canadian Naval Leadership*

P. Whitney Lackenbauer, *Battle Grounds: The Canadian Military and Aboriginal Lands*

Cynthia Toman, *An Officer and a Lady: Canadian Military Nursing and the Second World War*

Shaw, Amy J., *Crisis of Conscience: Conscientious Objection in Canada during the First World War*

James G. Fergusson, *Canada and Ballistic Missile Defence: Déjà Vu All Over Again*

Benjamin Isitt, *From Victoria to Vladivostok: Canada's Siberian Expedition, 1917-19*

James Wood, *Militia Myths: Ideas of the Canadian Citizen Soldier, 1896-1921*

Printed and bound in Canada by Friesens

Set in Myriad and News Gothic by Artegraphica Design Co. Ltd.

Text design: Irma Rodriguez

Copy editor: Sarah Wight

Proofreader and Indexer: Dianne Tiefensee